Cancer Nursing:
A Solid Foundation for Practice

2nd Edition

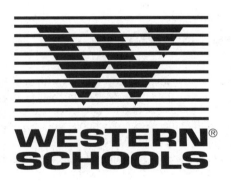

WESTERN® SCHOOLS

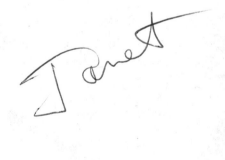

By
Ellen Carr, RN, MSN, AOCN

36 contact hours will be awarded upon successful completion of this course.

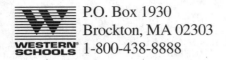 P.O. Box 1930
Brockton, MA 02303
1-800-438-8888

ABOUT THE AUTHOR

Ellen Carr, RN, MSN, AOCN, has been a health care and medical writer for more than 20 years. She specializes in assignments about clinical nursing, therapeutic and diagnostic technologies, and patient advocacy. She earned her bachelor's degree in journalism from the University of Colorado in 1976 and her master's degree in oncology nursing from the MGH Institute of Health Professions in Boston in 1988. Since 1997, she has been an advanced certified oncology nurse. Ms. Carr is currently a medical and surgical oncology case manager at the Rebecca and John Moores University of California, San Diego (UCSD) Cancer Center. Ms. Carr continues to participate in local and national Oncology Nursing Society projects.

Ellen Carr has disclosed that she has no significant financial or other conflicts of interest pertaining to this course book.

ABOUT THE SUBJECT MATTER REVIEWER

Vanna M. Dest, MSN, APRN, BC, AOCN, is an oncology nurse practitioner for the Radiation Oncology Associates of Southern Connecticut at the Hospital of Saint Raphael in New Haven, CT. She has been practicing in the field of oncology for the past 23 years. She received her bachelor's degree from Southern Connecticut State University in 1984, earned her master's degree from Yale University in 1992 and, most recently, earned a post-master's certificate from Yale University in 2002. She is a courtesy faculty member at Yale School of Nursing and a member of the editorial board for *RN* magazine. She has written many articles on various cancer topics. She is an active member in the Oncology Nursing Society and the American Society of Therapeutic Radiation Oncology.

Vanna Dest has disclosed that she is on the MedImmune speaker's bureau for cytoprotection.

Nurse Planner: Amy Bernard, RN, BSN, MS

Copy Editor: Jaime Stockslager Buss, MSPH, ELS

Indexer: Sylvia Coates

ISBN 978-1-57801-211-4

COURSE INSTRUCTIONS
IMPORTANT: Read these instructions *BEFORE* proceeding!

COMPLETING THE FINAL EXAMINATION

Enclosed with your course book you will find a FasTrax® answer sheet. Use this answer sheet to respond to all the final exam questions that appear in this course. If the course has less than 100 questions, leave any remaining answer circles on the FasTrax answer sheet blank.

Be sure to fill in circles completely using **blue or black ink.** The FasTrax grading system will not read pencil. If you make an error, you may use correction fluid (such as White Out) to correct it.

FasTrax answer sheets are preprinted with your name and address and the course title. If you are completing more than one course, be sure to record your answers on the correct corresponding answer sheet.

A PASSING SCORE

The final exam is a multiple choice exam. You must score 70% or better in order to pass this course and receive a certificate of completion. Should you fail to achieve the required score, an additional FasTrax answer sheet will be sent to you so that you may make a second attempt to pass the course. You will be allowed three chances to pass the same course without incurring additional charges. After three failed attempts, your file will be closed.

RECORDING YOUR HOURS

Use the Study Time Log provided in this course book to monitor and record the time it takes to complete this course. Upon completion, tally your total time spent and use this information to respond to the final question of the course evaluation.

COURSE EVALUATIONS

The Course Evaluation provided in this course book is a critical component of the course and must be completed and submitted with your final exam. Responses to evaluation statements should be recorded in the lower right hand corner of the FasTrax answer sheet, in the section marked "Evaluation." Evaluations provide Western Schools with vital feedback regarding courses. Your feedback is important to us; please take a few minutes to complete the evaluation.

To provide additional feedback regarding this course, Western Schools services, or to suggest new course topics, use the space provided on the Important Information form found on the back of the FasTrax instruction sheet included with your course. Return the completed form to Western Schools with your final exam.

SUBMITTING THE COMPLETED FINAL EXAM

For your convenience, Western Schools provides a number of exam grading options. Full instructions and complete grading details are listed on the FasTrax instruction sheet provided with this course. If you are mailing your answer sheet(s) to Western Schools, we recommend you make a copy as a back-up.

EXTENSIONS

You have two (2) years from the date of purchase to complete this course. If you are not able to complete the course within 2 years, a six (6) month extension may be purchased. If you have not completed the course within 30 months from the original enrollment date, your file will be closed and no certificate will be issued.

CHANGE OF ADDRESS?

In the event that your address changes prior to completing this course, please call our customer service department at 1-800-618-1670, so that we may update your file.

WESTERN SCHOOLS GUARANTEES YOUR SATISFACTION

If any continuing education course fails to meet your expectations, or if you are not satisfied for any reason, you may return the course materials for an exchange or a refund (less shipping and handling) within 30 days. Software, video, and audio courses must be returned unopened. Textbooks must not be written in or marked up in any other way.

Thank you for using Western Schools to fulfill your continuing education needs!

WESTERN SCHOOLS
P.O. Box 1930
Brockton, MA 02303
(800) 438-8888
www.westernschools.com

WESTERN SCHOOLS
STUDY TIME LOG

CANCER NURSING: A SOLID FOUNDATION FOR PRACTICE

INSTRUCTIONS: Use this log sheet to document the amount of time you spend completing this course. Include the time it takes you to read the instructions, read the course book, take the final examination, and complete the evaluation.

| | Time Spent | |
Date	Hours	Minutes
_____	_____	_____
_____	_____	_____
_____	_____	_____
_____	_____	_____
_____	_____	_____
_____	_____	_____
_____	_____	_____
_____	_____	_____
_____	_____	_____
_____	_____	_____
_____	_____	_____
_____	_____	_____
_____	_____	_____
_____	_____	_____
_____	_____	_____

TOTAL*

Hours	Minutes

* Please use this total study time to answer the final question of the course evaluation.

WESTERN SCHOOLS
COURSE EVALUATION

CANCER NURSING: A SOLID FOUNDATION FOR PRACTICE

INSTRUCTIONS: Using the scale below, please respond to the following evaluation statements. All responses should be recorded in the lower right-hand corner of the FasTrax answer sheet, in the section marked "Evaluation." Be sure to fill in each corresponding answer circle completely using blue or black ink. Leave any remaining answer circles blank.

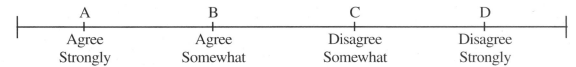

A	B	C	D
Agree Strongly	Agree Somewhat	Disagree Somewhat	Disagree Strongly

OBJECTIVES: After completing this course, I am able to

1. Describe cancer trends in the United States and worldwide.

2. Describe the characteristics and behavior of cancer cells.

3. Identify cancer prevention and detection strategies.

4. Discuss major treatment modalities for cancer.

5. Describe nursing care associated with venous access devices.

6. Discuss bone marrow and stem cell transplants.

7. Identify side effects of cancer treatment and appropriate interventions.

8. Recognize oncology emergencies and their management.

9. Describe risk factors, screening, symptoms, and management of specific cancers.

10. Describe complementary and alternative therapies used in cancer treatments.

11. Identify psychosocial stressors and support strategies for cancer patients and families.

12. Recognize the needs of special populations of cancer patients.

13. Discuss the elements of palliative care.

14. Describe the internet as a source of cancer information.

15. Identify professional issues relevant to oncology nursing.

COURSE CONTENT: Using the scale above, please evaluate the course content:

16. The course materials were well-organized and clearly written.

17. The course expanded my knowledge and understanding of the subject matter.

18. This offering met my professional educational needs.

19. The final examination was well-written and at an appropriate level for the content of the course.

ATTESTATION

20. By submitting this answer sheet, I certify that I have read the course materials and personally completed the final examination based on the material presented. Mark "A" for Agree and "B" for Disagree.

COURSE HOURS

21. Please select the response that best reflects the total number of hours that it took to complete this course.

A. More than 38 hours   C. 29–33 hours

B. 34–38 hours   D. Fewer than 29 hours

Note: To provide additional feedback regarding this course, Western Schools services, or to suggest new course topics, use the space provided on the Important Information form found on the back of the FasTrax instruction sheet included with your course.

CONTENTS

FIGURES AND TABLES

PRETEST

1. Begin this course by taking the pretest. Circle the answers to the questions on this page, or write the answers on a separate sheet of paper. Do not log answers to the pretest questions on the FasTrax test sheet included with the course.

2. Compare your answers to the PRETEST KEY located in the back of the book. The pretest answer key indicates the course chapter where the content of that question is discussed. Make note of the questions you missed, so that you can focus on those areas as you complete the course.

3. Complete the course by reading each chapter and completing the exam questions at the end of the chapter. Answers to these exam questions should be logged on the FasTrax test sheet included with the course.

1. Hyperplasia is defined as an abnormal
   a. increase in cell size.
   b. increase in the number of cells.
   c. number of less-mature cells.
   d. decrease in the number of cells.

2. Americans, on the whole, have poor nutrition habits because they
   a. have underlying diseases that make them eat.
   b. are educated in school to eat as much as they want.
   c. eat out a lot.
   d. have no other alternative but to eat poorly.

3. Experts recommend using a sunblock with a sun protection factor rating of at least
   a. 10.
   b. 15.
   c. 30.
   d. 35.

4. A sign of chronic toxicity from radiation therapy is
   a. dry mouth.
   b. moist mouth.
   c. radiation erythema.
   d. salty taste.

5. An example of an antimetabolite chemotherapy agent is
   a. cisplatin (Platinol).
   b. vincristine (Oncovin).
   c. thiotepa (Thioplex).
   d. methotrexate (Mexate).

6. An example of an antitumor antibiotic chemotherapy agent is
   a. cyclophosphamide (Cytoxan).
   b. idarubicin (Idamycin).
   c. 5-fluorouracil (5-FU).
   d. procarbazine (Mutalane).

7. During a bone marrow and peripheral stem cell transplant, the process of harvesting blood stem cells begins
   a. after consolidation treatment.
   b. within an hour of blood typing.
   c. after the blood has been centrifuged.
   d. before chemotherapy administration.

8. An intervention to relieve hot flashes is
   a. using oil-based lotions.
   b. taking hot baths.
   c. using antidepressants for a brief time.
   d. joining a support group.

9. A symptom that could be related to chemo brain is

   a. forgetfulness.

   b. nausea.

   c. constipation.

   d. hoarseness.

10. Early signs of cardiac tamponade include

    a. nausea and vomiting.

    b. fidgeting.

    c. weakness in the legs.

    d. dyspnea.

11. One treatment strategy for pleural effusion is

    a. brachytherapy.

    b. antibiotics.

    c. hydration.

    d. pleurodesis.

12. Most breast cancers in the United States occur in

    a. women under age 50.

    b. women over age 50.

    c. women over age 70.

    d. women over age 80.

13. A tumor marker used to evaluate breast cancer treatment is

    a. blood urea nitrogen.

    b. creatinine.

    c. prostate-specific antigen.

    d. CA 27.29.

14. A population at high risk for developing prostate cancer is

    a. African American males.

    b. Asian American males.

    c. men with no known history of prostate cancer in their family.

    d. men between ages 30 and 50.

15. In 2006 in the United States, the relative survival rate for non-Hodgkin's lymphoma at 1 year is

    a. 63%.

    b. 73%.

    c. 83%.

    d. 93%.

16. Leukemia is a disease of the

    a. lung.

    b. blood.

    c. skin.

    d. brain.

17. A chemotherapy agent included in an induction protocol for acute myelogenous leukemia (AML) is

    a. etoposide

    b. doxorubicin (adriamycin).

    c. cyclophosphamide.

    d. capecitabine (xeloda).

18. When a patient is under stress, the nurse's communication style with the patient should be

    a. limited.

    b. detailed.

    c. clear.

    d. emotional.

19. A possible cause of childhood cancer is exposure to

    a. radiation.

    b. animals.

    c. protein.

    d. other sick children.

20. A symptom of burnout is

    a. multitasking.

    b. flexibility.

    c. enthusiasm.

    d. indifference.

INTRODUCTION

The diagnosis of cancer touches everyone. We all know family members and friends challenged by the disease. And, of course, our patients—who fight this disease—remain the focus of our care, which includes an amazing and comprehensive set of knowledge and skills that need to be current and relevant.

Everyone who is part of the health care system faces the daunting task of providing ever more effective care for cancer patients. Our larger, aging population means that the incidence of cancer as a chronic illness will continue to rise significantly (Yancik, 2005). In providing some signposts for the task at hand, the National Cancer Institute has published its strategic initiatives for 2015 (see Table i). These initiatives provide a framework to improve care for cancer patients as well as those who live on to become long-term survivors of cancer from their time of diagnosis.

The pressure on researchers and scientists to rein in cancer continues to be intense. Responding to the challenge, researchers are bringing exciting new cancer diagnostic strategies and therapies to the clinical arena. The standard modalities of treatment—surgery, radiation therapy, chemotherapy—are being expanded to include targeted therapies, which build on advances in biotherapy and molecular biology. Typically, these modalities of therapy are used in combination with one another—providing a complementary and synergistic attack against cancer cells. So, driven by these multi-approach strategies, cancer care continues to be more complex and costly—a challenge that impacts the economic health of our society (Edwards et al., 2005; Williams-Brown & Singh, 2005).

Although the focus on breakthroughs and novel technologies continues, the underlying fears and personal, intimate trials associated with a cancer diagnosis do not change for the patient or family members. Thus, nursing care remains grounded in meeting that elusive goal each day—providing quality care for the patient (Given & Sherwood, 2005).

The purpose of this course is to provide nurses with a solid foundation for caring for patients with cancer. The course is intended for registered and licensed practical and vocational nurses who care for cancer patients or whose goal is to become specialized in cancer patient care. It can also be a useful resource for certification preparation.

TABLE i: NCI's 2015 GOAL—ELIMINATE THE SUFFERING AND DEATH DUE TO CANCER

STRATEGIC INITIATIVES TO MEET THE CHALLENGE GOAL

Understand the Causes and Mechanisms of Cancer

We will conduct and support basic, clinical, and population research to gain a more complete understanding of the genetic, epigenetic, environmental, behavioral, and sociocultural determinants of cancer and the biological mechanisms underlying cancer resistance, susceptibility, initiation, regression, progression, and recurrence.

Accelerate Progress in Cancer Prevention

We will accelerate the discovery, development, and delivery of cancer prevention interventions by investing in research focused on systems biology, behavior modifications, environmental and policy influences, medical and nutritional approaches, and training and education for research and health professionals.

Improve Early Detection and Diagnosis

We will support the development and dissemination of interventions to detect and diagnose early-stage malignancy.

Develop Effective and Efficient Treatments

We will support the development and dissemination of interventions to treat malignancy by either destroying all cancer cells or modulating and controlling metastasis, both with minimal harm to healthy tissue.

Understand the Factors that Influence Cancer Outcomes

We will support and conduct studies to increase our understanding of and ability to measure the environmental, behavioral, sociocultural, and economic influences that affect the quality of cancer care, survivorship, and health disparities.

Improve the Quality of Cancer Care

We will support the development and dissemination of quality improvement interventions and measure their success in improving health-related outcomes across the cancer continuum.

Improve the Quality of Life for Cancer Patients, Survivors, and Their Families

We will support the development and dissemination of interventions to reduce the adverse effects of cancer diagnosis and treatment and improve health-related outcomes for cancer patients, survivors, and their families.

Overcome Cancer Health Disparities

We will study and identify factors contributing to disparities, develop culturally appropriate approaches, and disseminate interventions to overcome those disparities across the cancer control continuum from disease prevention to end-of-life care.

Note. From *NCI Challenge Goal 2015,* by National Cancer Institute, 2005. Retrieved October 31, 2006, from http://www.cancer.gov/aboutnci/2015

REFERENCES

Edwards, B., Brown, M., Wingo, P., Howe, H., Ward, E., Ries, L., et al. (2005). Annual report to the nation on the status of cancer, 1975-2002, featuring population-based trends in cancer treatment. *Journal of the National Cancer Institute,* 97(19), 1407-1427.

Given, B. & Sherwood, P. (2005). Nursing-sensitive patient outcomes – A white paper. *Oncology Nursing Forum,* 32(4), 773-784.

National Cancer Institute. (2005). *NCI challenge goal 2015.* Retrieved October 31, 2006, from http://www.cancer.gov/aboutnci/2015

Williams-Brown, S. & Singh, G. (2005). Epidemiology of cancer in the United States. *Seminars in Oncology Nursing,* 21(4), 236-242.

Yancik, R. (2005). Population aging and cancer: A cross-national concern. *Cancer Journal,* 11(6), 437-441.

CHAPTER 1

EPIDEMIOLOGY

CHAPTER OBJECTIVE

After completing this chapter, the reader will be able to describe cancer trends in the United States and worldwide based on epidemiological statistics.

LEARNING OBJECTIVES

After studying this chapter, the reader will be able to

1. recognize cancer as the second leading cause of death in the United States.

2. list the most common cancer sites in men in the United States.

3. identify the most common cancer sites in women in the United States.

4. recognize the reasons for increases in death due to lung cancer.

INTRODUCTION

Cancer is a group of diseases characterized by uncontrolled growth and spread of abnormal cells. *Cancer* is a term for more than 100 disorders in which cells grow and multiply uncontrollably. Yet each cancer diagnosis has its own set of risk factors, disease trajectory, treatment plan, and expected outcomes.

Epidemiology terms used in discussions about cancer include:

*   incidence—the number of new cases occurring per year

*   mortality—the number of deaths occurring annually

*   mortality rate—for the population, the average risk of dying from cancer

*   prevalence of disease—the number of persons alive at a particular time with the disease.

(National Cancer Institute [NCI], 2005a, 2005b)

During 2006 in the United States, an estimated 1,399,790 new cancer cases were diagnosed. One-half of new cases of cancer occur in people ages 65 and older (American Cancer Society [ACS], 2006; Jemal et al., 2006) (see Figure 1-1).

In 2006, approximately 564,830 people died from a cancer diagnosis—more than 1,500 people per day. Following cardiovascular disease, cancer is the second leading cause of death in the United States (see Table 1-1). Death due to cancer in the United States is about one in four deaths, or about 23%.

Between 2002 and 2003, net cancer death rates declined slightly. This was the first recorded decrease in death rates since national mortality records were first compiled in 1930 (Jemal et al., 2006). Death rates for all cancers have decreased. For men, since 1993, the rate of decline has been about 1.5% per year. For women, since 1992, the

FIGURE 1-1: LEADING SITES OF NEW CANCER CASES AND DEATHS – 2006 ESTIMATES

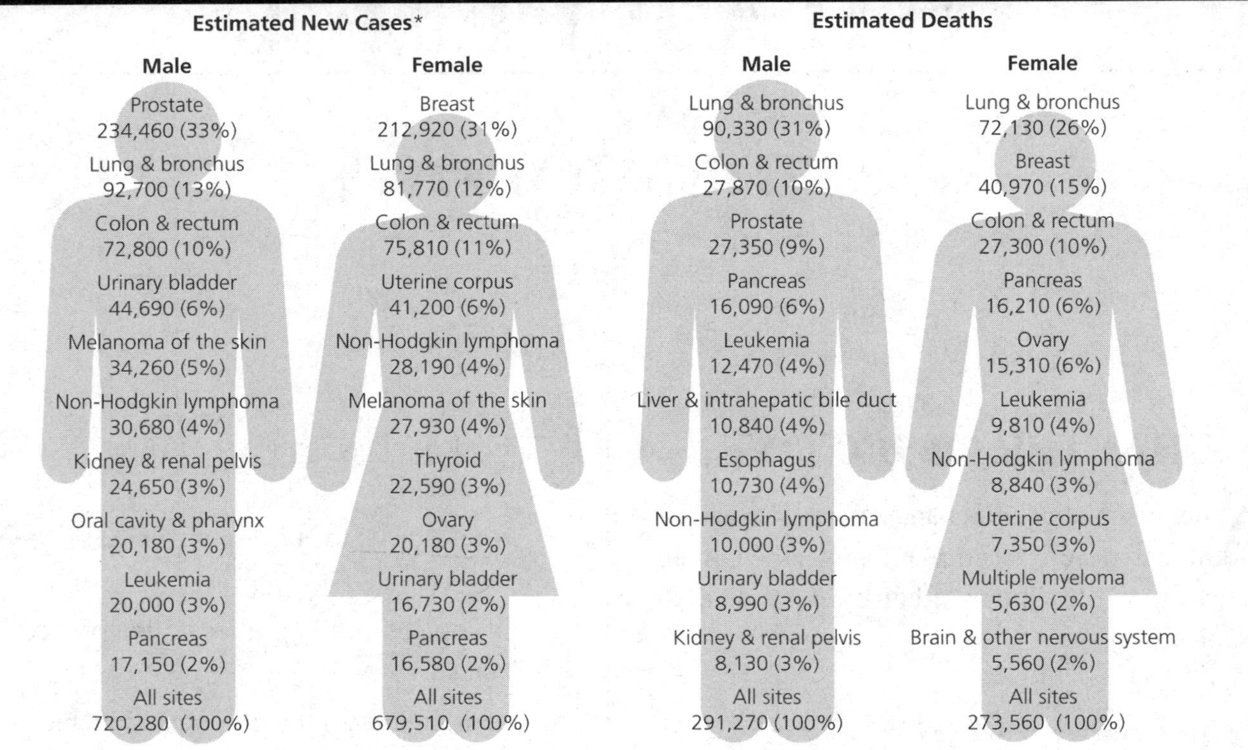

Estimated New Cases*

Estimated Deaths

Male	Female
Prostate 234,460 (33%)	Breast 212,920 (31%)
Lung & bronchus 92,700 (13%)	Lung & bronchus 81,770 (12%)
Colon & rectum 72,800 (10%)	Colon & rectum 75,810 (11%)
Urinary bladder 44,690 (6%)	Uterine corpus 41,200 (6%)
Melanoma of the skin 34,260 (5%)	Non-Hodgkin lymphoma 28,190 (4%)
Non-Hodgkin lymphoma 30,680 (4%)	Melanoma of the skin 27,930 (4%)
Kidney & renal pelvis 24,650 (3%)	Thyroid 22,590 (3%)
Oral cavity & pharynx 20,180 (3%)	Ovary 20,180 (3%)
Leukemia 20,000 (3%)	Urinary bladder 16,730 (2%)
Pancreas 17,150 (2%)	Pancreas 16,580 (2%)
All sites 720,280 (100%)	All sites 679,510 (100%)

Male	Female
Lung & bronchus 90,330 (31%)	Lung & bronchus 72,130 (26%)
Colon & rectum 27,870 (10%)	Breast 40,970 (15%)
Prostate 27,350 (9%)	Colon & rectum 27,300 (10%)
Pancreas 16,090 (6%)	Pancreas 16,210 (6%)
Leukemia 12,470 (4%)	Ovary 15,310 (6%)
Liver & intrahepatic bile duct 10,840 (4%)	Leukemia 9,810 (4%)
Esophagus 10,730 (4%)	Non-Hodgkin lymphoma 8,840 (3%)
Non-Hodgkin lymphoma 10,000 (3%)	Uterine corpus 7,350 (3%)
Urinary bladder 8,990 (3%)	Multiple myeloma 5,630 (2%)
Kidney & renal pelvis 8,130 (3%)	Brain & other nervous system 5,560 (2%)
All sites 291,270 (100%)	All sites 273,560 (100%)

*Excludes basal and squamous cell skin cancers and in situ carcinoma except urinary bladder.

Note: Percentages may not total 100% due to rounding.

©2006, American Cancer Society, Inc., Surveillance Research

Note. From American Cancer Society. *Cancer Facts & Figures 2006,* Atlanta: American Cancer Society, Inc. Reprinted with permission.

rate of decline has been about 0.9% per year. (See Figure 1-2 and Figure 1-3.)

CANCER SITES AND DEMOGRAPHICS

The most common cancer sites in men—lung, color and rectum, and prostate—account for 56% of new cancer cases. Prostate cancer alone accounts for one-third of new cancer cases in men, or one out of every six men over their lifetime.

For women, lung, breast, and colorectal cancers account for 54% of new cases. Breast cancer alone accounts for 31% of new cancer cases, or one of every eight women over their lifetime. For women, mortality rates for breast and colorectal cancer have slightly decreased. Yet cases of lung cancer in women continue to slightly rise (Jemal et al., 2006). Since 1987, lung cancer surpassed breast cancer as the leading cause of cancer death in women. In 2006, lung cancer was the cause of death in 26% of women who died from cancer.

African American men have a 40% higher death rate from cancer than the rate for Caucasian men. African American women have an 18% higher death rate from cancer than the rate for Caucasian women (Jemal et al., 2006) (see Table 1-2).

For the four major cancer sites—lung, breast, color and rectum, and prostate—cancer incidence and death rates are lower in certain ethnic groups (Asian-American/Pacific Islander; American Indian/Alaskan Native, Hispanic/Latino) than for Caucasians and African Americans. However, cancer rates for liver, stomach, and cervical cancers are generally higher in these other ethnic groups than in Caucasians (Jemal et al., 2006). In addition, those from minority populations are more

TABLE 1-1: LEADING CAUSES OF DEATH – 2005

[Data are based on the 10th revision of the International Classification of Disease (ICD). Rates per 100,000 population in specified group. Numbers are based on weighted data rounded to the nearest individual, so categories may not add to total.]

Age	Number	Rate	Age	Number	Rate
All Ages			Malignant neoplasms	16,085	35.8
All Causes	2,443,387	847.3	Diseases of the heart	13,688	30.5
Diseases of the heart	696,947	241.7	Intentional self-harm	6,851	15.3
Malignant neoplasms	557,271	193.2	Human immunodeficiency virus (HIV) disease	5,707	12.7
Cerebrovascular disease	162,672	56.4	45-54 years		
Chronic lower respiratory disease	124,616	43.3	All causes	172,385	430.1
Accidents (unintentional injuries)	106,742	37.0	Malignant neoplasms	49,637	123.8
1-4 years			Diseases of the heart	37,570	93.7
All causes	4,858	31.2	Accidents	14,675	36.6
Accidents (unintentional injuries)	1,641	10.5	Chronic liver disease and cirrhosis	7,216	18.0
Congenital malformations	530	3.4	Intentional self-harm (suicide)	6,308	15.7
Assault (homicide)	423	2.7			
Malignant neoplasms	402	2.6	55-64 years		
Diseases of the heart	165	1.1	All causes	253,342	952.4
5-14 years			Malignant neoplasms	93,391	351.1
All causes	7,150	17.4	Diseases of the heart	64,234	241.5
Accidents (unintentional injuries)	2,718	6.6	Chronic lower respiratory disease	11,280	42.4
Malignant neoplasms	1,072	2.8	Diabetes mellitis	10,022	37.7
Congenital malformations	417	1.0	Cardiovascular disease	9,897	37.2
Assault (homicide)	356	0.9	65-74 years		
Diseases of the heart	265	0.6	All causes	422,990	2,314.7
Intentional self-harm (suicide)	264	0.6	Malignant neoplasms	144,757	792.1
15-24 years			Diseases of the heart	112,547	615.9
All causes	33,046	91.4	Cerebrovascular disease	29,788	163.0
Accidents (unintentional injuries)	15,412	39.0	Chronic lower respiratory disease	21,992	120.3
Assault (homicide)	5,219	12.9	Diabetes mellitis	16,709	91.4
Intentional self-harm (suicide)	4,010	9.9	75-84 years		
Malignant neoplasms	1,790	4.3	All causes	707,654	5,556.9
Diseases of the heart	1,022	2.5	Diseases of heart	213,581	1,677.2
25-34 years			Malignant neoplasms	167,062	1,311.9
All causes	41,355	103.6	Cerebrovascular diseases	54,889	431.0
Accidents	12,569	31.5	Chronic lower respiratory disease	49,241	386.7
Intentional self-harm (suicide)	5, 046	12.6	Diabetes mellitis	23,282	182.8
Assault (homicide)	4,489	11.2	85 years and older		
Malignant neoplasms	3,872	9.7	All causes	681,076	14,828.3
Diseases of the heart	3,165	7.9	Diseases of the heart	250,173	5,446.8
			Malignant neoplasms	79,182	1,723.9
25-44 years			Cerebrovascular disease	66,412	1,445.3
All causes	91,140	202.9	Alzheimer's disease	34,552	752.3
Accidents	16,710	37.2	Influenza and pneumonia	31,995	696.6

Note. From Deaths: Leading causes for 2002 by R.N. Anderson & B.L. Smith, *National vital statistics reports;* vol 53 no 17. Hyattsville, Maryland: National Center for Health Statistics. 2005. Retrieved April 3, 2007, from http://www.cdc.gov/nchs/data/nvsr/nvsr53/nvsr53_17.pdf

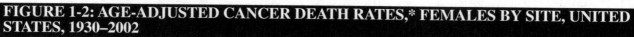

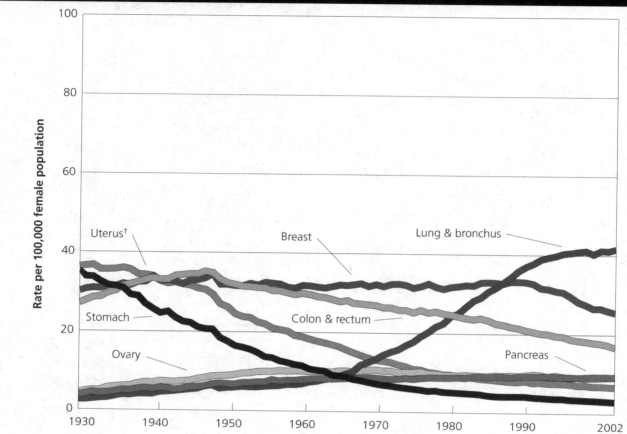

FIGURE 1-2: AGE-ADJUSTED CANCER DEATH RATES,* FEMALES BY SITE, UNITED STATES, 1930–2002

*Per 100,000, age-adjusted to the 2000 US standard population. †Uterus cancer death rates are for uterine cervix and uterine corpus combined.

Note: Due to changes in ICD coding, numerator information has changed over time. Rates for cancer of the lung and bronchus, colon and rectum, and ovary are affected by these coding changes.

Source: US Mortality Public Use Data Tapes 1960 to 2002, US Mortality Volumes 1930 to 1959, National Center for Health Statistics, Centers for Disease Control and Prevention, 2005.

American Cancer Society, Surveillance Research, 2006

Note. From American Cancer Society. *Cancer Facts & Figures 2006,* Atlanta: American Cancer Society, Inc. Reprinted with permission.

commonly diagnosed with later stage disease than Caucasians (Jemal et al., 2006) (see Table 1-3).

For many cancer sites—including the pancreas, liver, esophagus, lung, and stomach—the 5-year survival rate for all sexes, ages, and ethnic groups is poor (less than 25%) (Jemal et al., 2006).

RISK FACTORS AND CAUSES OF CANCER

Tobacco smoking is the primary risk factor for cancer. It causes an estimated 30% of all cancer deaths. In 2006, 170,000 cancer deaths were caused by tobacco use (ACS, 2006). Tobacco use

has declined slightly in the past 20 years (see Figure 1-4), although the number of women and young people who smoke has increased (see Chapter 3). Efforts to establish legislation that curbs tobacco use include taxes on tobacco products, restrictions in marketing and advertising of tobacco products, and agreements between the states and tobacco companies that earmark monies toward state tobacco-control programs. Many states, however, have shifted tobacco legislation settlement monies away from comprehensive programs to prevent and reduce tobacco use (National Center for Tobacco-Free Kids, 2006).

Following tobacco use, poor nutrition and inactivity are the next highest risk factors leading to a

FIGURE 1-3: AGE-ADJUSTED CANCER DEATH RATES,* MALES BY SITE, UNITED STATES, 1930–2002

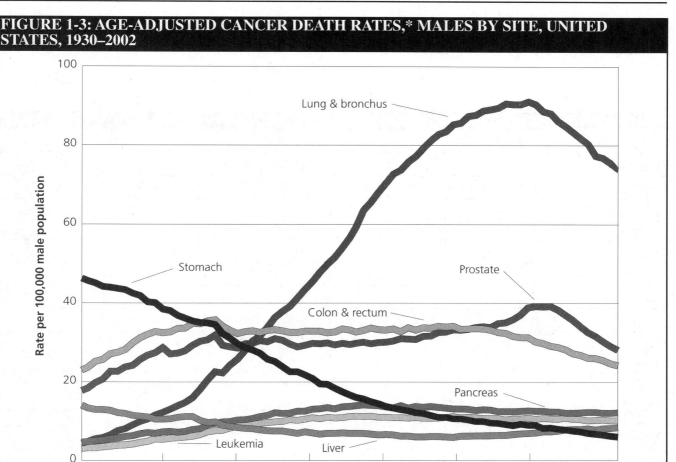

*Per 100,000, age-adjusted to the 2000 US standard population.

Note: Due to changes in ICD coding, numerator information has changed over time. Rates for cancer of the liver, lung and bronchus, and colon and rectum are affected by these coding changes.

Source: US Mortality Public Use Data Tapes 1960 to 2002, US Mortality Volumes 1930 to 1959, National Center for Health Statistics, Centers for Disease Control and Prevention, 2005.

American Cancer Society, Surveillance Research, 2006

Note. From American Cancer Society. *Cancer Facts & Figures 2006,* Atlanta: American Cancer Society, Inc. Reprinted with permission.

cancer diagnosis. Approximately one-third of cancer deaths is attributed to poor nutrition, physical inactivity, and overweight or obesity (ACS, 2006).

Other factors also play a role. In 2006, more than one million diagnosed skin cancers could have been prevented by using protection from the sun (ACS, 2006). Other cancers are known to be triggered by environmental exposure to toxins and infectious agents, such as hepatitis B virus (HBV) and human immunodeficiency virus. Inherited cancers are estimated to account for 5% to 10% of all cancers.

The ACS estimates that regular screening exams for cervical, colorectal, breast, prostate, oral cavity, and skin cancers can detect those specific cancers at an early stage. Cancers that can be detected early account for 50% of all new cancers. The 5-year survival rate for these cancers is about 86%, when detected early and treated promptly (ACS, 2006).

In 2006, the NCI estimated that approximately 10.1 million Americans with a history of cancer were alive in January 2002, the latest statistics available. For the period 1995 to 2001, the 5-year relative survival rate from cancer was 65%. This was an increase in survival from the period 1974 to 1976, which was 50% (NCI, 2005c).

Among the factors that are attributed to longer survival rates are:

- Moderate reduction in tobacco use
- Screening programs, especially those for breast and colorectal cancers

- Education about wearing sunscreen, protective clothing, and hats or caps as protection from sun exposure

TABLE 1-2: MORTALITY 2002

Cancer	All Races			Whites			Blacks		
	Total	Males	Females	Total	Males	Females	Total	Males	Females
All cancers	190.1	234.1	160.5	188.3	230.6	159.7	234.5	311.4	188.2
Lung and bronchus	54.2	71.9	41.2	54.5	71.2	42.2	61.2	93.1	40.3
Breast	14.2	0.3	25.2	13.8	0.3	24.6	20.2	0.5	34.1
Cervix uteri	2.5	–	2.5	2.2	–	2.2	4.7	–	4.7
Colorectal	19.0	23.0	16.1	18.5	22.4	15.5	26.4	32.1	22.7
Prostate	26.6	26.6	–	24.5	24.5	–	58.0	58.0	–
Non-Hodgkin lymphoma	7.3	9.3	5.9	7.6	9.7	6.1	4.9	5.8	4.3
Melanoma of skin	2.7	3.9	1.7	3.0	4.4	2.0	0.4	0.4	0.4

Source: National Center for Health Statistics data as analyzed by NCI. Data are age-adjusted to the 2000 standard using age groups: < 1, 1-4, 5-14, 15-24, 25-34, 35-44, 45-54, 55-64, 65-74, 75-84, 85+. Analysis uses the 2000 Standard Population as defined by NCHS (http://www.cdc.gov/nchs/data/statnt/statnt20.pdf).
– Statistic not shown. Rate based on less than 25 cases for the year 2002.

Note. From *Cancer Trends Progress Report – 2005 Update*, National Cancer Institute, NIH, DHHS, 2005, Bethesda, MD, December 2005. Retrieved October 31, 2006, from http://progressreport.cancer.gov

TABLE 1-3: INCIDENCE 2002

Cancer	All Races			Whites			Blacks		
	Total	Males	Females	Total	Males	Females	Total	Males	Females
All cancers	459.6	540.0	404.1	467.6	541.3	417.3	499.4	650.4	397.6
Lung and bronchus	62.7	78.5	51.3	63.6	77.1	53.9	78.5	115.5	53.5
Breast	67.5	1.5	124.2	69.1	1.5	128.5	69.5	2.0	120.5
Cervix uteri	7.1	–	7.1	6.6	–	6.6	10.5	–	10.5
Colorectal	49.5	58.0	42.8	49.0	57.1	42.4	60.4	72.6	52.5
Prostate	164.9	164.9	–	160.0	160.0	–	247.0	247.0	–
Non-Hodgkin lymphoma	19.8	23.6	16.9	20.8	24.7	17.7	15.4	18.5	13.1
Melanoma of skin	18.7	23.0	15.8	22.3	26.9	19.2	0.8	–	–

Source: SEER Program, National Cancer Institute. Incidence data are from the SEER 9 areas (http://seer.cancer.gov/registries/terms.html). Data are age-adjusted to the 2000 standard using age groups: < 1, 1-4, 5-9, 10-14, 15-19, 20-24, 25-29, 30-34, 35-39, 40-44, 45-49, 50-54, 55-59, 60-64, 65-69, 70-74, 75-79, 80-84, 85+. Analysis uses the 2000 Standard Population (Census P25-1130) as defined by NCI (http://seer.cancer.gov/stdpopulations/).
– Statistic not shown. Rate based on less than 25 cases for the year 2002.

Note. From *Cancer Trends Progress Report – 2005 Update*, National Cancer Institute, NIH, DHHS, 2005, Bethesda, MD, December 2005. Retrieved October 31, 2006, from http://progressreport.cancer.gov

FIGURE 1-4: DECREASED SMOKING LINE GRAPH

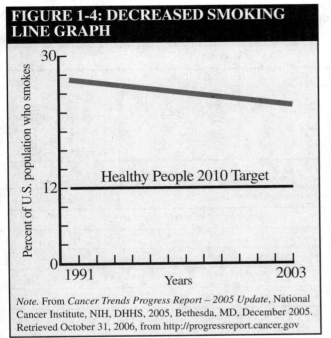

Note. From *Cancer Trends Progress Report – 2005 Update*, National Cancer Institute, NIH, DHHS, 2005, Bethesda, MD, December 2005. Retrieved October 31, 2006, from http://progressreport.cancer.gov

- Immunization against HBV and development of a vaccine against hepatitis C virus (both can lead to liver cancer)

- Improved use of effective but underutilized screening tools for colorectal and breast cancers

- Improvements in nutritional lifestyle

- Development of agents that reduce the risk of developing specific cancers—also called *chemoprevention* (for example, tamoxifen for breast cancer)

- Development of molecularly targeted agents, which specifically target cancer cells and cause fewer side effects than conventional chemotherapy or radiation therapy

- Increased enrollment in clinical trials to speed up evaluation of new approaches to treatment

- Identification of and reduction of disparities across ethnic, racial, gender, and socioeconomic groups.

(CDC, 2007; ACS, 2006; Jemal et al., 2006; NCI, 2005a, 2005b; Miller-Murphy et al., 2005)

INTERNATIONAL CANCER TRENDS

According to the International Union Against Cancer (UICC), one in every eight deaths worldwide is due to cancer. Cancer claims twice as many lives as acquired immunodeficiency syndrome (AIDS) (UICC, 2006).

During 2002 (the latest date for available statistics), 10.9 million new cases of cancer were diagnosed worldwide, with 6.7 million deaths. The most commonly diagnosed cancers are lung cancer (1.3 million, or 12.4% of all new cancers), breast cancer (1.15 million), and colorectal cancer (1 million) (Parkin, Bray, Ferlay, & Pisani, 2005) (see Table 1-4).

Cancer deaths worldwide are most commonly lung, stomach, and liver cancers. The most widespread cancer in the world is breast cancer. It accounts for 23% of cancer cases in women (Parkin et al., 2005) (see Figure 1-5).

Since 1985, lung cancer has been the most common cancer in the world and lung cancer cases have increased by 51% (44% in men, 76% in women). The rise is largely attributable to the aging population and population growth. In 2002, lung cancer was the cause of approximately 17.6% of all cancer patient deaths. The highest rates of death are among men, with most diagnosed from North America and Europe (especially Eastern Europe). Those from Australia, New Zealand, and eastern Asia (China and Japan) have a moderately high rate of death from lung cancer (Parkin et al., 2005).

The worldwide risk for cancers varies, depending on geography and exposure to selected risk factors—especially those related to lifestyle and environment (Parkin et al., 2005).

People from developing countries who are diagnosed with cancer make up almost half of all people in the world who die from cancer. This statistic is a major change from 1980, when it was estimated that 69% of those dying from cancer

TABLE 1-4: INCIDENCE AND MORTALITY BY SEX AND CANCER SITE, WORLDWIDE, 2002

| | INCIDENCE | | | | | | MORTALITY | | | | | |
| | MALES | | | FEMALES | | | MALES | | | FEMALES | | |
	Cases	ASR (World)	Cumulative risk (age 0–64)	Cases	ASR (World)	Cumulative risk (age 0–64)	Deaths	ASR (World)	Cumulative risk (age 0–64)	Deaths	ASR (World)	Cumulative risk (age 0–64)
Oral cavity	175,916	6.3	0.4	98,373	3.2	0.2	80,736	2.9	0.2	46,723	1.5	0.1
Nasopharynx	55,796	1.9	0.1	24,247	0.8	0.1	34,913	1.2	0.1	15,419	0.5	0.0
Other pharynx	106,219	3.8	0.3	24,077	0.8	0.1	67,964	2.5	0.2	16,029	0.5	0.0
Esophagus	315,394	11.5	0.6	146,723	4.7	0.3	261,162	9.6	0.5	124,730	3.9	0.2
Stomach	603,419	22	1.2	330,518	10.3	0.5	446,052	16.3	0.8	254,297	7.9	0.4
Colon/rectum	550,465	20.1	0.9	472,687	14.6	0.7	278,446	10.2	0.4	250,532	7.6	0.3
Liver	442,119	15.7	1.0	184,043	5.8	0.3	416,882	14.9	0.9	181,439	5.7	0.3
Pancreas	124,841	4.6	0.2	107,465	3.3	0.1	119,544	4.4	0.2	107,479	3.3	0.1
Larynx	139,230	5.1	0.3	20,011	0.6	0	78,629	2.9	0.2	11,327	0.4	0.0
Lung	965,241	35.5	1.7	386,891	12.1	0.6	848,132	31.2	1.4	330,786	10.3	0.5
Melanoma of skin	79,043	2.8	0.2	81,134	2.6	0.2	21,952	0.8	0.0	18,829	0.6	0.0
Kaposi sarcoma*												
Breast				1,151,298	37.4	2.6				410,712	13.2	0.9
Cervix uteri				493,243	16.2	1.3				273,505	9.0	0.7
Corpus uteri				198,783	6.5	0.4				50,327	1.6	0.1
Ovary				204,499	6.6	0.5				124,860	4.0	0.2
Prostate	679,023	25.3	0.8				221,002	8.2	0.1			
Testis	48,613	1.5	0.1				8,878	0.3	0.0			
Kidney	129,223	4.7	0.3	79,257	2.5	0.1	62,696	2.3	0.1	39,199	1.2	0.1
Bladder	273,858	10.1	0.4	82,699	2.5	0.1	108,310	4.0	0.1	36,699	1.1	0.0
Brain, nervous system	108,221	3.7	0.2	81,264	2.6	0.2	80,034	2.8	0.2	61,616	2.0	0.1
Thyroid	37,424	1.3	0.1	103,589	3.3	0.2	11,297	0.4	0.0	24,078	0.8	0.0
Non-Hodgkin lymphoma	175,123	6.1	0.3	125,448	3.9	0.2	98,865	3.5	0.2	72,955	2.3	0.1
Hodgkin disease	38,218	1.2	0.1	24,111	0.8	0.1	14,460	0.5	0.0	8,352	0.3	0.0
Multiple myeloma	46,512	1.7	0.1	39,192	1.2	0.1	32,696	1.2	0.1	29,839	0.9	0.0
Leukemia	171,037	5.9	0.3	129,485	4.1	0.2	125,142	4.3	0.2	97,364	3.1	0.2
All sites but skin	5,801,839	209.6	10.3	5,060,657	161.5	9.5	3,795,991	137.7	6.4	2,927,896	92.1	4.9

*Africa only.

Note. From "Global Cancer Statistics, 2002," by M. Parkin, F. Bray, J. Ferlay, & P. Pisani, 2005, *CA Cancer J Clin 2004; 55*:74-108. Reprinted with permission of Lippincott Williams & Wilkins (http://lww.com).

FIGURE 1-5: INCIDENCE, MORTALITY, AND PREVALENCE BY LOCATION

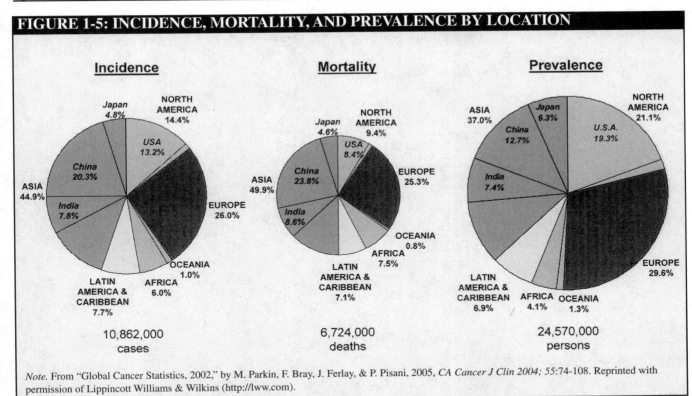

Note. From "Global Cancer Statistics, 2002," by M. Parkin, F. Bray, J. Ferlay, & P. Pisani, 2005, *CA Cancer J Clin 2004; 55:*74-108. Reprinted with permission of Lippincott Williams & Wilkins (http://lww.com).

were from developing countries (Parkin et al., 2005). Worldwide statistics show that the high rate of cancer in developing countries can be linked to affluence and lifestyle, which are linked to such risk factors as tobacco use and obesity.

More specifically, in 2002, the number of new cancer cases in China was 2.2 million (20.3% of the world total). In 2002 in North America, new cancer cases were 1.6 million, or 14.4% of the world total. The cancer death ratio, men to women, is 1:3; the incidence rate, men to women, is 1:15 (Parkin et al., 2005).

In sub-Saharan Africa, the AIDS epidemic has created a cancer problem with Kaposi sarcoma (KS) and AIDS-associated lymphomas. In 2004, the death rate from KS-associated AIDS was 52,000 (Parkin et al., 2005).

SUMMARY

Although cancer death rates have declined slightly in the United States, cancer remains the second most common cause of death. The most common cancer sites in men—lung, colorectal, and prostate—account for 56% of new cases. Prostate cancer alone accounts for one-third of new cancer cases in men. For women, lung, breast, and colon and rectum, cancer account for 54% of new cases, with breast cancer responsible for one-third of new cases. Internationally, lung cancer is the most commonly diagnosed cancer. Worldwide, the leading causes of cancer deaths are lung, stomach, and liver cancers.

EXAM QUESTIONS

CHAPTER 1
Questions 1-4

Note: Choose the option that BEST answers each question.

1. Based on U.S. statistics reported in 2005, cancer is

    a. the first leading cause of death.

    b. the second leading cause of death.

    c. the third leading cause of death.

    d. the most frequently reported illness.

2. In the United States, the most common sites of cancer in men are

    a. brain, colon and rectum, and prostate.

    b. lung, colon and rectum, and prostate.

    c. lung, bladder, and skin.

    d. oral cavity, prostate, and lung.

3. In the United States, the most common sites of cancer in women are

    a. brain, colon and rectum, and breast.

    b. lung, breast, and uterus.

    c. lung, skin, and uterus.

    d. breast, lung, and colon and rectum.

4. Death due to lung cancer is still primarily attributed to

    a. age.

    b. diet.

    c. tobacco use.

    d. viruses.

REFERENCES

American Cancer Society. (2006). *Cancer facts & figures 2006.* Atlanta: Author.

Anderson, R.N. & Smith, B.L. (2005). *Deaths: Leading causes for 2002.* National vital statistics reports; vol. 53 no. 17. Hyattsville, MD: National Center for Health Statistics. Retrieved April 3, 2007, from http://www.cdc.gov/nchs/data/nvsr/nvsr53/nvsr53_17.pdf

Centers for Disease Control and Prevention. (2007). *Preventing and controlling cancer: The nation's second leading cause of death: At a glance 2007.* Retrieved April 17, 2007 from http://www.cdc.gov/nccdphp/publications/aag/dcpc.htm

International Union Against Cancer. (2006). *National cancer control planning.* Retrieved October 31, 2006, from http://www.uicc.org/index.php?id=1257&L=0

Jemal, A., Siegel, R., Ward, E., Murray, T., Xu, J, Smigal, C., et al. (2006). Cancer statistics, 2006. *CA: Cancer Journal for Clinicians, 56*(2), 106–130.

Miller-Murphy, C., Ballon, L., Culhane, B., Mafrica, L., McCorkle, M., & Worrall, L. (2005). Oncology Nursing Society environmental scan 2004. *Oncology Nursing Forum, 32*(4), 742.

National Cancer Institute. (2005a). *Cancer mortality maps & graphs.* Available from http://www3.cancer.gov/atlasplus

National Cancer Institute. (2005b). *Cancer trends progress report—2005 update.* Available from http://progressreport.cancer.gov

National Cancer Institute. (2005c). *Cancer trends progress report—2005 update. Trends at a glance.* Available from http://progress-report.cancer.gov/trends-glance.asp

National Center for Tobacco-Free Kids. (2006). *Executive Summary and key findings of the multistate settlement agreement* (MSA). Retrieved April 17, 2007, from http://tobaccofreekids.org/reports/settlements/

Parkin, D., Bray, F., Ferlay, J., & Pisani, P. (2005). Global cancer statistics, 2002. *CA: Cancer Journal for Clinicians, 55*(2), 74–108.

CHAPTER 2

BIOLOGY OF CANCER

CHAPTER OBJECTIVE

After completing this chapter, the reader will be able to describe what is currently known about carcinogenesis and cell biology, which provide the foundation for cancer prevention, detection, and treatment.

LEARNING OBJECTIVES

After studying this chapter, the reader will be able to

1. list prefixes that describe the tissue origins for cell types (e.g., *sar-*, *adeno-*, *osteo-*).

2. identify three characteristics of cancerous cells.

3. describe how tumor doubling time can be controlled.

4. identify a type of cancer that can have familial and genetic traits.

INTRODUCTION

The biology of cancer provides answers about how to treat a particular tumor. This chapter reviews how cancer cells grow, how their growth becomes uncontrolled, and how treatments improve as more is learned about how cancer cells behave on a molecular level.

OVERVIEW

The term *cancer* refers to a group of diseases that allow uncontrolled cell growth. All forms of cancer involve out-of-control growth and spread of abnormal cells, coupled with a decrease in the body's immune system surveillance.

All cells in the body go through a cycle of development and proliferation. Cell cycle growth is shown in Figure 2-1. All normal body cells grow, divide, and die. Normal cells in children divide more rapidly than normal adult cells. But in adults, normal cells of most tissues divide only to replace worn-out or dying cells and to repair injuries.

A cancer cell—in its out-of-control state—grows, divides, and spreads to other parts of the body. When cells spread, the process of cell growth and division goes unchecked. These out-of-control cells accumulate and form tumors that can compress, invade, and destroy normal tissue. If cancer cells break away from the malignant tumor, they can travel throughout the body via the bloodstream or the lymph system, taking root in new areas of the body. This spreading of malignant cells to sites distant from their origin is called *metastasis* (Volker, 2005).

Terminology

Even though research continually further clarifies the malignant process, standard terms and processes are still used to describe cancer and

FIGURE 2-1: THE FOUR PHASES OF THE CELL CYCLE

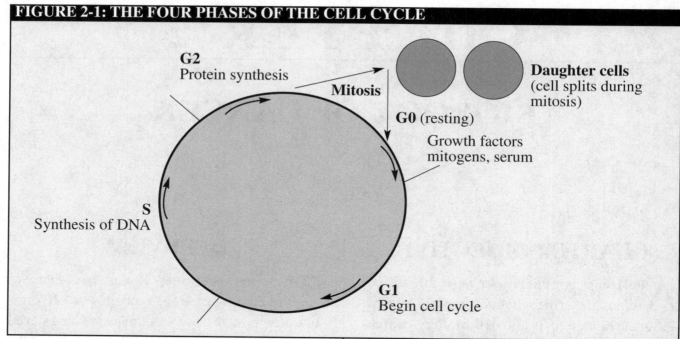

malignancy. *Neoplasia* is the abnormal growth of new tissue. When a tumor grows because of the size of cells, the growth is called *hypertrophy*. When the growth increase is due to an increase in the number of cells, it is called *hyperplasia*. Neoplasia can refer to benign or malignant growth. *Benign* tumors grow but consist of normal cells. Benign tumors do not spread to other parts of the body.

A *neoplasm*—or *tumor*—is not malignant unless it has the characteristics of malignant lesions or abnormal, out-of-control cells. Neoplastic growth may be *metaplastic*—in which one mature cell type is replaced by another mature type—or it may be *dysplastic*—in which a mature type of cell is replaced by a less mature type of cell. The replacement cell may also be a precursor to precancerous cells (in situ) or invasive cancer cells.

Carcinogenesis is the process by which cancer cells congregate to become a malignant tumor. It is also known as *oncogenesis* or *malignant transformation*. To become transformed into malignancies, tumors need to have an *initiator*, or primary change, in the cells from normal to abnormal. When the cells first start to grow, they need a *promoter*, or a secondary cause, activity, or force that induces a malignancy. Then, as the tumor grows— expanding

and spreading—it becomes more virulent and out of control (CancerSource, 2004).

Primary Diagnosis

Cancerous tumors may be described as "solid." Examples of solid tumors are cancers of the breast, lung, and colon. Examples of hematologic cancers, or those based in blood or lymph fluid, include some forms of leukemia and lymphoma. In leukemia, the cancer cells involve the blood and blood-forming organs (bone marrow, lymphatic system, and spleen) and circulate throughout the body.

The origin of the cancer cell gives the cancer its name and the primary diagnosis. Thus, breast cancer starts with malignant cells in the breast; colon cancer starts in the colon. An estimated 10% to 12% of all patients have more than one primary diagnosis (Merkle & Loescher, 2006). Secondary diagnoses involve tumors identified in the areas to which the primary cancer has spread. For example, a patient with a breast tumor could develop a secondary breast tumor in the contralateral breast or a patient may have breast cancer and develop second primary thyroid cancer (Volker, 2005).

Classification

Tumors are classified, which allows precision in diagnosis and treatment. Classification is based on both the tumor's tissue of origin and the malignant or benign nature of the tumor's growth. For example, the suffix *-oma* is used for both benign tumors (papilloma, cystoma) and malignant tumors (sarcoma, carcinoma). Sarcomas originate from connective tissue, such as bone and muscle; carcinomas originate from the epithelium.

Hematologic malignancies have their origin in the hematopoietic system, or the blood and lymph. They start developing in stem cells in the bone marrow. Terms such as *lympho-* and *myelo-* describe the origins of hematologic cancers (e.g., acute myeloblastic leukemia) (Merkle & Loescher, 2006).

Staging of tumors is based on standards developed for that type of tumor. Many tumor staging methods exist, but there is consistency in the staging used for most individual solid tumor types, such as staging for lung, breast, and colon cancers.

TNM definitions are a basic framework for many staging schemas. TNM represents:

T = the size of the primary tumor

N = lymph node involvement

M = degree of spread, or metastasis.

Numbers added to these letters establish the degree, number, size, and spread of the tumor, allowing further definition of the malignancy. Table 2-1 presents a staging schema for lung cancer. For example, for a lung cancer in this TNM schema, a T1, N2, M0 means that the tumor is 3 cm or less in dimension (T1) and has metastasized to the ipsilateral mediastinal lymph nodes (N2) but has not metastasized to distant sites (M0) (American Joint Committee on Cancer, 2002).

CANCER CELL CHARACTERISTICS

Volker (2005) explains that cancerous cells have several distinct characteristics:

- **Loss of proliferative control.** Proliferation is the rapid increase of cells. In normal cells, the need for cell replacement stimulates cell production. This results in a balance between cell loss and cell production. In a cancerous cell, no control mechanism stops production once a stimulus has signaled cell production to begin. Moreover, cell growth continues unabated.

- **Loss of the ability to differentiate.** A cell's specific structure, function, and rate of division establish its ability to differentiate. Low-grade tumors have well-differentiated cells that deviate least from the normal cells from which they arise; high-grade tumors, which are more aggressive, have poorly differentiated cells and less closely resemble normal cells. Anaplastic cells have an atypical tissue structure and growth pattern and bear little resemblance to normal cells of the involved tissue. Tumors that have poorly differentiated cancer cells usually have a poorer prognosis; they are more aggressive and more resistant to treatment.

- **Biochemical changes.** If a cell lacks differentiation, some biochemical characteristics also may be missing because the cell exists in an immature form. Cancer cells also may develop new biochemical characteristics because of changes in enzyme patterns or deoxyribonucleic acid (DNA).

- **Chromosomal instability.** Normal cells have an extremely stable chromosome structure. Cancer cells have unstable chromosomes and tend to mutate often. As cancer cells reproduce, they create new malignant variations of themselves. These constant mutations can cause a tumor to have a small group of malignant cells that resists cancer therapies.

TABLE 2-1: STAGING OF LUNG CANCER

Lung cancer is the most common cause of cancer-related death in men and women; approximately 174,470 new cases were diagnosed in 2006. This disease is one of the most difficult cancers to treat; 5-year survival rates are approximately 15% (ACS, 2006). Bronchoscopy is an important procedure for accurate staging prior to therapy. Surgery and radiation therapy are the primary modalities of treatment for localized or regional disease. The primary tumor may be squamous cell carcinoma or adenocarcinoma. Metastatic spread occurs to intrathoracic lymph nodes, followed by the cervical lymph nodes, liver, brain, bones, adrenal glands, kidneys, and contralateral lung.

Primary Tumor (T)

TX   Primary tumor cannot be assessed

T0   No evidence of primary tumor

Tis Carcinoma in situ

T1   Tumor ≤ 3 cm without invasion more proximal than the lobar bronchus

T2   Tumor > 3 cm in size; involves main bronchus ≥ 2 cm distal to the carina; invades visceral pleura

T3   Direct invasion of chest wall, diaphragm, pericardium; involves main bronchus, < 2 cm distal to the carina

T4   Tumor invades mediastinum, heart, great vessels, trachea, esophagus, vertebral body, carina; or separate tumor nodules in the same lobe; or tumor with a malignant pleural effusion

Regional Lymph Nodes (N)

NX   Regional lymph nodes cannot be assessed

N0   No regional lymph node metastasis

N1   Metastasis in ipsilateral peribronchial and/or ipsilateral hilar lymph nodes

N2   Metastasis in ipsilateral mediastinal and/or subcarinal lymph nodes

N3   Metastasis in contralateral mediastinal, contralateral hilar, ipsilateral or contralateral scalene, or supraclavicular lymph node(s)

Distant Metastasis (M)

MX   Distant metastasis cannot be assessed

M0   No distant metastasis

M1   Distant metastasis

Stage Grouping

Stage	T	N	M
Stage 0	Tis	N0	M0
Stage IA	T1	N0	M0
Stage lB	T2	N0	M0
Stage IIA	T1	N1	M0
Stage IIB	T2	N1	M0
	T3	N0	M0
Stage IIIA	T1	N2	M0
	T2	N2	M0
	T3	N1, N2	M0
Stage IIIB	Any T	N3	M0
	T4	Any N	M0
Stage IV	Any T	Any N	M1

Note. Used with the permission of the American Join Committee on Cancer (AJCC), Chicago, Illinois. The original source for this material is the *AJCC Cancer Staging Manual,* Sixth Edition (2002) published by Springer-New York, www.springeronline.com.

- **Ability to metastasize.** As a tumor's cells repeatedly mutate, the cells increase and spread. Metastasis is the spread and growth of a primary malignant tumor. About 30% of patients with solid tumors have detectable metastasis at the time of diagnosis. Cancers often have a set pattern of metastasis based on the organ of origin. For example, lung cancer tends to spread to the liver, bones, and brain. The most common sites of metastasis from solid tumors are the lungs, liver, central nervous system (brain and spine), and bone (see Table 2-2).

TABLE 2-2: SITES OF METASTASIS FOR COMMON TUMORS

Cancer	Sites of Metastasis
Lung cancer	Lymph nodes, brain, bone, liver, pancreas
Colorectal cancer	Adjacent lymph nodes, liver
Breast cancer	Bone, brain, lung, liver
Leukemia	Visceral organs, brain
Prostate cancer	Bone, adjacent lymph nodes, lung

Factors that can contribute to increased metastatic spread include the initial stage of the tumor when diagnosed, a high rate of tumor growth, the initial site of spread, trauma, necrotic tissue, heat, and radiation (Volker, 2005).

Characteristics of Malignant Tumors

Cell growth alone is not sufficient to classify a tumor as malignant, because benign lesions can also grow. Malignant changes include these characteristics:

- **Invasiveness.** Malignant neoplasms can expand, invade, and destroy normal adjacent tissue.

- **Rapid growth.** Although benign and even normal cells can grow and divide rapidly, malignant cells are highly proliferative.

- **Decreased contact inhibition.** Even when normal cells grow and divide quickly, they are able to stop growing when they reach adjacent tissue. Malignant cells do not stop growing; they invade surrounding tissues.

- **Dissemination.** Usually, malignant cells spread or metastasize throughout the body through known patterns of dissemination, such as via contiguous spread, the lymphatic system or bloodstream, transabdominal seeding and, to a lesser degree, transplantation during surgical procedures (Volker, 2005).

Alterations in Cell Biology

A cell's carcinogenic changes can be anatomic, biochemical, or kinetic. Anatomic changes in the cell include the abnormal size and shape of cells, increased rates of mitosis (cell division) in malignant cells, and modification of the cell structure itself, including the cell membrane and organelles (mitochondria and, in particular, the nucleus). Malignant cells commonly have enlarged nuclei, chromosomal changes, or multiple mitoses.

To evaluate these cell changes, researchers can conduct histopathologic examinations involving stains that show the changes; consequently, cancer cells often appear blue on microscopic examination. Biochemical changes to the cell can include increases in the concentrations of enzymes on the cell surface, an increased number of prostaglandins on the cell surface, and decreases in the concentrations of certain growth factors or oxygen concentrations needed for cell division.

Kinetic changes include changes in the growth and division of cells. Proliferation rates may vary from tumor to tumor and from one patient to another. The cancer doubling time indicates the length of time for division of all tumor cells present; the doubling time may range from hours to months or even years. On average, a tumor requires approximately 30 doubling times to become clinically detectable (1 cm) (Volker, 2005).

Tumor doubling time—a manifestation of cancer growth—can be controlled by:

- vascularization of the tumor (development of a blood supply), so that the cells have adequate nutrition for growth

- the presence of a necrotic tumor or dead cells, which may interfere with uptake of nutrients and with growth

- expression of tumor antigens, which influence escape from immune surveillance

- genetic factors, which enhance or suppress tumor growth.

(CancerSource, 2006; Chen & Hunter, 2005; Viele, 2005).

TARGETED THERAPIES

Individual cancer types have different growth rates, spreading patterns, and treatment responses. The specific characteristics of a cancer provide the basis for targeted treatment strategies. The wealth of knowledge now accumulating from research in microbiology and genetics is the basis for more and more targeted therapies that focus on specific cancer cell characteristics (CancerSource, 2005; Merkle & Loescher, 2006). (See Chapter 7.)

One of the main advantages of molecular targeted therapies is a reduction in the side effects associated with traditional cancer treatments such as chemotherapy. Because these targeted therapies avoid any action on healthy cells, side effects from treatment can be minimized (CancerSource, 2005).

The clinical application of targeted therapies covers many areas of investigation—some of them producing agents that will become the treatments of the future. Figure 2-2 shows some of the targets for non-small-cell lung cancer (NSCLC), which include growth factors and receptors, signal transduction pathways, tumor-associated antigens and markers, angiogenic pathways, and cell survival pathways. Here is a brief review of the foundation of these therapies.

Role of the Immune System

Researchers continue to learn about the role of the host's immune system in carcinogenesis, metastasis, and response to therapy. In the past, the theory of immune surveillance argued that, although transformation of cells occurs often, an intact, fully operational immune system can still detect abnormal cells and destroy them. However, in both the very

FIGURE 2-2: BIOLOGIC TARGETS FOR NSCLC THERAPY

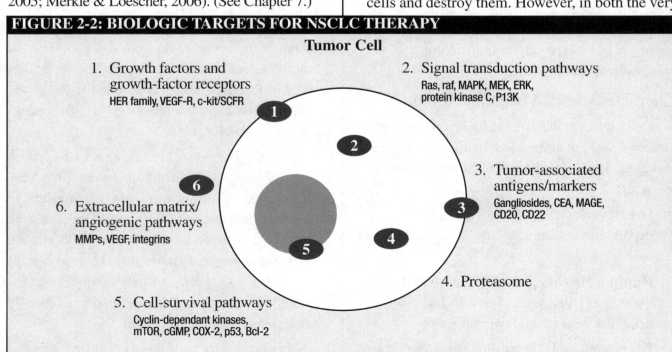

Tumor Cell

1. Growth factors and growth-factor receptors
   HER family, VEGF-R, c-kit/SCFR

2. Signal transduction pathways
   Ras, raf, MAPK, MEK, ERK, protein kinase C, P13K

3. Tumor-associated antigens/markers
   Gangliosides, CEA, MAGE, CD20, CD22

4. Proteasome

5. Cell-survival pathways
   Cyclin-dependant kinases, mTOR, cGMP, COX-2, p53, Bcl-2

6. Extracellular matrix/angiogenic pathways
   MMPs, VEGF, integrins

Note. From *New Advances in the Management of Advanced NSCLC: The Expanding Role of Targeted Therapies* by R. Perez-Soler & V. Miller, 2005. Retrieved April 17, 2007 from http://www.medscape.com/viewprogram/3929 © 2005 Medscape. Reprinted with permission from Medscape.

young and the very old, the immune system operates at less-than-optimal levels. It is in these age-groups that increased rates of cancer occur. Now researchers are discovering that the body's immune system is a powerful force or adjunct therapy in fighting cancer cell occurrence and spread.

One category of targeted immunotherapies (biologic response modifiers) is monoclonal antibodies. Antibodies, normal mechanisms of the immune system, protect cells from foreign invaders and infectious agents, such as bacteria. The strategy of monoclonal antibodies is to program the antibodies to remember previous invaders so they can effectively and quickly destroy the invaders when they attack the cell again (CancerSource, 2005). (See Chapter 7 for more information on some of the monoclonal antibodies that the U.S. Food and Drug Administration [FDA] has approved as treatments.)

Cell-mediated immunity, another role of the immune system in cancer, provides protection from cellular antigens, which invade the body and transform cells while doing damage. Cells that fight off these antigens come in a variety of forms and actions. The three types of lymphocytes that mobilize cell-mediated immunity are the helper/inducer T-lymphocytes, cytotoxic T-lymphocytes, and natural killer cells. These lymphocytes either directly attack unhealthy cells or are integral to the process of destroying those cells (CancerSource, 2005; Volker, 2005).

Small Molecule Compounds

Another class of targeted therapies are small-molecule compounds, which seek out molecules found only in cancer cells. Among the mechanisms of these compounds is to inhibit growth of certain proteins found within or on the cell surface, thus controlling cell growth or destroying the cell. An example of these molecular targeted therapies is epidermal growth factor receptor (EGFR) inhibitors. EGFRs are produced in excessive

amounts by many tumors, such as those of the lung, breast, and colon.

EGFR signal transduction occurs in normal and abnormal cells and is the result of a receptor being bound by a ligand. (A ligand is a substance that binds to certain immune cells and may suppress tumor growth.) When ligand transmission is interrupted, tumor growth is affected. Because many of these molecular defects—such as those affecting EGFRs—can contribute to tumor growth, more than one drug or agent is used in treatments to effectively attack or destroy tumor growth (CancerSource, 2005; National Cancer Institute [NCI], 2006; Viele, 2005).

Vascular endothelial growth factors (VEGFs) involve the targeted pathway of angiogenesis, which brings a consistent and complicated blood supply (carrying oxygen and nutrients) to cells. VEGFs include a family of proteins that contribute to the cascade of events that supports angiogenesis. Angiogenesis inhibitors—a promising area of treatment—are further described in Chapter 7 (Viele, 2005).

Role of Oncogenes in Tumor Growth

As background, similar genes may be lost or mutated in different types of cancer. An ordered or sequential loss of tumor-suppressor genes is also possible as cells progress from predisposed to overtly cancerous. Finally, several chromosomal regions can harbor oncogenes. Oncogenes, when activated, can lead to the transformation of normal cells into cancer cells.

Selected genetic alterations are thought to cause carcinogenesis, creating the cell changes that affect initiation, promotion, and transformation of normal cells to cancer cells. Researchers have established that these genetic alterations affect two types of genes. The first, oncogenes, called *proto-oncogenes* when they are a mutated form of activated normal genes, affect normal cell growth. Proto-oncogenes promote uncontrolled cellular proliferation by disrupting the cell's grow/no-grow signaling network. The second type, anti-oncogenes, or tumor suppressor genes, block tumor development by regulating the oncogenes involved in cell growth (CancerSource, 2004, 2005; NCI, 2006).

Oncogenes can dominate a change in the cell. When activated, a single mutant area on one chromosome is sufficient to change the function of the cell from normal to malignant. With the presence and activity of oncogenes, the body appears to have an increased susceptibility to specific cancers or groups of cancers or to the precursors of malignancy. More than 50 different proto-oncogenes are now known and, of these, about 20 have actually been found in mutant form in human tumors. Table 2-3 lists selected proto-oncogenes. These oncogenes appear to express themselves through mutations, chromosomal deletions, or other genetic changes (CancerSource, 2004, 2005; NCI, 2006).

Tumor Suppressor Genes

Because epithelial cells affect the largest number of cancers (breast, colon, lung, prostate), limiting the growth of a specialized cell type is key to stopping carcinogenesis. The normal role of a tumor-suppressor gene is to stop out-of-control cell proliferation. Tumor-suppressor genes are a built-in braking system against runaway cell proliferation. Therefore, a mutation in a tumor-suppressor gene—causing it to malfunction—can lead to a loss of the brake on the cell's growth. Cell proliferation and the cascade of malignancy can follow.

Tumor-suppressor genes are also involved in the progression of several common, noninheritable forms of cancer, such as breast and colorectal cancer. The number of tumor-suppressor genes that have been discovered is small in number but is growing. This area of exploration is thought to be rich with possibility (CancerSource, 2005, 2006; Volker, 2005).

In clinical practice so far, none of the known dominant oncogenes has been implicated in an inherited human cancer. However, both recessive tumor-suppressor genes and DNA mismatch repair gene defects have demonstrated that they are involved in cells that have an inherited predisposition to cancer (CancerSource, 2006; Volker, 2005).

TABLE 2-3: SELECTED LIST OF PROTO-ONCOGENES (ONCOGENES)		
Proto-oncogenes	**Classification**	**Activated in…**
ab1	Signal transducer	Chronic myelogenous leukemia
erbB-1	Growth factor receptor	Squamous cell carcinoma, astrocytoma
erbB-2 (Her2/neu)	Growth factor receptor	Adenocarcinoma of breast, ovary, and stomach
myc	Transcription factor	Burkitt's lymphoma; carcinoma of lung, breast, and cervix
H-ras	G-protein (guanine nucleotide-binding protein)	Carcinoma of colon, lung, and pancreas; melanoma
sis	Growth factor	Astrocytoma
src	Non-receptor tyrosine kinase	Colon carcinoma, breast adenocarcinoma
bcl-2	Programmed cell death regulator	Lymphoma
(American Cancer Society, 2006; Merkle & Loescher, 2006; Volker, 2005)		

FAMILY PREDISPOSITION

The most common cancers—even when showing familial traits—are not inherited. Individuals may not always inherit a "cancer gene." Instead, they may inherit a susceptibility, as well as a possible resistance, to certain cancers. A large number of genes may be involved in tumorigenesis, and several different cancer genes may be involved in the same tumor. Certain genes have been associated with the occurrence of colon, prostate, breast, and ovarian cancers. Also, genetics appear to be involved in leukemia and other cancers (NCI, 2006).

Still, a strong family history of certain cancers may be the basis for what some see as one of the most accessible breakthroughs of cancer care. The opportunity may exist to seek genetic counseling that is accurate, meaningful, and life saving. The promise of such genetic counseling is that it would target individuals so that they seek specific screening protocols, engage in certain behaviors, and avoid certain risks factors for cancer.

Hereditary Cancers

Genetics can provide clues about chromosome abnormalities because almost all solid human malignant tumors have abnormalities. Discoveries about genetics and chromosome heredities are leading to ways to identify a cancer's predisposition in families (Sifri, Gangadharappa, & Acheson, 2004). For example, researchers have identified the contributing gene causing the development of retinoblastoma. In another example, families with a genetic predisposition for familial polyposis coli have a prevalence of colon cancer that is estimated at 100%. Armed with knowledge about the family's genetic heredity for certain colon cancers, practitioners can begin early screening for family members and start treatments early to be more effective (CancerSource, 2006; Chen & Hunter, 2005; Sifri et al., 2004).

In many common cancers, such as colon, breast, lung, and bladder cancer, the tumor suppressor gene p53 has been found to be mutated. Once this gene is mutated, the cancerous cell becomes resistant to chemotherapy and radiation. For example, mutations of p53 genes have been identified in 30% to 79% of epithelial ovarian cancers. Researchers hope that knowledge about this gene may help predict whether a specific malignancy will respond to particular treatments, such as chemotherapies and biologics (Volker, 2005).

Another example of the genetic basis for cancer is the discovery of two major genes responsible for the inherited predisposition to breast cancer: BRCA1 and BRCA2. The BRCA1 gene has been shown in studies to increase the risk of breast and ovarian cancer. Women who have mutations of BRCA1 generally have a risk of breast cancer of 85% by age 70, in contrast to the lifetime risk of 12% for the general population. A mutation of the BRCA1 gene produces an ovarian cancer risk of 26% to 85% by age 70. BRCA1 gene susceptibility is more prevalent in the Ashkenazi Jewish population (Chen & Hunter, 2005; NCI, 2006).

Mutations of the BRCA2 gene are thought to account for approximately 35% of mutations in families with histories of multiple cases of breast cancer. The BRCA2 gene is also associated with male breast cancer, ovarian cancer, prostate cancer, and pancreatic cancer (Chen & Hunter, 2005; NCI, 2006).

Genetics and the theories being researched about carcinogenesis are very complex. In a gross oversimplification, the development of a malignancy only requires the activation of a proto-oncogene or the loss of function of a DNA repair gene or both copies of a tumor-suppressor gene. Tumors form because of a multistep, highly interactive set of processes, involving a succession of genetic changes in the evolving tumor cell population. Loss or inactivation of the same gene may contribute to the development of several different common cancers (CancerSource, 2006).

VIRUSES ASSOCIATED WITH HUMAN CANCER

Like the emerging roles of the immune system, genetic factors, and environmental factors in tumor growth, the role of viruses in cancer development is not entirely clear. Connections between tumor growth and viruses continue to be studied.

Specific viruses—for example, herpes simplex virus (types 1, 2, and 6), cytomegalovirus, Epstein-Barr virus, and human T-cell leukemia virus—are targets of study. The family of papova viruses, which includes human papilloma virus, has been strongly linked to cervical cancer and a vaccine is now available as preventive treatment (FDA, 2006). Human immunodeficiency virus is known to be associated with the development of malignant tumors. In certain countries, such as China, the prevalence of hepatitis B virus (HBV) has been correlated with a high incidence of primary hepatomas (CancerSource, 2005).

The relationship between viruses and human cancers appears to be strong, although many of the mechanisms of action are still unknown. One way to determine a direct causal link between agent and host is to attempt to prevent the disease through vaccination. Over the next several decades, use of the HBV vaccine will contribute important information about the connection between HBV infection and the development of hepatomas. If HBV contributes to the development of certain cancers, the hope is that the prevention of hepatitis B through vaccines may also prevent selected cancers (CancerSource, 2005).

SUMMARY

Understanding the biology of cancer helps researchers and clinicians decide the best treatment for a particular tumor when it is diagnosed. Armed with knowledge about the characteristics and behaviors of tumor cells, researchers and clinicians can better understand and successfully treat malignant tumors. Increased knowledge in this area can lead to better strategies that target tumor cells and will revolutionize the way that cancer cells can be controlled and patients treated.

EXAM QUESTIONS

CHAPTER 2
Questions 5-8

Note: Choose the option that BEST answers each question.

5. A malignant tumor arising from connective tissue is called a(n)

    a. adenocarcinoma.

    b. adenoma.

    c. lipoma.

    d. sarcoma.

6. One of the characteristics of a cancer cell is

    a. increased ability to differentiate.

    b. loss of proliferative control.

    c. loss of photosensitivity.

    d. stable chromosomes.

7. Tumor doubling time can be controlled by

    a. pressure from other organs.

    b. necrotic tumor, or dead cells.

    c. time.

    d. reduced blood supply.

8. Researchers have found a familial, genetic link in cancers of the

    a. brain.

    b. testes.

    c. lung.

    d. colon.

REFERENCES

American Cancer Society. (2006). *Oncogenes and tumor suppressor genes.* Retrieved October 31, 2006, from http://www.cancer .org/ docroot /ETO/content/ETO_1_4x_oncogenes_and _tumor _suppressor_genes.asp

American Joint Committee on Cancer. (2002). *AJCC cancer staging manual* (6th ed.). New York: Springer-Verlag.

CancerSource. (2004). *Understanding cancer.* Retrieved April 17, 2007, from http://www .cancersource.com/Search/34,16407-6

CancerSource. (2005). *Targeted therapies take aim at cancer.* Retrieved April 17, 2007, from http://www.cancersource.com/Search/34,27737

CancerSource. (2006). *Cancer genetic overview.* Retrieved April 17, 2007, from http://www .cancersource.com/Search/48,CDR0000062838

Chen, Y., & Hunter, D. (2005). Molecular epidemiology of cancer. *CA: Cancer Journal for Clinicians, 55*(1), 45–54.

Medscape. (2005). *New advances in the management of advanced NSCLC. The expanded role of targeted therapies.* Retrieved April 17, 2007, from http://www.medscape.com/viewarticle /504206_2

Merkle, C., & Loescher, L. (2006). Biology of cancer. In C. Yarbro, M. Frogge, & M. Goodman (Eds.), *Cancer nursing: Principles and practice* (6th ed., pp. 3–25). Sudbury, MA: Jones & Bartlett.

National Cancer Institute. (2006). *Prevention, genetics, causes.* Available from http://www .cancer.gov/cancertopics/prevention-genetics-causes

Perez-Soler, R., & Miller, V. (2005). *New advances in the management of advanced NSCLC: The expanding role of targeted therapies.* Retrieved April 17, 2007, from http://www.medscape .com/viewprogram/3929

Sifri, R., Gangadharappa, S., & Acheson, L. (2004). Identifying and testing for hereditary susceptibility to common cancers. *CA: Cancer Journal for Clinicians, 54*(6), 309–326.

U.S. Food and Drug Administration. (2006). *FDA licenses new vaccine for prevention of cervical cancer and other diseases in females caused by human papillomavirus.* Retrieved April 17, 2007, from http://www.fda.gov/bbs/topics /NEWS/2006/NEW01385.html

Viele, C. (2005). Keys to unlock cancer: Targeted therapy. *Oncology Nursing Forum, 32*(5), 935–940.

Volker, D. (2005). Biology of cancer and carcinogenesis. In J. K. Itano & K. N. Taoka (Eds.), *Core curriculum for oncology nursing* (4th ed., pp. 443–464). St. Louis: Elsevier.

CHAPTER 3

PREVENTION AND DETECTION

CHAPTER OBJECTIVE

After completing this chapter, the reader will be able to discuss the latest developments in cancer prevention and detection strategies for selected cancers.

LEARNING OBJECTIVES

After studying this chapter, the reader will be able to

1. recognize the American Cancer Society (ACS) 2015 challenge goals to prevent and detect cancer.

2. identify interventions that help people quit smoking.

3. describe the ACS guidelines for cancer screening.

4. indicate factors that may genetically predispose a person to developing cancer.

INTRODUCTION

Prevention and detection strategies are important reasons for progress in reducing the incidence and mortality rates of cancer. The American Cancer Society (ACS) is one of the leading public advocates for prevention and detection efforts. It has published challenge goals and nationwide objectives, which concretely establish targets for cancer reduction by the year 2015 (see Table 3-1). The ACS emphasizes that any progress in cancer prevention is due to the combined efforts of government agencies, private companies, other nonprofit organizations, health care providers, policymakers, insurers, and the American public (ACS, 2006a; CancerSource, 2006b; National Cancer Institute [NCI], 2005a).

As progress continues in cancer reduction efforts, nurses are on the front lines in most cancer prevention activities. Their access to the public and their status as recognized sources of credible knowledge make nurses an important component in cancer prevention.

PREVENTION AND RISK FACTORS

Risk factors increase a person's chance of developing a disease, such as cancer. Different cancers have different risk factors. Even though they are identified as risks, these factors do not necessarily cause cancer directly. Many people with one or more risk factors never develop cancer, whereas others with cancer may have no known, recognized risk factors. Still, data suggest that known risk factors can be addressed, mobilizing cancer-prevention strategies (Mahon, 2005b; NCI, 2005b, 2006a). For example, smoking—a known precursor to lung cancer and other cancers—is a risk that can be addressed by quitting smoking (NCI, 2005a).

According to the ACS, the risk factors of smoking, diet, and infectious diseases contribute to about 75% of all cancer cases in the United States

TABLE 3-1: AMERICAN CANCER SOCIETY 2015 GOALS

2015 Challenge Goals

- A 50% reduction in age-adjusted cancer mortality rates.
- A 25% reduction in age-adjusted cancer incidence rates.
- A measurable improvement in the quality of life (physical, psychological, social, and spiritual) from the time of diagnosis and for the balance of life, of all cancer survivors.

2015 Nationwide Objectives

Adult Tobacco Use

- Reduce to 12% the proportion of adults (18 and older) who are current cigarette smokers.
- Reduce to 0.4% the proportion of adults (18 and older) who are current users of smokeless tobacco.

Youth Tobacco Use

- Reduce to 10% the proportion of high school students (under 18) who are current cigarette smokers.
- Reduce to 1% the proportion of high school students (under 18) who are current users of smokeless tobacco.

Nutrition & Physical Activity

- The trend of increasing prevalence of overweight and obesity among U.S. adults and youth will have been reversed, and the prevalence of overweight and obesity will be no higher than it was in 2005.
- Increase to 70% the proportion of adults and youth who follow American Cancer Society guidelines with respect to the appropriate level of physical activity, as published in the *American Cancer Society Guidelines on Nutrition and Physical Activity for Cancer Prevention.*
- Increase to 75% the proportion of persons who follow American Cancer Society guidelines with respect to consumption of fruits and vegetables as published in the *American Cancer Society Guidelines on Nutrition and Physical Activity for Cancer Prevention.*

Comprehensive School Health Education

- Increase to 50% the proportion of school districts that provide a comprehensive or coordinated school health education program.

Sun Protection

- Increase to 75% the proportion of people of all ages who use at least two or more of the following protective measures that may reduce the risk of skin cancer: Avoid the sun between 10 a.m. and 4 p.m., wear sun-protective clothing when exposed to sunlight, use sunscreen with an SPF of 15 or higher, and avoid artificial sources of ultraviolet light (e.g., sun lamps, tanning booths).

Breast Cancer Early Detection

- Increase to 90% the proportion of women aged 40 and older who have breast cancer screening consistent with American Cancer Society guidelines (by 2010).

Colorectal Cancer Early Detection

- Increase to 75% the proportion of people aged 50 and older who have colorectal cancer screening consistent with American Cancer Society guidelines.

Prostate Cancer Early Detection

- Increase to 90% the proportion of men who follow age-appropriate American Cancer Society detection guidelines for prostate cancer.

Note. From American Cancer Society. *Cancer Prevention & Early Detection Facts & Figures 2007.* Atlanta: American Cancer Society, Inc. Reprinted with permission.

(ACS, 2006c). Smoking is a risk factor for cancers of the lung, mouth, throat, larynx, bladder, head and neck, esophagus, and kidneys. Many health care experts believe that cancers caused by cigarette smoking and heavy use of alcohol would decrease in incidence if people quit smoking and drinking. For its part, the ACS estimates that in the year 2006 about 170,000 cancer deaths are expected to be caused directly by tobacco use. When excessive alcohol consumption combines with tobacco use, the combination causes a synergistic effect for some cancers, especially head and neck cancers (U.S. Department of Health and Human Services [HHS], 2004).

The risk factor of poor or inappropriate diet is related to many preventable cancers. Scientific evidence suggests that between 20% and 40% of cancer deaths are related to nutrition and other preventive lifestyle factors (ACS, 2006b; Olsen, 2005). In addition, certain cancers are related to preventable viral infections, such as hepatitis B virus, human papillomavirus, human immunodeficiency virus, and human T-cell leukemia/lymphoma virus-I.

Another preventable domain is sun exposure. Applying protection from the sun's rays can prevent as many as one million incidents of skin cancer each year in the United States. (Olsen, 2005).

Nevertheless, the direct cause-effect of cancer is not as clear for many other environmental risk factors. For most people, tobacco smoke, poor nutritional habits, and sedentary lifestyles have a larger effect on personal cancer risk than do pollutants in food, drinking water, and air (ACS, 2006c; NCI 2005a).

The risks of voluntary and involuntary environmental exposure depend on the hazard's concentration and intensity and the amount of exposure time. We now have a body of knowledge that suggests a substantially increased risk for workers exposed to high concentrations of certain chemicals, metals, and other exposures. We also know that environmental risk factors include radiation exposure and some drugs used in therapies (Olsen, 2005).

Studies continue to establish risk profiles for low-dose or event exposures. For example, we now know that secondhand tobacco smoke represents a significant public health hazard (NCI, 2006c). To minimize the risk, nurses in their advocacy role are part of efforts to establish safe occupational practices, drug testing, and consumer product safety. Chemical or radiation exposure safety standards develop from federal regulatory and risk management standards at the U.S. Food and Drug Administration (FDA), Environmental Protection Agency (EPA), and the Occupational Safety and Health Administration.

For most potential carcinogens, data are only available from high-dose experiments in animals or highly exposed occupational groups. To set human safety standards, regulators sometimes base their standards on animal study data and conditions that address low- to high-dose exposure. Because of this uncertainty, regulators make conservative assumptions to err on the side of safety. Table 3-2 lists what is known about selected environmental exposures.

TABLE 3-2: SELECTED ENVIRONMENTAL EXPOSURES (1 OF 2)

Chemicals

Various chemicals (for example, benzene, asbestos, vinyl chloride, arsenic, aflatoxin) show definite evidence of human carcinogenicity; others are considered probable human carcinogens based on evidence from animal experiments (for example, chloroform, dichlorodiphenyl-trichloroethane [DDT], formaldehyde, polychlorinated biphenyls [PCBs], polycyclic aromatic hydrocarbons). Often in the past, direct evidence of human carcinogenicity has come from studies of workplace conditions involving sustained, high-dose exposures. Occasionally, risks are greatly increased when particular exposures occur together (for example, asbestos exposure and cigarette smoking).

TABLE 3-2: SELECTED ENVIRONMENTAL EXPOSURES (2 OF 2)

Radiation

Only high-frequency radiation—ionizing radiation (IR) and ultraviolet (UV) radiation—has been proven to cause human cancer. Exposure to sunlight (UV radiation) causes almost all cases of basal and squamous cell skin cancer and is a major cause of skin melanoma. Disruption of the earth's ozone layer by atmospheric chemical pollution (the "ozone hole") may lead to rising levels of UV radiation.

Evidence that high-dose IR (e.g., X-rays, radon, etc.) causes cancer comes from studies of atomic bomb survivors, patients receiving radiotherapy, and certain occupational groups (for example, uranium miners). Virtually any part of the body can be affected by IR, but especially bone marrow and the thyroid gland. Diagnostic medical and dental X-rays are set at the lowest dose levels possible to minimize risk without losing image quality. Radon exposures in homes can increase lung cancer risk, especially in cigarette smokers; remedial actions may be needed if radon levels are too high.

Unproven Risks

Public concern about environmental cancer risks often focuses on risks for which no carcinogenicity has been proven or on situations where known carcinogen exposures are at such low levels that risks are negligible. For example:

Pesticides. Many kinds of pesticides (e.g., insecticides, herbicides) are widely used in producing and marketing our food supply. Although high doses of some of these chemicals cause cancer in experimental animals, the very low concentrations found in some foods are generally well within established safety levels. However, environmental pollution by slowly degraded pesticides such as DDT, a result of past agricultural practices, can lead to food-chain bioaccumulation and to persistent residues in body fat. Such residues have been suggested as a possible risk factor for breast cancer. Studies have shown that concentrations in tissue are low, however, and the evidence has not been conclusive.

Continued research regarding pesticide use is essential for maximum food safety, improved food production through alternative pest control methods, and reduced pollution of the environment. In the meantime, pesticides play a valuable role in sustaining our food supply. When properly controlled, the minimal risks they pose are greatly overshadowed by the health benefits of a diverse diet rich in foods from plant sources.

Nonionizing radiation. Electromagnetic radiation at frequencies below ionizing and UV levels has not been shown to cause cancer. While some epidemiologic studies suggest associations with cancer, others do not, and experimental studies have not yielded reproducible evidence of carcinogenic mechanisms. Low-frequency radiation includes radiowaves, microwaves, and radar as well as power frequency radiation arising from the electric and magnetic fields associated with electric currents (extremely low-frequency radiation).

Toxic wastes. Toxic wastes in dump sites can threaten human health through air, water, and soil pollution. Although many toxic chemicals contained in such wastes can be carcinogenic at high doses, most community exposures appear to involve very low or negligible dose levels. Clean-up of existing dump sites and close control of toxic materials in the future are essential to ensure healthy living conditions in our industrialized society.

Nuclear power plants. IR emissions from nuclear facilities are closely controlled and involve negligible levels of exposure for communities near such plants. Although reports about cancer clusters in such communities have raised public concern, studies show that clusters do not occur more often near nuclear plants than they do by chance elsewhere in the population.

(ACS, 2006c; NCI, 2005a)

Tobacco Use

Tobacco use is a major preventable cause of disease and premature death in the United States (Mahon, 2004b; NCI, 2006c). Tobacco use is associated with cancers of the lung, mouth, larynx, pharynx, esophagus, pancreas, kidney, bladder, and uterine cervix. Tobacco use also contributes to comorbid conditions such as chronic obstructive pulmonary disease, peripheral vascular disease, arteriosclerosis, and coronary artery disease.

Cigarette consumption in the United States increased in the 1940s, peaking in 1963, but has decreased since 1964, when the first U.S. Surgeon General reported that cigarette smoking was linked to lung cancer (ACS, 2006c; NCI, 2005a, 2006c).

Among men, the lung cancer death rate peaked approximately 30 years after 1963 and has decreased since 1990. The lung cancer death rate among women, who began regular cigarette smoking about 20 years after men (the "Virginia Slims Era"), has not yet peaked (see Figures 3-1 and 3-2). However, the age-adjusted rate appeared to be leveling off in the mid-1990s (NCI, 2005a, 2006c).

Compared to nonsmokers, men who smoke are about 23 times more likely to develop lung cancer; women who smoke are about 13 times more likely to develop lung cancer (HHS, 2004).

The death toll from tobacco use is expected to double by 2020 (Olsen, 2005). Tobacco use accounts for 30% of all cancer deaths and 90% of all lung

FIGURE 3-1: AGE-ADJUSTED CANCER DEATH RATES,* FEMALES BY SITE, UNITED STATES, 1930-2002

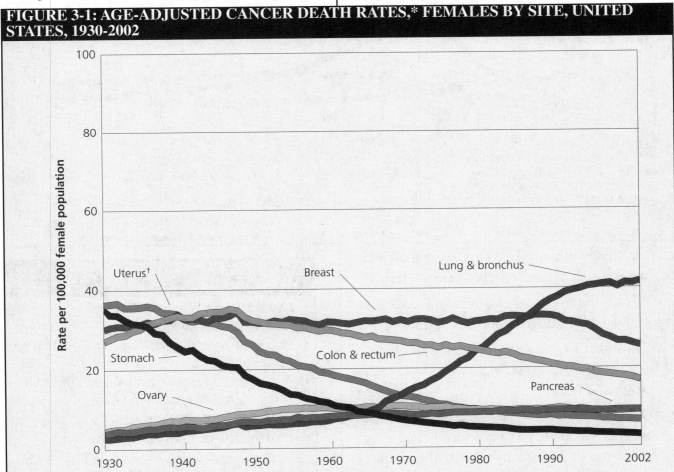

*Per 100,000, age-adjusted to the 2000 US standard population. †Uterus cancer death rates are for uterine cervix and uterine corpus combined.

Note: Due to changes in ICD coding, numerator information has changed over time. Rates for cancer of the lung and bronchus, colon and rectum, and ovary are affected by these coding changes.

Source: US Mortality Public Use Data Tapes 1960 to 2002, US Mortality Volumes 1930 to 1959, National Center for Health Statistics, Centers for Disease Control and Prevention, 2005.

American Cancer Society, Surveillance Research, 2006

Note. From American Cancer Society. *Cancer Facts & Figures 2006b*, Atlanta: American Cancer Society, Inc. Reprinted with permission.

FIGURE 3-2: AGE-ADJUSTED CANCER DEATH RATES,* MALES BY SITE, UNITED STATES, 1930-2002

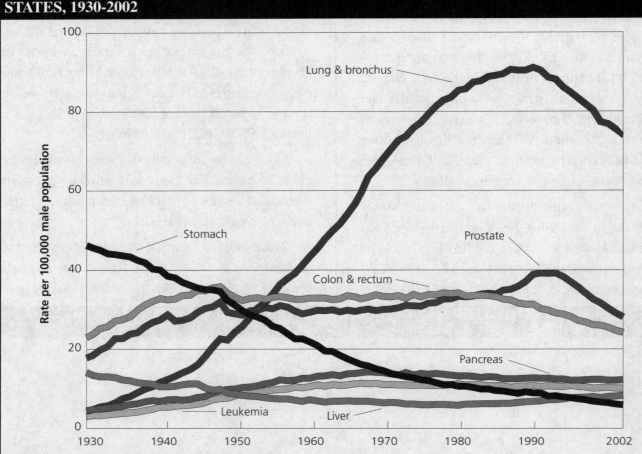

*Per 100,000, age-adjusted to the 2000 US standard population.

Note: Due to changes in ICD coding, numerator information has changed over time. Rates for cancer of the liver, lung and bronchus, and colon and rectum are affected by these coding changes.

Source: US Mortality Public Use Data Tapes 1960 to 2002, US Mortality Volumes 1930 to 1959, National Center for Health Statistics, Centers for Disease Control and Prevention, 2005.

American Cancer Society, Surveillance Research, 2006

Note. From American Cancer Society. *Cancer Facts & Figures 2006b*, Atlanta: American Cancer Society, Inc. Reprinted with permission.

cancer deaths in men. In women, tobacco use accounts for 80% of cancer deaths (Olsen, 2005).

According to the 2004 Surgeon General's report about the health consequences of smoking:

- Smoking harms nearly every organ of the body, causing many diseases, and affects the general health of smokers.

- Quitting smoking has immediate and long-term benefits, reducing risks for diseases caused by smoking. (Table 3-3 lists strategies to quit smoking.)

- Smoking cigarettes with lower machine-measured yields of tar and nicotine (i.e., menthol cigarettes) provide no clear benefit to health.

TABLE 3-3: STRATEGIES TO QUIT SMOKING

- Standard self-help materials
- Individual counseling
- Social support interventions, such as "buddy systems"
- Group therapy and behavioral modification
- Nicotine-replacement products
- Antidepressant therapy
- Varenicline tartrate (Chantix), a medication approved by the FDA in 2006 to help smokers stop smoking

(Mahon, 2005a)

Malignancies caused or contributed to by smoking have expanded to include acute myeloid leukemia, cervical cancer, kidney cancer, pancreatic cancer, and stomach cancer. These diagnoses expand the well-known list of cancer diagnoses or other conditions caused or worsened by smoking: bladder, esophageal, laryngeal, lung, oral, and throat cancers; chronic lung disease; and coronary heart and cardiovascular disease (HHS, 2004).

Youth Tobacco Use

An estimated 3,000 young people begin smoking each day. Historical data show that smoking in youths peaked in 1976 at 39%, declined about one-quarter between 1976 and 1981 to 29%, and remained at this level until 1992. Current cigarette smoking among U.S. 12th graders began to increase sharply in 1993, rose by one-third in the mid-1990s, peaked in 1997 (37%), but has declined in recent years (ACS, 2006b; NCI, 2005b). In 2004, approximately 28% of high-school students reported using some form of tobacco product (Centers for Disease Control and Prevention [CDC], 2005). This level was unchanged from estimates in 2002.

In 2004, among middle-school students, approximately 11.7% report using a tobacco product (cigarettes, smokeless tobacco, cigars). In 2002, 13.3% of middle-schoolers reported use of tobacco products. Both high-school and middle-school students reported seeing fewer actors using tobacco on television and in movies (CDC, 2005).

In determining whether progress is being made in reducing youth cigarette smoking, these statistics are important:

- From 1997 to 2002, the retail price of cigarettes increased approximately 80%; from spring 2002 to spring 2004, the price only increased 4%.

- Funding for smoking-reduction campaigns directed at youths has drastically decreased; statewide quit-smoking campaigns had a 28% decline in financial support, FY 2002 to FY 2004.

- Tobacco industry expenditures for advertising and promotion in 1997 were $5.7 billion; in 2002, expenditures were $12.5 billion. (CDC, 2005)

The reasons people start smoking are complex. Previous studies indicate that youths who smoke are generally from low socioeconomic families, have friends who smoke (peer pressure), have lower scholastic achievements, and have lower self-esteem than their peers.

Marketing and popular culture messages remain the powerful impetus for adolescents to start or continue smoking. To make long-term progress in reducing tobacco use and tobacco-related deaths, studies show that effective ways to curb smoking include increasing the cost of tobacco products through taxes, prohibiting the sale of tobacco products to anyone under age 18, and developing counter-marketing campaigns against tobacco use (NCI, 2005c; Giarelli, Ledbetter, Mahon, & McElwain, 2004; Mahon, 2005b).

Nutrition

Being overweight or obese is estimated to account for 20% of all cancer deaths in women and 14% of cancer deaths in men (Olsen, 2005). In 2000, an estimated 64% of U.S. adults were overweight or obese. In addition, the percentage of children considered overweight continues to climb; for children ages 6 to 19 years old, the recent estimate of obesity is 15%.

After cigarette smoking, dietary choices and physical activity are the primary cancer risk behaviors that people can change. No matter how old a person is, a healthy diet can promote health and reduce cancer risk. Although no diet guarantees full protection against any disease, sound nutritional strategies can reduce the risk of developing cancer.

Many dietary factors can affect cancer risk: types of foods, food preparation methods, portion sizes, food variety, and overall caloric balance. Cancer risk can be reduced by an overall dietary pattern that includes a high proportion of plant foods (fruits, vegetables, grains, and beans); limited amounts of meat, dairy, and other high-fat foods; and a balance of caloric intake and physical activity.

Although nutritional and activity deficiencies plague adult Americans, trends showing poor diet and exercise affect the health of children as well. These trends include—but are not limited to—an increase in caloric intake, greater use of high-fat convenience foods, and a decline in physical activity, due in part to shifts toward more eating out, more sedentary lifestyles, and advertisement of high-calorie foods (NCI, 2005a; Olsen, 2005).

Table 3-4 reviews the NCI's dietary guidelines.

TABLE 3-4: NCI DIETARY GUIDELINES

- Reduce fat intake to 30% of calories or less.
- Increase fiber to 20 to 30 g/day, with an upper limit of 35 g.
- Include a variety of fruits and vegetables in the daily diet.
- Avoid obesity.
- Consume alcoholic beverages in moderation, if at all.
- Minimize consumption of salt-cured, salt-pickled, and smoked foods.

Note: These cancer prevention guidelines are consistent with the USDA/DHHS *Dietary Guidelines for Americans*.

(NCI, 2005a)

Sun Exposure

The evidence against exposure to the sun, sunlamps, and tanning salons is accumulating. All generate harmful UV radiation that, in the least, cause sunburn and, over the long term, may lead to unsightly skin blemishes, premature aging of the skin, cataracts and other eye problems, skin cancer, and a weakened immune system (Olsen, 2005).

Sun exposure is also a known cancer risk factor. Moreover, it is known that sun exposure is getting worse. According to the most recent estimates from the National Aeronautics and Space Administration, the Earth's ozone layer, the thin shield in the stratosphere that protects life from UV radiation, is being depleted at a rate of 4% to 6% each decade. According to reports from the EPA, chemicals used since the 1980s are depleting the ozone layer. A depleted ozone layer means that additional UV radiation reaches Earth's surface (CancerSource, 2006b; Olsen, 2005).

Although people with light skin are more susceptible to sun damage, darker-skinned people—including African Americans and Hispanic Americans—also can be damaged by the sun. The American Academy of Dermatology, American Academy of Ophthalmology, Skin Cancer Foundation, American Academy of Pediatrics, National Weather Service, and FDA have joined in recommending ways to protect against the sun. Table 3-5 provides recommendations to protect against sun exposure.

SCREENING AND DETECTION

Combined with early treatment, the ACS estimates that regular screening examinations can detect (and save lives) in early or asymptomatic stages of cancers of the breast, colon, rectum, cervix, and prostate. Screening and early detection can also save lives for those diagnosed with cancers of the testes, oral cavity, and skin.

The ACS bases its recommendations on scientific research and expert opinion. Some cancers included in the ACS recommendations can be found early by self-examinations (e.g., breast), physical examinations by a health professional (e.g., breast, thyroid gland, skin, colon, rectum, testicle, and prostate), and by X-ray or laboratory tests (e.g., mammography, Papanicolaou [Pap] test, and prostate-specific antigen [PSA] blood test). In many cases, the best screening strategy is a combination of two or more early-detection approaches (e.g., mammography, clinical breast examination

TABLE 3-5: SUN PROTECTION TIPS
• Limit the time you are exposed to the sun.
• Avoid exposure to the high-noon sun, from 10 a.m. to 3 p.m.
• Wear protective clothing, such as a hat, long sleeves, and sunglasses.
• Use sunscreen.
– A sun protection factor (SPF) of 30 or greater offers the maximum protection from the sun by blocking 96% of UV exposure; sunscreen with an SPF of 15 blocks out 93% of all UV rays. (An SPF of 30 allows an individual to stay out in the sun twice as long as an SPF of 15 with the same protection.)
– For those with light complexions, apply sunscreen frequently (every 20 minutes) Also apply sunscreen after swimming, sweating, or showering. Otherwise, standard recommendation is to apply sunscreen no less than every 2 hours.
– Apply sunscreen 15 to 20 minutes before sun exposure. This allows the sunscreen to soak into deeper layers of the outer skin.
– On average, an adult should use about two tablespoons of sunscreen for a single application.
(Maltzman, 2004)

[CBE] by a health professional, and breast self-examination [BSE]) (Fields & Chevlen, 2006; Mahon, 2004a, 2004b; Morrison, 2005; Smith, Cokkinides, & Eyre, 2006).

The ACS reports that those who follow specific early detection recommendations for the most prevalent cancers have a 5-year relative survival rate of about 81%. (These cancers—accounting for about half of all new cancer cases—are breast, colon, rectum, cervix, prostate, testis, oral cavity, and skin.) Survival for people with these cancers is greatly improved by early detection. Moreover, the ACS estimates that if all Americans participated in regular cancer screenings, the cancer survival rate could increase to 95% (ACS, 2006b).

Many screening guidelines exist. As an example, Table 3-6 lists an ACS summary of screening guidelines for the most common cancer diagnoses. Who should be screened and at what age, what screening tests should be used, and what are the proper intervals of screening remain topics of discussion and disagreement. Choice of screening guidelines may be influenced by differences in populations of interest and considerations of screening effectiveness as well as a family history of cancer. Of the many barriers that prevent widespread screening, the paramount barrier is cost. Studies have attempted to show cost-benefit ratios of cancer screening programs, especially for breast, colon, and prostate cancer.

In addition to cost, other barriers to screening include a lack of general health care and preventive care, lack of a regular health care provider, lack of physician recommendations, and personal and cultural inhibitions. Methods to establish effective screening will continue to be a major focus in cost of care analyses of cancer prevention and detection (Fields & Chevlen, 2006; Mahon, 2004a, 2004b).

Genetics and Cancer Risk

Although genetics is a factor in the development of cancer, cancer cannot be explained by heredity alone. Approximately 5% to 10% of cancers are linked to a genetic mutation (Olsen, 2005). The recent explosion in genetics information suggests many promising avenues for prevention and treatment. Still, the science of establishing a genetic predisposition to cancer, based on an understanding of the cancer surveillance and risk-management options, is in its infancy (CancerSource, 2006a; NCI, 2006b; Sifri, Gangadharappa, & Acheson, 2004).

Clarity on the substance and impact of genetic information, based on scientific breakthroughs, will change all aspects of health care, including cancer prevention, detection, and treatment. In 2000, completion of the first draft of the Human Genome

TABLE 3-6: RECOMMENDATIONS FOR THE EARLY DETECTION OF CANCER IN ASYMPTOMATIC PEOPLE

Site	Recommendation
Cancer-related checkup	A cancer-related checkup is recommended every 3 years for people ages 20 to 40 and every year for people ages 40 and older. This exam should include health counseling and, depending on a person's age, might include examinations for cancers of the thyroid, oral cavity, skin, lymph nodes, testes, and ovaries, as well as for some nonmalignant diseases.
Breast	Women age 40 and older should have an annual mammogram and an annual clinical breast examination (CBE) by a health care professional and should perform monthly breast self-examination (BSE). The CBE should be conducted close to the scheduled mammogram. Women ages 20 to 39 should have a CBE by a health care professional every 3 years and should perform monthly BSE.
Colon and rectum	Beginning at age 50, men and women should follow one of the examination schedules below: • A fecal occult blood test every year and a flexible sigmoidoscopy every 5 years.* • A colonoscopy every 10 years.* • A double-contrast barium enema every 5 to 10 years.* * A digital rectal exam should be done at the same time as sigmoidoscopy, colonoscopy, or double-contrast barium enema. People who are at moderate or high risk for colorectal cancer should talk with a doctor about a different testing schedule.
Prostate	The ACS recommends that both the PSA blood test and the digital rectal examination be offered annually, beginning at age 50, to men who have a life expectancy of at least 10 years and to younger men who are at high risk. Men in high-risk groups, such as those with a strong familial predisposition (i.e., two or more affected first-degree relatives) and blacks, may begin at a younger age (i.e., 45 years).
Uterus	*Cervix:* All women who are or have been sexually active or who are 18 and older should have an annual Pap test and pelvic examination. After three or more consecutive satisfactory examinations with normal findings, the Pap test may be performed less frequently. Discuss the matter with your physician. *Endometrium:* Women at high risk for cancer of the uterus should have a sample of endometrial tissue examined when menopause begins.

(ACS, 2006b)

Project's 3-billion base-pair sequence of the human genome propelled investigators to focus on genetics-based origins of disease and care.

Genetic testing may be appropriate when parents or other family members also have a specific cancer diagnosis or when several extended members of the family have the same cancer diagnosis.

In time, patients will be offered a genetic foundation for patient care. Nurses will be at the forefront of integrating laboratory breakthroughs into public and clinical settings. The basics of cancer genetics will become a framework for practice, used to identify cancers from multiple genetic defects or mutations in the cell regulation process. The start of these defects may be inherited causes, age, or internal controls of growth undermining normal and malignant cells (CancerSource, 2006a; NCI, 2006b; Washburn et al., 2005).

In addition to providing basic patient education about genetics, nurses should incorporate genetics into the health assessment, recognizing that inherited factors may be involved in a patient's disease. Nurses can then help decide whether a referral to a genetic counselor is warranted (Washburn et al., 2005).

SUMMARY

The rationale for cancer prevention and screening is well known, with the biggest "bang for the buck" focused on reducing tobacco use, eating a better diet, limiting exposure to the sun, and following ACS guidelines for screening and detection. Prevention and detection efforts are also focusing on what is known about a person's genetic heritage and whether that heritage increases the risk of developing malignancies. Early detection and prevention efforts correlate with better survival rates.

EXAM QUESTIONS

CHAPTER 3
Questions 9-12

Note: Choose the option that BEST answers each question.

9. One of the ACS's 2015 challenge goals is

    a. 30% reduction in overall age-adjusted cancer mortality.

    b. 40% reduction in overall age-adjusted cancer mortality.

    c. 50% reduction in overall age-adjusted cancer mortality.

    d. 60% reduction in overall age-adjusted cancer mortality.

10. To help a person quit smoking, the nurse can best emphasize

    a. eating.

    b. resting.

    c. long-range goals.

    d. diversionary behaviors.

11. For early detection of colorectal cancer, the ACS recommends asymptomatic persons ages 50 and older have a colonscopy every

    a. 2 years.

    b. 3 years.

    c. 5 years.

    d. 10 years.

12. Genetic defects that predispose some people to develop cancer may be triggered by

    a. age.

    b. geography.

    c. depression.

    d. level of intelligence.

REFERENCES

American Cancer Society. (2007). *Cancer Prevention & Early Detection Facts & Figures 2007*. Atlanta: Author.

American Cancer Society. (2006a). *ACS 2015 nationwide objectives*. Retrieved April 17, 2007, from http://www.facs.org/cancer/coc/acschallengegoals.pdf

American Cancer Society. (2006b). *Cancer facts & figures 2006*. Atlanta: Author.

American Cancer Society. (2006c). *Environmental carcinogens*. Available from http://www.cancer.org/docroot/PED/ped_1_1.asp

CancerSource. (2006a). *Cancer genetics overview*. Available from http://www.cancersource.com/Search/48,CDR0000517309

CancerSource. (2006b). *Prevention, risk, and screening*. Available from http://www.cancersource.com/CancerBasics/PreventionScreening/

Centers for Disease Control and Prevention. (2005). Tobacco use, access, and exposure to tobacco in media among middle and high school students—United States, 2004. *Morbidity and Mortality Weekly Report, 54*(12), 297–301.

Fields, M., & Chevlen, E. (2006). Screening for disease: Making evidence-based choices. *Clinical Journal of Oncology Nursing, 10*(1), 73–76.

Giarelli, E., Ledbetter, N., Mahon, S., & McElwain, D. (2004). "Not lighting up": A case study of a woman who quit smoking. *Oncology Nursing Forum, 31*(3), E54–63

Mahon, S. (2004a). Colorectal cancer screening: A review of the evidence. *Clinical Journal of Oncology Nursing, 8*(5), 536–540.

Mahon, S. (2004b). Screening for lung cancer: What is the evidence? *Clinical Journal of Oncology Nursing, 8*(2), 188–189.

Mahon, S. (2005a). Review of selected approaches to promoting smoking cessation. *Clinical Journal of Oncology Nursing, 9*(6), 745–747.

Mahon, S. (2005b). Screening for prostate cancer: Informing men about their options. *Clinical Journal of Oncology Nursing, 9*(5), 625–627.

Maltzman, J. (2004). *Be sun smart and cancer smart*. Available from http://www.oncolink.org/resources/article.cfm?c=3&s=38&ss=164&id=824

Morrison, C. (2005). Early detection of cancer. In J. K. Itano & K. N. Taoka (Eds.), *Core curriculum for oncology nursing* (4th ed., pp. 861–876). St. Louis: Elsevier.

National Cancer Institute. (2005a). *Cancer prevention overview*. CancerNet (PDQ®) web sites for health professionals. Retrieved April 17, 2007, from http://wwwicic.nci.nih.gov/cancertopics/pdq/prevention/overview/healthprofessional

National Cancer Institute. (2005b). *Cancer trends progress report—2005 update. Trends at a glance*. Retrieved April 17, 2007, from http://progressreport.cancer.gov/trends-glance.asp

National Cancer Institute. (2006a). *Lung cancer (PDQ®): Prevention*. Retrieved April 17, 2007, from http://wwwicic.nci.nih.gov/cancertopics/pdq/prevention/lung/healthprofessional

National Cancer Institute. (2006b). *Prevention, genetics, causes.* Available from http://www.cancer.gov/cancertopics/prevention-genetics-causes

National Cancer Institute. (2006c). Smoking and cancer. Available from http://www.cancer.gov/cancertopics/smoking

Olsen, S. (2005). Epidemiology and prevention of cancer. In J. K. Itano & K. N. Taoka (Eds.), *Core curriculum for oncology nursing* (4th ed., pp. 839–860). St. Louis: Elsevier.

Sifri, R., Gangadharappa, S., & Acheson, L. (2004). Identifying and testing for hereditary susceptibility to common cancers. *CA: Cancer Journal for Clinicians, 54*(6), 309–326.

Smith, R., Cokkinides, V., & Eyre, H. (2006). American Cancer Society guidelines for the early detection of cancer, 2006. *CA: Cancer Journal for Clinicians, 56*(1), 11–25.

Washburn, N., Sommer, V., Spencer, S., Simmons, S., Adkins, B., Rogers, M., et al. (2005). Outpatient genetic risk assessment in women with breast cancer: One center's experience. *Clinical Journal of Oncology Nursing, 9*(1), 49–53.

U.S. Department of Health and Human Services. (2004). *The health consequences of smoking: A Report of the Surgeon General.* Washington, DC: U.S. Department of Health and Human Services, Centers for Disease Control and Prevention, National Center for Chronic Disease Prevention and Health Promotion, Office on Smoking and Health.

CHAPTER 4

SURGERY

CHAPTER OBJECTIVE

After completing this chapter, the reader will be able to describe surgery as means to diagnose, stage, and treat malignancies.

LEARNING OBJECTIVES

After studying this chapter, the reader will be able to

1. recognize a diagnostic surgical procedure in cancer care.

2. identify early-stage tumor sites that are initially treated with surgery.

3. recognize a surgical procedure that is considered preemptive in cancer care.

4. cite two goals of nursing care for surgical cancer patients.

INTRODUCTION

Surgery is a major component of cancer therapy and has many goals. Surgical procedures provide the means to establish a diagnosis, determine the staging of the disease, and treat the disease or allow other treatments to be delivered (by implanting tubes, catheters, hardware, or implants). Table 4-1 lists the roles of surgery in cancer care.

TABLE 4-1: ROLES OF SURGERY IN CANCER CARE

- Diagnostic
- Staging
- Screening
- Curative
- Restorative/Reconstructive
- Preemptive/Prophylactic
- Placement of treatment conduits
- Monitoring
- Palliative

SURGERY, DIAGNOSIS, AND STAGING

Surgical procedures provide a means to obtain tissue for a definitive diagnosis. Biopsy types performed by surgeons include incisional biopsies, excisional, biopsies, and needle biopsies. Needle biopsies include fine needle aspirations, core biopsies, and sentinel node biopsies. (Table 4-2 highlights surgical diagnostic techniques and examples of information the procedures provide.)

Surgery can determine the extent of disease, thereby providing essential information for staging. For example, during surgery, the spread of a tumor can be established by the surgeon by marking the tumor's borders or noting residual disease on adjacent organs. A tissue sample can also be obtained. This sample is sent to a pathologist for evaluation. That tissue evaluation leads to staging of the tumor.

TABLE 4-2: SURGICAL TECHNIQUES USED FOR DIAGNOSIS

Type of Procedure	Use	Example of info provided
Incisional biopsy	Removes partial sample for evaluation when entire tumor cannot be removed	Breast cancer: Diagnosis
Excisional biopsy	Removes entire tumor	Skin cancer: Diagnosis
Needle biopsy	21-22 gauge needle, removes fluid or cells	
• Fine needle aspiration (FNA)	Initial sample for pathologic diagnosis	Thyroid cancer: Diagnosis
• Core biopsy	Larger sample than FNA for pathologic diagnosis	Breast cancer: Hormonal status
• Sentinel node biopsy	Targets first (sentinel) node that drains primary tumor site and tumor drainage system; lower risk of lymphedema	Breast cancer: Lymph node status establishes extent (metastasis) of disease
Diagnostic laparotomy	Visualized via lighted scope	Prostate cancer: Determines stage and extent of disease

(For examples of cancer staging made possible by tissue excised during surgical procedures, see Chapter 13, Table 13-1, and Chapter 14, Table 14-3.)

SURGERY AS TREATMENT

This section reviews surgery as a form of cancer treatment. Subsequent chapters review other cancer treatment modalities, including radiation therapy (RT), chemotherapy (and hormonal therapy), and biotherapy/targeted therapy. In most treatment plans for cancer, more than one modality is used.

General Treatment Terms

Before reviewing surgery as a treatment modality, one must understand certain terms that are used when discussing cancer care treatment.

Adjuvant treatment. Treatment given in addition to primary treatment. (Example: Chemotherapy is added after surgery to increase the likelihood of cancer cure or control.)

Neoadjuvant treatment. Treatment given before the main treatment. (Example: Radiation therapy given before surgery can shrink the tumor burden.)

Sequential treatment. Treatment modalities that follow one another. (Example: Chemotherapy and RT are followed by hormonal therapy.)

Concurrent treatment. Treatment modalities scheduled at the same time. (Example: Chemotherapy and RT are scheduled during the same treatment period [e.g., 6 weeks].

Surgical Procedures

Surgery is the oldest form of treatment for cancer. When surgery is the preferred treatment for a cancer diagnosis, the tumor is solid and either contained or responsive to debulking (reduction).

Surgery can be:

* primary treatment—removing the tumor and a margin of adjacent normal tissue.

* adjuvant treatment—removing tissues to decrease the risk of cancer incidence, progression, or recurrence.

* prophylactic treatment—removing nonvital organs that can have a high risk of subsequent cancer.

* palliative treatment—removing tissues or organs that reduce the patient's pain but do not cure the disease.

• used in combination as treatment—for example, preoperative chemotherapy can reduce a tumor burden before primary surgery; surgery has become a common component of multimodality treatment strategies for lung, breast, colon, and ovarian cancers.

Traditionally, surgery has been a first-line treatment for early stage or nonmetastasized breast, lung, pancreatic, and colon tumors (Manser et al., 2005). Table 4-3 lists other common tumors for which surgery is used as an early-stage treatment strategy.

TABLE 4-3: SELECTED TUMORS TREATED WITH SURGICAL RESECTION
(as a first-line treatment strategy in early-stage malignancy)

Brain	Ovarian
Breast	Pancreatic
Cervical	Prostate
Colorectal	Skin
Endometrial	Melanoma
Esophageal	Sarcoma
Gastric	Stomach
Head and neck	Testicular
Lung	Thyroid
Small-cell	Uterine
Non-small-cell	

Table 4-4 lists some of the surgical procedures that serve as treatments to anticipate or avoid further malignancy or cancer spread. The focus of these surgeries is primarily to assess the status of the disease and determine the effectiveness of previous treatment.

TABLE 4-4: SELECTED PREEMPTIVE SURGICAL PROCEDURES
• Mastectomy
• Oophorectomy
• Colectomy
• Endoscopic polypectomy
• Routine skin surveillance with lesion removal

Surgical techniques have progressed with so-called minimal access surgery. For oncology patients, minimal access surgery allows adequate tissue biopsies for accurate diagnosis of malignancy to determine the degree of spread, to stage the disease, and to assess operability. In addition, minimal access surgery may be a way to treat the malignancy itself, such as with tumors of the brain, lung, stomach, liver, pancreas, gallbladder, kidney, colon, ovary, endometrium, and cervix (Szopa, 2005).

An example of minimal access surgery is the laparoscopic procedure. As a novel surgical procedure, laparoscopic cholecystectomy was first reported in 1989. In 1992, more than 20% of all cholecystectomies were performed using minimal access techniques (Gillespie, 2006). Studies continue to determine the advantages of these surgical techniques, evaluating morbidity, mortality, convalescence, and cost. These studies attempt to establish whether minimal access techniques should be the standard of care rather than traditional, more extensive surgeries.

In gynecology, routine laparoscopy is a preferred option to treat interval tubal ligations, resections of ectopic (tubal) pregnancies, fulguration of endometriosis, and selected ovarian cystectomies.

Other surgical methods include electrosurgery (use of electrical current to destroy cells), cryosurgery (use of liquid nitrogen to freeze tissue and destroy cells), laser surgery (a method that amplifies light to stimulate radiation emission to destroy cells), stereotactic surgery (a method to locate a surgical target using three-dimensional coordinates), and robotics (a method using computer imaging and technology with robotic arms to improve dexterity, access, and control).

Surgical Care

Care of surgical cancer patients is based on goals of preoperative and postoperative care (see Table 4-5). Nurses provide education, manage

TABLE 4-5: GOALS OF NURSING CARE DURING SURGICAL TREATMENT

Assessment, interventions, and evaluation
- Pain
- Skin integrity and wound care
- Infection
- Airway maintenance
- Metabolic balance
- Fluid balance
- Nutrition

Psychological and emotional support
- Anxiety
- Fear

complications and symptoms, and offer support and comfort care.

An important component of surgical care of the patient is pain control, which includes administration of pain medication during the immediate post-operative period (Gillespie, 2006). Methods to manage pain immediately after surgery include short-acting, IV-administered pain medication (e.g., meperidine [Demerol]) or patient-controlled analgesia pumps, which allow the patient to self-deliver safe doses of analgesia via a pump.

After surgery, physicians prescribe oral pain medications for lingering pain. These pain medications are reviewed in Chapter 22.

ESTABLISHING ACCESS FOR TREATMENT

Chapter 8 reviews vascular access devices (VADs), a means to deliver IV chemotherapy or biologic therapy. Other surgically placed devices to provide access for treatment include the Ommaya reservoir and feeding tubes.

Ommaya Reservoir

The Ommaya reservoir is surgically implanted in the patient's cranium and has a catheter that feeds the patient's ventricle. This device allows direct infusion of chemotherapy, antibiotics, or pain medication to the brain, which is necessary because regular IV access through the venous system does not penetrate the blood-brain barrier.

Accessing an Ommaya reservoir requires sterile procedure, using a small-gauge needle. Drug instillation is preceded and followed by sampling of cerebrospinal fluid to confirm positioning. Drugs instilled are well diluted to prevent irritation of brain cells. In addition, they do not contain any preservative that would inadvertently damage brain cells (Hayden & Goodman, 2006).

Feeding Tubes

When a patient cannot maintain nutrition—due to treatment in the oral cavity or throat or because of anorexia related to cancer treatment—a feeding tube is surgically placed. Feeding tubes allow the patient to receive liquid nutrition. Nutritional products designed for tube feeding are formulated to provide the patient with all the necessary protein, carbohydrates, vitamins, and minerals. Some even contain dietary fiber and other nonnutritional elements.

Types of tubes are:

- nasogastric (NG) tube—inserted through the nasal passageway for short-term use

- percutaneous endoscopic gastrostomy (PEG) tube—inserted directly into the stomach through the abdominal wall, with the tube exiting outside the body; also called G-tube (gastrostomy tube)

- J-tube—similar in operation to the PEG tube; inserted into the jejunum and, because of its placement, may decrease the risk of aspiration; smaller in diameter than PEG tubes.

Table 4-6 reviews the care of patients with feeding tubes.

SUMMARY

Surgery has many roles in cancer diagnosis, treatment, and care. It is the preferred treatment for

TABLE 4-6: GENERAL GUIDELINES FOR FEEDING TUBES

- Pay attention to the skin around the entry site. For NG tubes, lubrication keeps nostril tissues from breaking down. For PEG tubes, watch for signs of infection, such as redness, swelling, and pain.

- After initial placement of the tube, the patient may experience some discomfort while getting used to the system (from gas or air or from adjusting to the liquid foods themselves).

- Before instilling nutrition, wash hands. Prepare the nutrition product for instillation. Check tube placement by aspirating for stomach contents through a syringe.

- Dilute nutrition products, as needed, to avoid clogging the tube.

- Instill nutrition slowly at room temperature. The pace and temperature help prevent abdominal cramping, nausea and vomiting, gastric distension, diarrhea, and aspiration.

- When a patient is receiving nutrition through a tube, keep him or her upright (no less than 30 degrees) to minimize the risk of regurgitation and aspiration. Continue to keep the patient upright for 30 to 60 minutes after feeding.

- To maintain patency, flush the tube with water before and after feeding. Carbonated cola can help flush some clogged tubes.

- If instilling nutrition by gravity method, schedule feedings every 4 to 6 hours. If instilling continuously through a feeding pump, flush the tube every 4 to 6 hours to maintain patency.

- If the patient becomes bloated after feedings, temporarily remove the adaptor feeding cap from the tube. Encourage the patient to cough.

(Cleveland Clinic, 2006; Oral Cancer Foundation, 2006)

malignant tumors that are solid and either contained or responsive to debulking (reduction). Tumors that can be treated surgically are diagnosed at an early stage. Among those tumors that can be treated surgically include breast, cervical, endometrial, gastric, head and neck, lung, prostate, thyroid, testicular, and skin tumors. Nursing care for patients following surgery focuses on wound care, metabolic balance, pain control, and airway maintenance during recovery. Surgery can also be used to establish conduits for other modality treatments, including VADs for chemotherapy and biotherapy, Ommaya reservoirs, and feeding tubes for nutrition.

EXAM QUESTIONS

CHAPTER 4
Questions 13-16

Note: Choose the option that BEST answers each question.

13. A purely diagnostic surgical procedure in cancer care is

    a. prostatectomy.

    b. placement of a feeding tube.

    c. oophorectomy.

    d. fine needle aspiration of a thyroid nodule.

14. An example of an early stage tumor that can be treated with surgery is

    a. non-Hodgkin's lymphoma.

    b. breast cancer.

    c. leukemia.

    d. multiple myeloma.

15. A surgical procedure that is considered preemptive in cancer care is

    a. colectomy.

    b. tracheostomy.

    c. thoracotomy.

    d. lymph node dissection.

16. Immediate postoperative nursing care for a surgical cancer patient would include

    a. administering chemotherapy.

    b. providing a list of support groups.

    c. administering consolidation therapy.

    d. administering pain medication.

REFERENCES

Cleveland Clinic. (2006). *Percutaneous endoscopic gastrostomy (PEG)*. Available from http://www.clevelandclinic.org/health/healthinfo/docs/2000/2000.asp?index=4911&src=news

Hayden, B., & Goodman, M. (2006). Chemotherapy: Principles of administration. In C. Yarbro, M. Frogge, & M. Goodman (Eds.), *Cancer nursing: Principles and practice* (6th ed., pp. 351–382). Sudbury, MA: Jones & Bartlett.

Gillespie, T. (2006). Surgical therapy. In C. Yarbro, M. Frogge, & M. Goodman (Eds.), *Cancer nursing: Principles and practice* (6th ed., pp. 212–228). Sudbury, MA: Jones & Bartlett.

Manser, R., Wright, G., Hart, D., Byrnes, G., & Campbell, D. A. (2005). Surgery for early stage non-small-cell lung cancer. *Cochrane Database of Systematic Reviews,* (1), Art. No.: CD004699. DOI: 10.1002/14651858.CD004699.pub2.

Oral Cancer Foundation. (2007). *Tube feeding.* Retrieved April 17, 2007, from http://www.oral-cancerfoundation.org/dental/tube_feeding.htm

Szopa, T. (2005). Nursing implications of surgical treatment. In J. K. Itano & K. N. Taoka (Eds.), *Core curriculum for oncology nursing* (4th ed., pp. 736–747). St. Louis: Elsevier.

CHAPTER 5

RADIATION THERAPY

CHAPTER OBJECTIVE

After completing this chapter, the reader will be able to describe radiation therapy as a treatment for malignancies.

LEARNING OBJECTIVES

After studying this chapter, the reader will be able to

1. list early-stage tumor sites that can be treated with radiation.

2. identify three components of radiation therapy (RT) that determine its effectiveness on targeted cancer cells.

3. identify three precautions used to protect caregivers of patients who are receiving brachytherapy.

4. describe two acute toxicities and two chronic toxicities common after RT.

INTRODUCTION

Radiation therapy (RT) can be used as a cancer treatment for some malignancies that respond to high-energy radiation. Other terms for RT include *radiotherapy* and *irradiation*. It is estimated that between 50% and 60% of cancer patients are treated with RT over the trajectory of their cancer treatment (National Cancer Institute [NCI], 2004; Witt, 2005).

RT is used as the only treatment modality for some tumors. It may also be the preferred treatment at a certain stage of diagnosis. Most frequently, RT is a component of multimodality therapy (with surgery, chemotherapy, targeted therapy, or a combination of all three) for localized or regional tumors. As with other cancer treatment modalities, the goals of RT are cancer cure, control, or palliation (relief of symptoms, such as pressure, bleeding, and pain) (Gosselin-Acomb, 2006).

For patients receiving RT, the primary focus of nursing care is education about and management of RT side effects. Side effects of RT generally correlate with the area of the body being treated. An exception to site-related side effects is fatigue, a general side effect of RT.

Background

RT is the use of high-energy radiation (ionizing radiation [IR]) to target tumor cells. IR interacts with molecules and atoms in tumor cells, killing them by damaging the cell's deoxyribonucleic acid (DNA). When damaged, the cell's DNA—the genetic information that controls the cell's reproduction—is altered. Thus, the cell cannot divide and grow as before, thus causing the tumor to shrink.

Cells that rapidly grow and multiply are especially sensitive to the effects of radiation. Among normal cells that are radiosensitive are the skin cells, mucous membranes, hair follicles, gastrointestinal (GI) cells, bone marrow, and reproductive cells. RT affects both tumor cells and normal cells.

Table 5-1 lists some of the tumor types for which RT is the primary treatment.

TABLE 5-1: SELECTED TUMORS AND MALIGNANCIES TREATED WITH RADIATION THERAPY AS PRIMARY THERAPY

- Localized breast cancers
- Unresectable bronchus and lung tumors
- Hodgkin's and non-Hodgkin's lymphomas
- Squamous cell tumors of the head and neck, bladder, skin, and cervix
- Adenocarcinomas of the alimentary tract
- Vascular tumors
- Connective tissue tumors
- Renal cell tumors
- Sarcomas: chondrosarcoma, osteogenic sarcoma, rhabdomyosarcoma, ganglioneurofibrosarcoma
- Thyroid and pituitary tumors
- Uterine tumors
- Brain tumors (benign and malignant)

(Witt, 2005)

PRINCIPLES OF RADIATION THERAPY

IR has biologic effects that cause damage to cellular DNA. It also alters the level of DNA damage, the degree to which the cell is deprived of oxygen (well-oxygenated tumors respond more to IR) and the cell's sensitivity to the radiation.

The degree to which radiation is absorbed in a tumor cell is affected by fractionation (dividing the dosing of radiation over time) and the rate at which the radiation is administered. The biologic effect of fractionation on tumor cells and normal cells is affected by the four R's of radiobiology:

- **Repair.** Divided doses of radiation better spare normal tissues because normal cells can repair and reproduce more effectively than tumor cells.

- **Reassortment or redistribution of cells.** Fractionated doses of radiation affect the cell's reproduction cycle. Redistribution—triggered by fractionated radiation doses—mobilizes more cells into mitosis, the most sensitive phase of a cell cycle for cell change or death.

- **Reoxygenation.** Cells deprived of oxygen die, thereby reducing the tumor burden.

- **Repopulation.** Cells multiply, replacing dead and dying cells.

Degree of Radiosensitivity

When used to treat cancer cells, IR is given in doses many times higher than those delivered by regular X-rays. All normal and tumor cells are susceptible to radiation effects, but cells vary in their sensitivity. Sensitivity to radiation depends on the rate of cell division; the more rapidly cells divide, the more sensitive to RT or radiosensitive, the cells or tissues are. Nondividing or slow-dividing cells are less sensitive to RT.

Therefore, when targeting cancer cells with RT, the effectiveness of RT depends on:

1. the timing of the therapy (radiation treatments are fractionalized-subdivided and repeated to decrease the size of the tumor and eliminate tumor cells)

2. the dose

3. the amount of radiation in the target field that is ultimately absorbed by the cell.

Sources of Ionizing Radiation

Therapeutic IR is emitted from highly energetic particles, such as:

- alpha particles—used in brachytherapy

- beta particles—similar to electrons, but less penetrating than gamma rays

- electromagnetic radiation—(X-rays and gamma rays).

Measurement and Dosing

Advances in treatment planning have decreased the effects of radiation on normal cells while allowing an increase in RT doses. RT is given in an absorbed dose called a *gray* (Gy). 1 Gy = 100 cGy = 100 rads (rad is the acronym for radiation absorbed dose). Doses are referred to as *low dose rate* or *high dose rate*. An example of a primary treatment target for a patient with a bronchial lesion is 16 Gy in eight fractions (divided doses) over approximately 2 weeks. An adjacent target area might have a dose of 44 Gy (in 22 fractions over approximately 5 weeks). A daily dose is usually 180 to 200 cGy/day.

RT Exposure

Depending on the type of radioactive element emitting particles or rays, the element's energies have various levels of penetration. The type of radioactive element determines the extent of shielding that is needed to absorb the radiation (Witt, 2005).

Another term associated with RT is sievert (Sv). The sievert is the unit of dose of IR equal to one joule per kilogram. The Sv (which replaced the term rem) is language used in safety and protection to quantify radiation exposure.

DELIVERY MODALITIES OF RADIATION THERAPY

Radiation oncologists and technicians use advanced equipment to target tumors with high-energy X-rays, electrons, or radioactive isotopes. RT can be delivered in various ways.

External Beam RT

The most common type of RT is external beam treatment, in which the RT source is outside of the patient's body. When cancer patients receive external RT, it is usually generated by a linear accelerator. The linear accelerator can deliver treatments such as X-rays (intermediate to deep treatments) or electron beams (more shallow treatments) (Gosselin-Acomb, 2006; Witt, 2005).

Another source of external beam radiation is the Cobalt-60 source. It emits gamma rays, which are more penetrating than the alpha and beta particle radiation emitted from X-rays and linear accelerator sources.

Before external beam treatments begin, the oncologist and the RT team plan the treatment, performing a simulation that determines the target areas for therapy. (Simulation sessions last 60 to 90 minutes.) Once treatment sessions begin, they are generally administered on an outpatient basis and last 15 to 30 minutes (for the session set-up, treatment, and posttreatment periods). The treatment itself lasts only a few minutes (Behrend, 2006). Typical courses of external beam RT are weekly for a period of weeks or daily for a period of weeks.

Patients are not radioactive at any time during external beam RT. Moreover, patients receiving external beam RT do not pose a threat to regular caregivers because the treatments are given in a shielded room with staff outside of the room (Gosselin-Acomb, 2006).

Internal RT (Brachytherapy)

For certain tumors, internal RT (also called *brachytherapy*) is used, in which the source of the high-energy rays is placed in a sealed or unsealed compartment inside the patient's body, giving off various amounts and intensities of energy. The source is placed as close as possible to the cancer cells—for example, on the surface, intracavitary, interstitial, or intraluminal. This treatment method allows higher and more intense doses of radiation to be targeted to the tumor area. Tumors treated with brachytherapy include those originating in the cervix, prostate, head and neck, breast, bronchus, brain, and bladder.

Radioactive substances used in brachytherapy include radium, cesium, and iodine. Depending on the tumor and therapy plan, brachytherapy may be implanted for only a short time or left in place over a longer period. The source of the radiation disintegrates at a given, predictable pace. This time is measured as the half-life. The half-life is an important metric for caregivers because it helps determine the amount and length of shielding needed for various radioactive elements.

In some selected cases, patients receiving internal RT may need to be isolated from visitors for a brief time so that visitors are not exposed to the radioactivity of the RT source. In those cases, after therapy is complete and the source of brachytherapy is removed, the patient poses no danger as a radioactive source. The concept of the therapy and the fact that the patient is no longer harboring an emitting radioactive source are important parts of patient and family teaching at discharge (Behrend, 2006; Gosselin-Acomb, 2006). Table 5-2 lists common radioactive elements and their half-lives and energy (Behrend, 2006; Gosselin-Acomb, 2006).

Principles of Radiation Safety for Brachytherapy

Three factors should be incorporated when providing care to a patient receiving internal RT:

1. **Time:** Minimize the amount of time the caregiver is in close range of the patient.

2. **Distance:** Maximize the amount of distance between the patient and the caregiver.

3. **Shield:** Use lead shielding or other methods instituted by the facility for caregiver protection during periods of direct care.

Table 5-3 provides a list of additional suggested precautions.

Systemic RT

Some RT protocols call for therapy to be delivered systemically. For example, thyroid cancers are treated with "unsealed" treatment protocols such as iodine. For bone pain, systemic strontium 89 and samarium 153 have been shown to be effective radiopharmaceutical agents.

RADIOSENSITIZERS AND RADIOPROTECTORS

Radiosensitizers make cancer cells more responsive to the effects of RT. Examples of radiosensitizing chemotherapies are 5-fluorouracil and cisplatin. Other agents and strategies being evaluated as radiosensitizers in clinical trials are:

• angiogenesis inhibitors—attempt to block the tumor's ability to create its own blood vessels

• growth factors—attempt to stop certain parts of the tumor from growing

• immunotherapy—enables chemotherapy to get to the targeted tumor, thus minimizing damage to surrounding normal tissue (NCI, 2004).

Agents called *radioprotectors* make RT less damaging to normal cells by promoting the repair of normal cells exposed to RT. For example, amifostine (Ethyol) helps reduce dry mouth from RT. Other agents are also being studied as radioprotectors (NCI, 2006).

TABLE 5-2: RADIOACTIVE ELEMENTS		
Element	**Half-life**	**Energy**
Cesium 137 (^{137}Cs)	30.0 years	0.66 MeV
Iridium 192 (^{192}Ir)	74.2 days	0.35 MeV
Iodine 131 (^{131}I)	8.0 days	0.36 MeV
Iodine 125 (^{125}I)	60.2 days	0.03 MeV
Strontium 89 (^{89}Sr)	50.5 days	1.46 MeV
MeV = million electron volts		

TABLE 5-3: SELECTED ISOLATION PRECAUTIONS FOR PATIENTS RECEIVING BRACHYTHERAPY

- Hang a sign on the door that radioactive indicates material is in use.
  - Place the patient in a private room.
  - Limit visitation (i.e., 1/2 hour/day).
  - Prohibit children and pregnant women from visiting.
- Limit the time nursing care is provided by each nurse (i.e., 1/2 hour per 8-hour shift).
  - Wear shielding as recommended by hospital protocol.
  - Orchestrate self-care for the patient as much as possible: place items within easy reach, including the call light and phone.
- Prepare for unexpected dislodgement of the radioactive source:
  - Forceps in the room
  - Accessible phone number for physician
  - Accessible phone number for radiation safety officer.

NURSING CARE FOR RADIATION THERAPY PATIENTS

The doses of radiation that damage or destroy cancer cells also can hurt normal cells, causing side effects. The scope of nursing care includes pretreatment, ongoing assessment, and posttreatment education interventions, with a focus on side effect management and comfort. Usually, side effects of RT are temporary and are limited to the field or area of radiation. In general, these effects disappear gradually when therapy ends, usually during the first weeks or months after RT (Maher, 2006; NCI, 2004).

Despite attempts during treatment sessions to shield normal, noncancerous cells, some normal cells are affected by RT. These healthy cells appear to recover more fully from the effects of radiation, because they can better repair cellular DNA damage. Still, the majority of side effects from radiation are the result of the irradiation of normal cells (Witt, 2005).

Acute and Chronic Side Effects

Acute side effects occur early in the course of RT, usually during the first weeks or months of RT. They typically pass shortly after the treatment course ends. Chronic or late side effects are permanent, occurring months to years after treatment. In general, rapidly dividing cells (such as those of the GI tract, mucosa, and bone marrow) within the targeted RT field are most susceptible to acute side effects. Slower-dividing cells (such as those of the spinal cord, peripheral nerves, kidneys, cartilage, and bone) can be the basis for chronic side effects.

Tables 5-4 and 5-5 review acute and long-term side effects of RT.

Fatigue

Fatigue—or a feeling of decreased energy—is one of the general side effects of RT. Fatigue is multifocal and subjective. Patients are not restricted from normal activity during RT, and many continue to work while undergoing treatment (Maher, 2006). However, they should balance normal activity with

TABLE 5-4: SELECTED ACUTE TOXICITIES FROM RT				
(Extent based on normal structures in RT field, dose, type of RT, and size of RT field)				
	Skin erythema	**Mucositis**	**Diarrhea**	**Alopecia**
Breast	X			
Chest/lung	X			
Central nervous system (Brain)	X			X
GI		X	X	
Head/Neck	X	X		X

TABLE 5-5: SELECTED LATE EFFECT TOXICITIES FROM RT

(Extent based on normal tissue tolerance, dose, type of RT, and size of RT field)

Eye
- Cataracts
- Dry eye
- Loss of sight

Small and large intestines
- Obstruction

Breast
- Lymphedema
- Breast fibrosis
- Subacute pneumonitis
- Pericarditis

Liver
- Liver failure

Cardiac
- Cardiomyopathy
- Pericarditis

Lung
- Subacute pneumonitis
- Pulmonary fibrosis

Esophagus
- Dysphagia
- Esophageal stricture

Stomach
- Gastritis

Head and neck
- Xerostomia
- Caries
- Osteoradionecrosis

Thyroid
- Hyperthyroidism or hypothyroidism
- Dysphagia

periods of rest. Strategies to address fatigue are listed in Chapter 11, Table 11-5.

Skin Reactions

In human skin, IR affects the rapidly dividing cells of the epidermis, hair follicles, and sebaceous glands and follows a predictive pattern of acute and late skin reactions. These reactions are normal and expected side effects of treatment, because the radi-ation must enter and, in some instances, exit through the skin in order to reach the target volume.

Time-dose-volume relationships of radiation influence the onset, duration, and intensity of skin reactions. The electron beam is superficially pene-trating and delivers high doses to the skin but can cause severe skin reactions. Linear accelerators as the source of RT have been more skin sparing.

As a result of RT, skin may redden and the area may become irritated, dry, or sensitive. The damage is similar to a sunburn. To manage skin problems from RT, nursing care includes skin evaluations before and during treatment to identify factors that may increase skin reactions. To manage skin reac-tions, the skin should be treated gently to avoid further irritation. The skin should be bathed care-fully using only warm water and mild soap. Acute reactions include erythema, hyperpigmentation, and dry desquamation that may proceed to moist desquamation. (When the reaction has progressed to moist desquamation, the skin's epithelial layer becomes thin and weeping, thus losing integrity.)

The most common sites of severe skin reactions with moist desquamation are areas where opposing skin surfaces touch or fold, such as the ear, neck, axilla, area under the breasts, perineum, and groin. Affected sites vary by treatment target. If the reac-tion is severe, a treatment break may be necessary to allow the skin to begin healing before completing the recommended total dose (resulting in a compro-mised treatment). Skin may return to normal and then undergo late effects, including scaling, finer hair, atrophy, and pigmentation changes.

A condition called *radiation recall* can occur with the concomitant use of chemotherapy agents, such as anthracyclines and selected chemotherapies (e.g., doxorubicin, daunorubicin, paclitaxel, methotrexate, hydroxyurea). The site that was irra-diated becomes inflamed and develops mucositis and erythema. Radiation recall can occur several months to a year after the initial irradiation. Hyperpigmentation of the skin can also follow and can be permanent. Skin reactions resulting from radiation recall are treated in the same way as other radiation skin reactions (Maher, 2006; NCI, 2004; Witt, 2005).

Hair Loss

Hair loss may occur in the treatment field. In most cases, the hair grows back following completion of RT. However, the return of hair usually depends on the dose. Complete and permanent hair loss can occur at skin doses of 45 Gy or more. Hair regrowth usually resumes at 2 to 3 months after treatments end, but usually at a slower rate of growth. New hair can continue to return for up to 1 year after treatment (Maher, 2006; NCI, 2004).

Mucositis and Stomatitis

Radiation can affect the membranes of the mouth and GI tract, causing mucositis, discomfort while swallowing, nausea, altered taste of foods, and diarrhea. The duration and intensity of the inflammatory response depend on the site of radiation, the total dose, the depth of penetration, and the number and frequency of treatments. The response usually begins 2 to 3 weeks after initiation of RT (at approximately 20 Gy) and persists for several weeks (3 to 6 weeks) after treatment is complete (Maher, 2006).

Late effects that correspond with irradiation of mucous membranes in various treatment fields include dry mouth (inability to produce saliva), inability to taste, dental caries, difficulty swallowing or pain when swallowing, bone necrosis, vaginal dryness, and pain during intercourse, urination, and elimination. These complications can affect an individual's quality of life (Maher, 2006; Witt, 2005).

Myelosuppression

During radiation treatments, the degree of bone marrow suppression depends on the amount of bone marrow included in the treatment field and previous exposure to chemotherapy.

Patient populations at risk for development of significant bone marrow suppression are those whose treatment fields include the whole body, the whole abdominal field, areas of the brain, pelvis, large limb bones, and iliac crest. When bone marrow is affected, the patient's neutrophil count declines rapidly, increasing the risk of infection, anemia, and thrombocytopenia. In severely immunocompromised patients, secondary infections are common, including infections by *Candida albicans*, *Candida tropicalis*, cytomegalovirus, and aspergillus.

Before treatment begins, an evaluation of the immune system should identify any factors that can increase the risk of radiation-induced neutropenia, thrombocytopenia, and anemia. Throughout treatment, complete blood count is monitored. Nurses should be on the alert for signs and symptoms of local or systemic infection, including recent fevers, chills, or night sweats (Maher, 2006).

When chemotherapy is given concurrently with RT, the patient should have frequent laboratory draws so that blood counts can be monitored and assessed for treatment side effects (Bucci, Bevan, & Roach, 2005)

ADVANCES IN RADIATION THERAPY

Over the past decade, RT treatments have improved as a result of better technologies with diagnostic tools (computed tomography, magnetic resonance imaging, positron-emission tomography, ultrasonography) and RT itself, using three-dimensional reconstruction in planning, computer-optimized algorithms, intensity modulated RT, and image-guided RT. These advances are attempting to overcome the challenges that continue to be associated with RT, including organ movement, targeted treatment to tumors while sparing normal tissue, and reduced treatment time (to reduce posttreatment side effects).

SUMMARY

RT is a treatment for localized or regional tumors, such of those of the breast, head and neck, lung, pancreas, and esophagus as well as metastatic disease to bone and brain. An individual's treatment plan includes adjustments to treatment field, dose, and timing. Among common side effects of RT are fatigue, skin burns, and mucositis. Although advances in treatment technology and planning may limit the severity of RT side effects, nursing care will continue to focus on acute and chronic side effect management.

EXAM QUESTIONS

CHAPTER 5
Questions 17-20

Note: Choose the option that BEST answers each question.

17. A tumor type that is treated with RT as a primary therapy is

    a. head and neck cancer.

    b. acute myelogenous leukemia.

    c. localized colon cancer.

    d. metastatic prostate cancer.

18. One factor that determines the effectiveness of RT on targeted cancer cells is

    a. amount of protection.

    b. dose.

    c. distance.

    d. shield.

19. For patients receiving brachytherapy, caregivers should protect themselves by limiting

    a. the dose.

    b. the angle on the targeted cells.

    c. exposure to advanced-stage tumors.

    d. time with the patient.

20. An acute toxicity from RT is

    a. constipation.

    b. skin erythema.

    c. myelosuppression.

    d. infection.

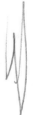

REFERENCES

Behrend, S. (2006). Radiation treatment planning. In C. Yarbro, M. Frogge, & M. Goodman (Eds.), *Cancer nursing: Principles and practice* (6th ed., pp. 250–282). Sudbury, MA: Jones & Bartlett.

Bucci, M., Bevan, A., & Roach, M. (2005). Advances in radiation therapy: Conventional to 3D, to IMRT, to 4D, and beyond. *CA: Cancer Journal for Clinicians, 55*(2), 117–134.

Gosselin-Acomb, T. (2006). Principles of radiation therapy. In C. Yarbro, M. Frogge, & M. Goodman (Eds.), *Cancer nursing: Principles and practice* (6th ed., pp. 229–249). Sudbury, MA: Jones & Bartlett.

Maher, K. (2006). Radiation therapy: Toxicities and management. In C. Yarbro, M. Frogge, & M. Goodman (Eds.), *Cancer nursing: Principles and practice* (6th ed., pp. 283–314). Sudbury, MA: Jones & Bartlett.

National Cancer Institute. (2004). *Radiation therapy for cancer: Questions and answers.* Retrieved April 17, 2007, from http://cancer.gov/cancertopics/factsheet/therapy/radiation

Witt, M. (2005). Nursing implications of radiation therapy. In J. K. Itano & K. N. Taoka (Eds.), *Core curriculum for oncology nursing* (4th ed., pp. 748–762). St. Louis: Elsevier.

CHAPTER 6

CHEMOTHERAPY

CHAPTER OBJECTIVE

After completing this chapter, the reader will be able to discuss chemotherapy agents—how they work, why they are ordered as part of treatment regimens, and how they should be safely handled.

LEARNING OBJECTIVES

After studying this chapter, the reader will be able to

1. name the phase of the cell cycle when deoxyribonucleic acid replication occurs.

2. differentiate the actions of four classifications of chemotherapy agents and give an example of each one.

3. identify a hormone used to treat breast cancer.

4. identify a bisphosphonate used to treat bone metastasis.

5. recognize steps to prevent extravasation.

INTRODUCTION

Chemotherapy has been a cornerstone of cancer care treatment for the past four decades. The term *chemotherapy* refers to any drug therapy and could be applied to agents used in cardiology, endocrinology, or any other medical specialty. Nevertheless, *chemotherapy* is a term that the lay public recognizes as a term for pharmaceuticals used to treat cancer. Other terms for chemotherapy in cancer care include *cytotoxic agents* and *antineoplastic agents* (Polovich, White, & Kelleher, 2005; Temple & Poniatowski, 2005).

HISTORY

During World War II, health care workers noticed that mustard gas, an agent used in chemical warfare, had a deleterious effect on the bone marrow of the soldiers who were exposed to it. Investigators theorized that if uncontrolled exposure to mustard gas could deplete the bone marrow, then controlled use of the agents might benefit patients as a treatment for hematologic tumors. Thus, nitrogen mustard became the first chemotherapeutic drug in modern times to be used successfully to treat cancer. Shortly after the discovery of nitrogen mustard's anticancer capabilities, the chemotherapy agents methotrexate (Mexate), cyclophosphamide (Cytoxan), and fluorouracil (5-FU) were developed and used as treatments for cancers (Polovich et al., 2005; Temple & Poniatowski, 2005).

Initially, chemotherapy was used as a method to palliate symptoms. But especially in the 1960s and 1970s, chemotherapy agents were shown to shrink tumors and better control cancer. Those improvements stemmed from the development and acceptance of combination chemotherapy, which targeted various biochemical processes. In some cases, chemotherapy administration prompted complete responses to treatment. Therefore, the goals of chemotherapy, as with other treatment modalities, continue to be cure, control, and palliation (Polovich et al., 2005; Temple & Poniatowski, 2005).

Chemotherapy-based protocols are the first-line treatment for most hematologic tumors and for cancers that have spread beyond the scope of local control. Combination chemotherapeutic protocols have resulted in legitimate cures and long-term control for some hematologic tumors (e.g., childhood leukemia, Hodgkin's disease) and advanced-stage solid tumors (e.g., testicular cancer) (Polovich et al., 2005; Temple & Poniatowski, 2005).

SCIENTIFIC FOUNDATION FOR CHEMOTHERAPY

Cell-Cycle Theory

Chemotherapy is a treatment strategy based on the effectiveness of cytotoxic drugs, which act on characteristics of individual tumor cells and cell-cycle kinetics. (For more information, see Chapter 2.)

It is known that both normal and malignant cells undergo a five-step process of cell growth between mitoses (see Figure 6-1). In gap 0 (G_0), cells are resting and out of cycle. When activated, the cells enter the cycle at gap 1 (G_1, or interphase), the period when cells prepare for deoxyribonucleic acid (DNA) synthesis and also synthesize ribonucleic acid (RNA) and certain proteins.

During S (synthesis) phase, DNA replication occurs. The gap between the end of S phase and mitosis is gap 2 (G_2), or premitotic phase, a pause for the cell to prepare for division. During mitosis (M), the chromosomes and nucleus move through the phases of prophase, metaphase, and anaphase to telophase, when the cell divides to become two distinct daughter cells. After mitosis, cells can leave the cycle and ultimately die or they return to a resting or dormant phase (G_0) and re-enter the cycle at G_1 (Polovich et al., 2005; Temple & Poniatowski, 2005).

The length of time a specific cell stays in each phase of the cell cycle is highly variable. The growth fraction is the portion of cells in the population that are actively cycling. Generally, cells in G_0 and G_1 are out of cycle, although many activities take place during these phases. These cells can actively synthesize RNA and proteins and differentiate; however, during the resting phase, they are typically resistant to the cytotoxic effects of chemotherapy.

The average time between mitoses (cycling time) is 1 to 2 days for most normal cells and 2 to 3 days for malignant cells (Temple & Poniatowski, 2005). Intermitotic time, however, does not describe the entire picture of tumor growth. For example, the length of the cell cycle of tumor cells in squamous cell carcinoma of the skin is somewhat longer than that of the tumor cells in acute myelogenous leukemia (AML). Despite this difference, AML cells spread quickly and become more lethal than squamous cell cancer because of the cell-cycle kinetics affecting the entire tissue.

Cells that have the fastest growing time, and therefore the fastest turnover in the body, respond most acutely to chemotherapy. Examples of fast-growing cells include those of the hair, gastrointestinal (GI) tract, bone marrow (hematopoietic), reproductive system, and skin (Polovich et al., 2005; Temple & Poniatowski, 2005). In patients undergoing chemotherapy, these cell types are also the targets of most of chemotherapy's toxicities (or side effects).

Table 6-1 provides a list of common cell-cycle-specific and nonspecific chemotherapy drugs.

FACTORS AFFECTING TUMOR RESPONSE TO CHEMOTHERAPY

Several factors combine to create the foundation for effective chemotherapy treatment. A brief review of these factors—debulking the tumor, pharmacokinetics, dosing and scheduling, pharmacology, and resistance—follows (Hayden & Goodman, 2006; Polovich et al., 2005; Temple & Poniatowski, 2005).

Debulking the Tumor

Because of tissue growth kinetics of tumor cells, tumors that have already begun to slow their growth rate are not as responsive to chemotherapy.

FIGURE 6-1: MECHANISM OF ACTION OF MAJOR CHEMOTHERAPY DRUGS

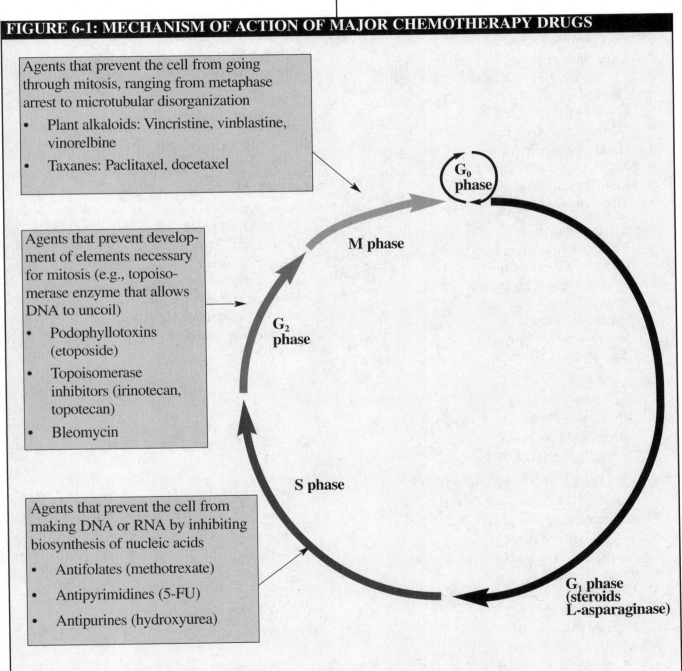

Agents that prevent the cell from going through mitosis, ranging from metaphase arrest to microtubular disorganization

- Plant alkaloids: Vincristine, vinblastine, vinorelbine
- Taxanes: Paclitaxel, docetaxel

Agents that prevent development of elements necessary for mitosis (e.g., topoisomerase enzyme that allows DNA to uncoil)

- Podophyllotoxins (etoposide)
- Topoisomerase inhibitors (irinotecan, topotecan)
- Bleomycin

Agents that prevent the cell from making DNA or RNA by inhibiting biosynthesis of nucleic acids

- Antifolates (methotrexate)
- Antipyrimidines (5-FU)
- Antipurines (hydroxyurea)

G_0 phase

M phase

G_2 phase

S phase

G_1 phase (steroids L-asparaginase)

Cell-cycle-nonspecific drugs, which are active throughout cell cycle:

- Alkylating agents (cyclophosphamide)
- Anthracycline antibiotics (doxorubicin)
- Nitrosoureas (carmustine)
- Miscellaneous (cisplatin, dacarbazine, mitomycin C)

TABLE 6-1: CLASSIFICATIONS OF COMMON CHEMOTHERAPIES: CELL CYCLE SPECIFIC AND CELL CYCLE NONSPECIFIC

CELL CYCLE SPECIFIC

Alkylating Agents
- Dacarbazine (DTIC-Dome)

Antimetabolite Agents
- Capecitabine (Xeloda)
- Cytarabine (Cytosar-U)
- Floxuridine/Fluorodeoxyuridine (FUDR)
- Fludarabine (Fludara)
- Fluorouracil
- Gemcitabine (Gemzar)
- Hydroxyurea (Hydrea)
- Mercaptopurine (Purinethol)
- Methotrexate (Mexate)
- Thioguanine

Antitumor Antibiotics
- Bleomycin (Blenoxane)
- Dactinomycin (Cosmegen)
- Daunorubicin (Cerubidine)
- Doxorubicin (Adriamycin)
- Idarubicin (Idamycin)
- Mitomycin (Mutamycin)
- Plicamycin (Mithracin)

Plant Alkaloids
- Etoposide (VePesid)
- Vinblastine (Velban)
- Vincristine (Oncovin)
- Vinorelbine (Navelbine)

CELL CYCLE NONSPECIFIC
- Busulfan (Myleran)
- Carboplatin (Paraplatin)
- Cisplatin (Platinol)
- Cyclophosphamide (Cytoxan, Neosar)
- Ifosfamide (Ifex)
- Chlorambucil (Leukeran)
- Mechlorethamine/nitrogen mustard (Mustargen)
- Melphalan (Alkeran)
- Streptozocin (Zanosar)
- Thiotepa (Thioplex)

Nitrosoureas
- Carmustine (BiCNU)
- Lomustine (CeeNU)

HORMONAL TREATMENTS

Adrenocorticoids
- Cortisone
- Hydrocortisone (Cortef)
- Dexamethasone (Decadron)
- Methylprednisolone (Solu-Medrol)
- Prednisone (Meticorten, Deltasone)

Antiestrogens
- Tamoxifen (Nolvadex)

Selective Estrogen Receptor Modulators
- Raloxifene (Evista)

MISCELLANEOUS AGENTS
- Asparaginase (Elspar)
- Dexrazoxane (Zinecard)
- Docetaxel (Taxotere)
- Paclitaxel (Taxol)
- Irinotecan (Camptosar)
- Mitotane (Lysodren)
- Mitoxantrone (Novantrone)
- Pamidronate (Aredia)
- Procarbazine

Another way to say this is that larger tumors have small growth fractions and are therefore less responsive to the cytotoxic effects of antineoplastic drugs. That is why these tumors are first debulked by surgery or radiation therapy, minimizing the tumor mass and thus lowering the tumor burden. Debulking also eliminates some of the blood supply to the tumor.

Pharmacokinetics

Clinical pharmacokinetic actions include:

- Absorption—The bioavailability of most anti-cancer drugs is unpredictable. As a result, many agents are given parenterally to ensure accurate dosing and optimal systemic exposure.

- Distribution—Distribution of drugs in the body is based on the drug's ability to penetrate different tissues and bind to plasma proteins. Drugs that are highly lipophilic tend to be more readily taken up by lipophilic tissues, such as bone marrow, fat, and cells in the central nervous system. For example, nitrosoureas such as carmustine and lomustine are useful for primary brain tumors and hematopoietic malignancies, such as Hodgkin's and non-Hodgkin's lymphomas.

  As a result of nutritional deficits, cancer patients can have decreased levels of plasma proteins, especially albumin. With that deficiency, the cytotoxic activity of highly protein-bound chemotherapy drugs, such as etoposide (VePesid, VP-16) and teniposide (Vumon), may be enhanced in these patients because a greater percentage of the drug is unbound and free to kill cancer cells.

- Metabolism—The liver provides the main mechanism for catabolism of drugs. Several chemotherapy drugs require activation intracellularly or systemically before they are able to exert their cytotoxic effects. When the liver is not compromised by disease, agents can act on tumors based on normal metabolic processes. If the liver is damaged or not functioning adequately, the agent's effectiveness is compromised. Therefore, liver function is key to the effectiveness of chemotherapy drugs.

- Excretion—Also known as *clearance,* excretion is one of the most important pharmacokinetic activities because it affects a drug's clinical side effects. Clearance determines the steady-state concentration and is independent of the half-lives of agents. Clearance is determined by blood flow to an organ, usually the kidney or liver, and the organ's efficiency in extracting the drug from the blood. Therefore, adequate kidney or liver function is key to clearing the agent and limiting toxicity. Agents cleared by the kidneys—whose toxic effects can result in renal insufficiency—include cyclophosphamide, etoposide, cisplatin, carboplatin, and methotrexate. These agents require dose modification when kidney function is compromised.

Dosing and Scheduling

Another factor that influences the number of tumor cells killed is the dose of chemotherapeutic drugs delivered. Generally, a selected dose of a chosen chemotherapeutic agent destroys a certain proportion of tumor cells. With each full dose of the drug, a certain proportion of tumor cells die. Between courses of chemotherapy, the tumor grows. Thus, repeat cycles of treatment steadily decrease the number of tumor cells that remain for the next course of treatment. This strategy is the foundation for protocols calling for aggressive dosing—as much as the patient can tolerate.

Dose-dense regimens use shorter times between courses of chemotherapy than the times between courses of conventional chemotherapy protocols. Typically in dose-dense regimens, chemotherapy courses are scheduled every 2 weeks rather than every 3 weeks. Dose-dense regimens are being used as treatments for breast and lung cancers. Data suggest that these regimens can prolong disease-free survival (National Cancer Institute, 2006). These dose-dense regimens can be considered if the chemotherapy side effects—especially periods of neutropenia—can be well managed by using supportive medications. Examples of supportive drugs that allow aggressive chemotherapy administration are the hematopoietic growth factors—granulocyte colony-stimulating factors, such as pegfilgrastim (Neulasta) and filgrastin (Neupogen), and granulocyte-macrophage colony-stimulating factors, such as sargramostin (Leukine) and erythropoetin (epoetin alfa, Procrit) (Hayden & Goodman, 2006; Polovich et al., 2005).

Adjuvant treatment, which occurs after primary treatments, boosts the effectiveness of the main treatment strategy. If no clinically detectable tumor is present but the risk of tumor recurrence is high, adjuvant chemotherapy administration can be effective. As an example, Figure 6-2 provides an adjuvant treatment strategy for rectal cancer that would begin after initial surgical resection.

Combination chemotherapy regimens capitalize on the additive, or synergistic, effects of chemotherapy on tumor cells. Specific agents affect the cell cycle at different phases, increasing the number of tumor cells exposed to the combined chemotherapies during a cycle. Combination regimens can modulate the toxicity of side effects because one agent can modulate the effect of another agent in the regimen. Combination regimens can also decrease the risk of drug resistance (Temple & Poniatowski, 2005).

Timing the administration of certain adjuvant chemotherapy agents can optimize the therapy's effectiveness. A shorter cell-cycle time, coupled with a higher percentage of tumor cells that are proliferating at one time (growth fraction), should lead to a greater number of cells killed by chemotherapeutic agents.

Pharmacology

The choice of specific chemotherapy agents to target specific tumors is based on many factors. Individual patient factors include anticipated toxicities from the agents, organ dysfunction (e.g., renal, hepatic), age, previous drug treatments, and subsequent protocols.

Some chemotherapy agents have a recommended maximum lifetime dose due to the cumulative toxic effect they have on patients. Examples of these include the anthracycline drugs doxorubicin (Adriamycin), daunorubicin (Cerubidine), and idarubicin (Idamycin). These drugs increase the risk of cardiomyopathy. Bleomycin (Blenoxane) also has a maximum lifetime dose recommendation. It is associated with an increased risk of pulmonary fibrosis.

If patients have preexisting neurologic deficits, neurotoxic drugs may need to be avoided. Previous bone marrow transplant or the use of severely marrow-toxic drugs may preclude patients from subsequent use of full doses of myelosuppressive drugs in cases of tumor recurrence or the development of new tumor types (Hayden & Goodman, 2006; Polovich et al.,

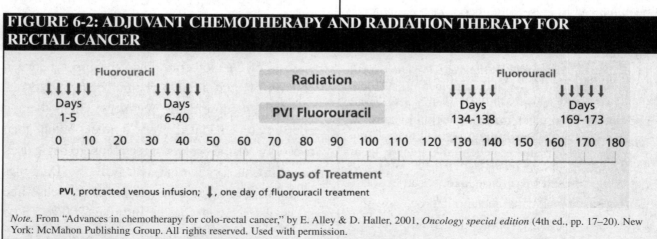

FIGURE 6-2: ADJUVANT CHEMOTHERAPY AND RADIATION THERAPY FOR RECTAL CANCER

PVI, protracted venous infusion; ↓, one day of fluorouracil treatment

Note. From "Advances in chemotherapy for colo-rectal cancer," by E. Alley & D. Haller, 2001, *Oncology special edition* (4th ed., pp. 17–20). New York: McMahon Publishing Group. All rights reserved. Used with permission.

2005; Temple & Poniatowski, 2005). Peripheral neuropathy is also dose-limiting.

Any antineoplastic drug can prompt toxicities. Some reasons for these toxicities stem from the tumor origin, drug resistance from alterations in protein binding, poor drug clearance, and the inability of a drug to reach its cellular target. For example, poorly lipophilic drugs administered systemically are ineffective for tumors found in the central nervous system, which are saturated with lipophilic tissue. Thus, they are unable to cross the blood-brain barrier. To circumvent this barrier, methotrexate (Mexate) or cytarabine (cytosine arabinoside, Ara-C) are among the few agents that can be administered directly to the intrathecal space. Additional agents are in development.

Tumors can be selective to certain types of chemotherapeutic agents. For example, 5-FU is most active in cancers of endodermal tissue, such as GI and breast neoplasms (Polovich et al., 2005).

Resistance

For some patients with tumors that are drug resistant, specific multiagent administration strategies capitalize on ways to better target the tumor. Still, using multiagent strategies may not overcome the tumor's resistance to therapy. Some of these strategies include scheduling the agents so that they are most effective when administered (e.g., at night, in certain sequences), aggressive dosing, and using new agents to augment the cytotoxic value of the main drugs in the protocol (Polovich et al., 2005; Temple & Poniatowski, 2005).

According to cell-cycle kinetics, as tumor burden decreases, the rate of proliferation increases. Thus, tumors treated with a chemotherapeutic regimen should become even more sensitive to the same therapy over time. Unfortunately, this is not the case. Many tumors respond at the beginning of chemotherapy and then recur or progress even though the same chemotherapy continues.

Why do agents become ineffective? Some theories suggest that the innate, vexing capabilities of the cancer cell are the cause. The cell's mechanisms of action allow it to mutate or navigate around the action of antineoplastic agents. Thus, in time, the tumor does not respond to the agent (Hayden & Goodman, 2006).

In summary, the optimal time to treat cancer is as soon as possible after diagnosis, when the tumor burden is at its lowest. In addition, protocols that are based on non-cross-resistant agents—given sequentially or in specific aggressive dosing—reduce the risk of multidrug resistance (Polovich et al., 2005; Temple & Poniatowski, 2005).

CLASSIFICATION OF CHEMOTHERAPY AGENTS

Chemotherapeutic agents are classified according to their mechanism of action or their derivation. Major chemotherapy classifications are alkylating agents, nitrosoureas (a subclass of alkylating agents), antimetabolites, antitumor antibiotics, plant alkaloids, hormonal agents, and miscellaneous agents.

The following sections highlight these classifications, identify their mechanisms of action, and point out specific characteristics of selected agents. (Check with recent chemotherapy or pharmacology texts or information from the pharmaceutical manufacturer for more complete information about each agent's targets, actions, and possible side effects. *Note*: When citing agents, this course lists the agent's generic name followed in parentheses by a representative brand name.)

Alkylating Agents

Alkylating agents alter the cell's DNA, leading to the incorrect pairing of purine and pyrimidine bases. Most are cell cycle nonspecific, acting at any time during the cell cycle or during the resting G_0 phase. Among toxicities of alkylating agents are hematologic (bone marrow suppression) and GI side effects.

The first alkylating agent used in cancer treatment was mechlorethamine (Mustargen), also called *nitrogen mustard*. It is a severe vesicant—an agent that can cause severe tissue damage if it extravasates or leaks into the perivascular or subcutaneous spaces. As with other vesicants, it must be handled with caution to prevent exposure to the clinician and to prevent extravasation during administration. The major therapeutic role of mechlorethamine in contemporary practice is in the MOPP protocol, a familiar chemotherapy regimen for Hodgkin's disease (Adams, DeRemer, & Holdsworth, 2005). This regimen consists of:

1. mechlorethamine (Mustargen)

2. vincristine (Oncovin)

3. procarbazine hydrochloride (Matulane)

4. prednisone.

The alkylating agents melphalan (Alkeran), busulfan (Myleran), and chlorambucil (Leukeran) are usually given orally. In addition to its use in chronic myelogenous leukemia, busulfan is also used in high-dose chemotherapy conditioning regimens for allogeneic or autologous bone marrow transplantation. Chlorambucil is well established in the treatment of chronic lymphocytic leukemia. Melphalan is a treatment for multiple myeloma.

Cyclophosphamide (Cytoxan) and ifosfamide (Ifex) rely on the kidneys and liver for elimination. Their toxicity may be prolonged in patients with compromised renal or hepatic failure. In approximately 2% to 40% of patients receiving cyclophosphamide, hemorrhagic cystitis occurs (Hayden & Goodman, 2006). This complication may be avoided by ensuring that the patient is adequately hydrated to clear cyclophosphamide from the system. Ifosfamide is associated with a higher incidence of urotoxicity than cyclophosphamide. A chemoprotectant—mesna (Mesnex)—is always given with ifosfamide to minimize the occurrence of hemorrhagic cystitis (Polovich et al., 2005).

Miscellaneous Agents

The platinum-containing compounds cisplatin (Platinol) and carboplatin (Paraplatin) require patients to have adequate renal function, because 90% of these drugs are excreted by the kidneys. Although cisplatin and other platinum analogues behave similarly to alkylators, their mechanisms of action are different—they inhibit DNA and protein synthesis, altering cell membrane transport and stopping mitochondrial function.

Although both cisplatin and carboplatin work in similar ways on tumors, they are dosed and administered differently. They also have different side effects. The dose-limiting toxicity of cisplatin is nephrotoxicity. Acute renal failure may occur within 24 hours of drug administration. To best address these toxicity risks, adequate hydration must be maintained. Also, with cisplatin, neurotoxicity, ototoxicity, and severe emesis can be side effects.

Carboplatin rarely necessitates aggressive hydration and diuresis, but nausea and vomiting are common. Dose-limiting myelosuppression is much more of an issue with carboplatin than with cisplatin (Hayden & Goodman, 2006).

Other agents with alkylating-like activity include dacarbazine (DTIC-Dome), temozolomide (Temodar), procarbazine (Matulane), and altretamine (Hexalen). Dacarbazine functions primarily as an alkylating agent but may also act as an antimetabolite by inhibiting purine nucleoside incorporation into DNA.

Dacarbazine is considered cell cycle specific and is extremely sensitive to light. Its most significant side effects are nausea and vomiting, which may decrease with repeated courses. Other toxicities include hepatic venoocclusive disease (appearing as fever and acute hepatic necrosis), a flu-like syndrome, myelosuppression, and photosensitivity (Polovich et al., 2005; Temple & Poniatowski, 2005).

Temozolomide is a new monofunctional alkylating agent that is similar to dacarbazine. It is administered orally and has significant activity in patients with malignant gliomas (glioblastoma multiforme, anaplastic astrocytoma) or advanced metastatic malignant melanomas.

Procarbazine is administered orally and is used in the treatment of Hodgkin's disease and brain tumors. Two drug interactions of procarbazine are important. The first is that use of the agent may lead to severe hypertension, headache, and sweating and coma. To prevent this drug interaction, patients should avoid eating foods high in tyramine, such as wine, ripe cheese, chocolate, and liver. The second interaction occurs when patients consume alcohol, which can result in nausea, vomiting, palpitations, and sweating (Polovich et al., 2005).

Nitrosoureas

A subclassification of alkylating agents, nitrosoureas are also cell cycle nonspecific. They disrupt DNA repair and duplication. Because they are non-cross-resistant with each other, nitrosoureas and alkylating agents are used together in multidrug regimens.

Nitrosoureas are lipid soluble and can cross the blood-brain barrier. They are used to treat tumors of the central nervous system, Hodgkin's and non-Hodgkin's lymphoma, and malignant melanoma. Major side effects of nitrosoureas include prolonged myelosuppression and GI reactions. Examples of nitrosoureas are carmustine (BiCNU), lomustine (CeeNU), and streptozocin (Zanosar).

Antimetabolites

Antimetabolites inhibit both protein and DNA synthesis. Because they are most effective during the S phase of the cell cycle, they are cell cycle specific. Their major toxicities are hematologic and GI side effects.

Antimetabolites used in cancer chemotherapy are structural analogues of nucleotide bases, which are the building blocks of DNA and RNA. The antifolate agent methotrexate (Mexate) is effective in the S phase, the phase that is most susceptible to an agent that reduces folate and thus prevents cells from proceeding with DNA synthesis. Large doses of methotrexate may be part of a treatment regimen for malignant lymphomas and sarcomas. Patients need to have adequate renal function to receive methotrexate-based treatment. Myelosuppression and mucositis also are side effects of methotrexate treatment. Doses are adjusted to address methotrexate toxicity (Polovich et al., 2005; Temple & Poniatowski, 2005).

One strategy is to follow high-dose methotrexate with leucovorin, also called *folinic acid*. Leucovorin "rescues" normal cells by providing them with the reduced folates they need for nucleic acid and protein synthesis. The rescue agent allows maximum tumor exposure to the chemotherapy agent while minimizing the toxicity of the agent on normal cells. (Leucovorin rescue is not required for lower dose methotrexate protocols.)

Fluorouracil (5-fluorouracil, 5-FU), a pyrimidine analogue, rapidly clears through the liver and therefore has a brief plasma half-life. The major dose-limiting toxicity of 5-FU depends on the schedule of administration. Myelosuppression is more prominent when the drug is given by rapid bolus injection. Mucositis and GI toxicity are more common with prolonged infusions over 4 to 5 days.

Capecitabine (Xeloda) is an oral agent that changes in the body to form 5-FU. It is approved by the U.S. Food and Drug Administration (FDA) for the treatment of metastatic breast cancer for which anthracyclines or paclitaxel (Taxol) is indicated. Capecitabine is also active in colorectal cancer. The major dose-limiting side effects of capecitabine include diarrhea, hand-and-foot syndrome, and stomatitis.

As with other antimetabolites, cytarabine (Cytosar-U) is most sensitive in the S phase. Cytarabine may be administered by continuous infusion or bolus depending on the tumor type and protocol. Side effects of cytarabine include myelosuppression and GI epithelial injury. When high-dose cytarabine is used for refractory acute myelogenous leukemia, patients may experience cerebellum dysfunction, conjunctivitis, and photosensitivity (Hayden & Goodman, 2006; Polovich et al., 2005; Temple & Poniatowski, 2005).

Antitumor Antibiotics

Antitumor antibiotics inhibit both RNA and DNA synthesis. Most are cell cycle nonspecific. Their most common side effects are hematopoietic and GI. Cumulative doses of some of these agents can lead to cardiac changes.

The anthracycline antibiotics—daunorubicin (Cerubidine), doxorubicin (Adriamycin), and idarubicin (Idamycin)—and the chemically related anthracenediones (mitoxantrone [Novantrone])—have multiple mechanisms of cytotoxicity. The anthracycline dose should be reduced in patients with hepatic dysfunction, especially if bilirubin is elevated. Dose adjustment is not necessary in patients with renal failure because renal clearance of anthracyclines is minimal (Polovich et al., 2005).

Cardiac toxicity from anthracyclines may appear as acute changes and arrhythmias on an electrocardiogram (ECG). The effects are more significant in patients with pre-existing heart disease. However, the more common and often therapy-limiting cardiotoxicity is the development of cardiomyopathy, which can lead to congestive heart failure. Up to 10% of patients receiving a cumulative dose of doxorubicin greater than 550 mg/m² develop this toxicity (Hayden & Goodman, 2006; Polovich et al., 2005; Temple & Poniatowski, 2005).

Cardiac function is usually monitored with serial measurements of left ventricular function and ECGs. Potential strategies to prevent or lessen cardiotoxicity include prolonged infusions of doxorubicin and cardioprotectant drugs such as dexrazoxane (Zinecard).

Mitoxantrone may be associated with less nausea, vomiting, and alopecia than other chemotherapy agents. Cardiac toxicity in patients treated with mitoxantrone appears to be less than that seen with doxorubicin. However, there may be no difference in the incidence of cardiomyopathy (Polovich et al., 2005).

Daunorubicin, doxorubicin, epirubicin (Ellence), and idarubicin are vesicants and can cause extravasation. Mitoxantrone is considered an irritant, but extravasation injury is much less common. Other toxicities of anthracyclines include mucositis, nausea, vomiting, and alopecia. The color of urine can also change (to pink or red) when patients receive these agents.

Liposomal encapsulation of doxorubicin and daunorubicin allow a longer half-life and increased uptake by tumor cells than do nonliposomal forms. Liposomal daunorubicin (DaunoXome) and liposomal doxorubicin (DOXIL) (pegylated form) are treatments for Kaposi sarcoma in patients with acquired immunodeficiency syndrome and in selected breast cancer and ovarian cancer protocols. Liposomal forms appear to lessen the side effects of alopecia, nausea, vomiting, hand-and-foot syndrome, and neurotoxicity. They are also not considered vesicants. Cardiac toxicity appears to be less dose-limiting. Doses greater than 1000 mg/m² have been given without significant changes in left ventricular function (Polovich et al., 2005; Temple & Poniatowski, 2005).

Bleomycin (Blenoxane), another antitumor antibiotic, is a cell-cycle-specific agent. Tumor cells are most sensitive to bleomycin in the G_2 phase or in the M phase of the cell cycle. Bleomycin has been used to synchronize cells into the G_2 and S phases so that other antineoplastic agents have a better kill rate. Bleomycin is also useful in combination chemotherapy regimens because of its lack of significant myelosuppression.

Bleomycin is highly dependent on renal clearance for elimination. Significant renal failure necessitates decreasing the dose by 50% to 75% of full dose. Pulmonary toxicity of bleomycin may initially present as cough, dyspnea, and pleuritic chest pain. Patients at higher risk for developing bleomycin-related pulmonary fibrosis include older patients (> 70 years), those with preexisting pulmonary disease, and those who have received mediastinal radiation therapy. Clinically significant pulmonary toxicity has been documented at cumulative doses of about 450 units or greater (Polovich et al., 2005). Flu-like symptoms, such as fever, chills, and myalgias, may present during the first 24 hours after bleomycin administration. Since anaphylaxis is possible, nurses should administer a test dose of bleomycin to the patient before the first dose and have emergency equipment and medications accessible.

Mitomycin (Mutamycin) is activated when added to an alkylating agent, the combination of which inhibits DNA synthesis and cell death. The drug works best in hypoxic tissues of solid tumors. Delayed and cumulative myelosuppression is seen with mitomycin (Hayden & Goodman, 2006).

Plant Alkaloids: Vinca Alkaloids and Taxanes

Common plant alkaloids include vinca alkaloids and the taxanes. Vinca alkaloids bind with microtubule proteins to stop the cell in metaphase, thereby inhibiting RNA and protein synthesis. These chemotherapeutic drugs are known to have neurotoxic effects (e.g., peripheral neuropathy) and effects on the hematopoietic, integumentary, and reproductive systems.

Vincristine (Oncovin) is used in protocols to treat leukemia, lymphoma, breast cancer, lung cancer, and multiple myeloma. It is neurotoxic but causes minimal myelosuppression. Dose modification should be considered in patients with hepatic dysfunction, particularly patients with biliary obstructions. Vincristine is a vesicant.

Vinblastine (Velban) is used primarily in germ cell tumors and advanced Hodgkin's disease. Vinblastine is myelotoxic and neurotoxic. Vinblastine is a vesicant.

Vinorelbine (Navelbine) is active in breast cancer and non-small-cell lung cancer and is both myelotoxic and neurotoxic. Vinorelbine is administered as a short infusion rather than an IV bolus and should be followed by a flush of 75 to 126 ml of isotonic solution to minimize injection site reactions (Polovich et al., 2005).

Vinblastine and vinorelbine have similar pharmacokinetic profiles, with excretion occurring primarily through the biliary tract. All the vinca alkaloids have a prolonged terminal elimination half-life of 1 to 4 days. Vinca alkaloids are known for their peripheral neurotoxicity, which is frequently a cumulative dose-limiting toxicity. The only effective management is discontinuation of therapy. The vinca alkaloids are vesicants that can extravasate.

The most recently approved plant alkaloids are the taxanes. Paclitaxel (Taxol), produced from the bark of the Western yew tree, stabilizes the mitotic spindle, causing disruption of cell division. Docetaxel (Taxotere) is produced from the leaves of the European yew tree and prompts different side effects than paclitaxel.

Until the early 1990s, extraction and isolation from plant material was the only source for paclitaxel. Then a semisynthetic process using a taxane precursor was developed. Because of the drug's poor water solubility, the injectable formulation must contain 50% polyoxyethylated castor oil (Cremophor EL) to maintain aqueous solubility (Temple & Poniatowski, 2005). Cremophor EL creates problems with administration because it can leach hepatotoxic plasticizer from polyvinyl chloride plastic, prompting hypersensitivity reactions in approximately 10% of patients. These allergic reactions include hypotension, bronchospasm, dyspnea, abdominal and leg pain, and severe facial flushing. Major hypersensitivity reactions can be prevented in most patients by the preinfusion administration of a corticosteroid (e.g., dexamethasone [Decadron]), an antihistamine (e.g., diphenhydramine [Benadryl]), and a histamine blocking drug (e.g., cimetidine [Tagamet] or ranitidine [Zantac]).

For routine use of paclitaxel with cisplatin or carboplatin, paclitaxel should be given first, followed by cisplatin or carboplatin. The taxanes also exhibit a high degree of protein binding (90% to 95%). Among the most significant toxicities associated with taxanes are myelosuppression, neurotoxicity, hypersensitivity, total body alopecia, and transient myalgias and arthralgias.

The toxicity profile of docetaxel is different from that of paclitaxel. The incidence of hypersensitivity reactions is lower with docetaxel, with severe reactions experienced in fewer than 1% of patients treated. Skin reactions—including pruritus, macular or papular lesions, erythema, and desquamation—are seen in 50% to 70% of patients treated with docetaxel (Polovich et al., 2005; Temple & Poniatowski, 2005). Signs of swelling and fluid overload with this agent include peripheral edema, generalized edema, pleural effusion, and cardiac tamponade. Treatment is corticosteroids.

Other Plant Alkaloids

Etoposide (VePesid, VP-16) and teniposide (Vumon, VP-26) are active against germ cell tumors and small-cell lung cancer, as well as other tumor types. The cytotoxic effects of etoposide exhibit a schedule dependency in the treatment of extensive small-cell lung cancer. These toxicities include myelosuppression and hypersensitivity, with infusion-related blood pressure changes being the most significant effect. Etoposide is available as an oral formulation, which has a bioavailability of approximately 50%. Thus, oral doses are usually two times the amount of IV doses (Temple & Poniatowski, 2005).

The semisynthetic analogues of topotecan (Hycamtin) and irinotecan (Camptosar) have undergone extensive clinical trials and have been approved by the FDA as single-agent therapy for refractory ovarian cancer (topotecan) and relapsed colon cancer (irinotecan). Myelosuppression is the major dose-limiting toxicity of topotecan, whereas diarrhea is the primary dose-limiting toxicity of irinotecan when administered on a once-weekly schedule. Topotecan is given as a multiple-day regimen. Irinotecan protocols typically have the agent given weekly or every 3 weeks.

Hormones

A variety of hormones, although not specifically classed as cytotoxic agents, are useful as single agents or part of multiagent therapies. The effect of each hormone is related to its particular mode of action. Treatments include estrogens, androgens, antiestrogens, and antiandrogens.

Steroids and steroid analogues are hormonal therapies used in cancer treatment. Their mechanism of action is thought to involve the inhibition of steroid-specific receptors located on the surface of cells. Blocking these receptors prevents the cell from receiving normal hormonal growth stimulation, thereby decreasing the growth fraction of the tumor (Vachani, 2005).

Tamoxifen citrate (Nolvadex) is an antiestrogen that is used for metastatic and adjuvant treatment for breast cancer with estrogen receptor–positive tumors. Tamoxifen is an estrogen antagonist (blocker) in breast tissue and an estrogen agonist (stimulator) in the endometrium, bone, and lipids. The most prominent toxicity is hot flashes, which affect approximately half of the women who use it. Other side effects include a slight risk of thromoembolism and a potential to cause endometrial cancer.

Another antiestrogen agent is toremifene (Fareston), which is thought to be a more pure antiestrogen. A trial comparing tamoxifen and toremifene indicated both were equally effective in treating metastatic breast cancer (Gerken, 2004b). However, toremifene appears to be less carcinogenic, at least in preclinical models. Megestrol (Megace) has also been used to treat metastatic breast cancer but more recently is primarily used for the treatment of anorexia-cachexia related to cancer (Gerken, 2004b).

Anastrozole (Arimidex) and letrozole (Femara) are aromatase inhibitors. They suppress post-menopausal estrogen synthesis by inhibiting the peripheral conversion of androgens to estrogens. They are used in the treatment of hormonally sensitive breast cancer in postmenopausal women or oophorectomized premenopausal women. Common side effects include weight gain, bone pain, hot flashes, and GI disturbances (Vachani, 2005; Gerken, 2004a; Viale, 2005).

Luteinizing hormone–releasing hormone agonists are synthetic analogues of the naturally occurring hormone. Castration levels of testosterone are achieved with leuprolide acetate (Lupron) and goserelin (Zoladex). They are used in the treatment of prostate cancer.

Antiandrogens are used in men with hormone-responsive metastatic prostate cancer, either as initial therapy or in combination with a gonadotropin-releasing hormone analogue. Flutamide (Eulexin) was the first antiandrogen approved by the FDA. Side effects include diarrhea, gynecomastia and, occasionally, hepatotoxicity.

Bisphosphonates

The bisphosphonates are an approved treatment for bone metastasis in advanced cancer (typically with the spread of breast or prostate cancer). They are also used in treatment and prevention of osteo-porosis. They are analogues of a naturally occurring compound called *pyrophosphate* that prevents bone breakdown. They are very effective in relieving bone pain associated with metastatic disease.

Bisphosphonates can be given orally or intra-venously. The latter is the preferred route of administration for many oncologists because it requires only a short infusion monthly. The two approved and commonly used IV bisphosphonates are pamidronate di-sodium (Aredia) and zolendronic acid (Zometa) (Maltzman, 2004; Maxwell & Viale, 2005).

Miscellaneous Agents

L-asparaginase (Elspar) is part of induction and consolidation therapy for acute lymphocytic leukemia. L-asparaginase is extracted from the bacteria *Escherichia coli*. Toxicities with L-asparaginase include hypersensitivity reaction, hyperglycemia, hypoprothrombinemia, and neurotoxicity.

Hydroxyurea (Hydrea) is an orally administered, DNA-selective antimetabolite that is used to treat acute and chronic leukemia and myeloma. Allopurinol (Zyloprim) with hydroxyurea (Hydrea) should be administered to prevent tumor lysis syndrome in acute leukemias.

Interferon alfa-2b (Intron A) is a manufactured form of interferon, a protein made naturally by the body to boost immunity and regulate other cell functions. It is an adjuvant treatment for adults with malignant melanoma who are at high risk for recurrence. It is also indicated—with anthracycline-combination chemotherapy—as an initial treatment for clinically aggressive follicular non-Hodgkin's lymphoma.

Interleukin-2, or IL-2, is a body protein produced by T lymphocytes as part of the immune system response. Aldesleukin is the commercial form of IL-2. It is indicated for treatment of some renal cell cancers and melanoma. Because it helps mobilize the immune system response, common side effects associated with IL-2 include pronounced flu-like symptoms, nausea and vomiting, compromised kidney function, skin changes, and fatigue.

FDA-approved chemotherapeutic drugs used to treat cancers are listed in Table 6-2.

NANOTECHNOLOGY-DRIVEN INNOVATIONS

The next few years will introduce more break-throughs in clinical practice related to the field of nanotechnology. Nanotechnology is an area of science that focuses on the manipulation of atoms and molecules. Nanotechnology methods have led

text continues on page 86

TABLE 6-2: SELECTED FDA-APPROVED ONCOLOGY DRUGS WITH INDICATIONS, JULY 2007 (1 OF 7)

Drug Generic Name	Drug Trade Name	Additional Information About Approved Use	Approval Date
abarelix	Plenaxis depot	For the palliative treatment of men with advanced symptomatic prostate cancer, in whom LHRH agonist therapy is not appropriate and who refuse surgical castration, and have one or more of the following: (1) risk of neurological compromise due to metastases, (2) ureteral or bladder outlet obstruction due to local encroachment or metastatic disease, or (3) severe bone pain from skeletal metastases persisting on narcotic analgesia	Nov 25 2003
aldesleukin	Prokine	Treatment of adults with metastatic melanoma	Jan 09 1998
Aldesleukin	Proleukin	Treatment of adults with metastatic renal cell carcinoma	May 05 1992
altretamine	Hexalen	Single agent palliative treatment of patients with persistent or recurrent ovarian cancer following first-line therapy with a cisplatin and/or alkylating agent based combination.	Dec 26 1990
anastrozole	Arimidex	Conversion to regular approval for the adjuvant treatment of postmenopausal women with hormone receptor positive early breast cancer	Sep 16 2005
asparaginase	Elspar	Therapy of patients with acute lymphocytic leukemia	Jan 10 1978
Asparaginase	Elspar	ELSPAR is indicated in the therapy of patients with acute lymphocytic leukemia. This agent is useful primarily in combination with other chemotherapeutic agents in the induction of remissions of the disease in pediatric patients.	Aug 01 2002
azacitidine	Vidaza	Indicated for treatment of patients with the following myelodysplastic syndrome subtypes: refractory anemia or refractory anemia with ringed sideroblasts (if accompanied by neutropenia or thrombocytopenia or requiring transfusions), refractory anemia with excess blasts, refractory anemia with excess blasts in transformation, and chronic myelomonocytic leukemia.	Jan 26 2007
bevacizumab	Avastin	FDA approved changed in the Avastin package insert regarding warning and dose and administration for Reversible Posterior Leukoencephalopathy Syndrome. Nasal septum perforation was also added as a serious adverse event.	Sep 21 2006
bevacizumab	Avastin	A first-line treatment of patients with locally advanced, metastatic or recurrent non-small cell lung cancer in combination with platinum-based chemotherapy	Oct 11, 2006
bexarotene capsules	Targretin	For the treatment by oral capsule of cutaneous manifestations of cutaneous T-cell lymphoma in patients who are refractory to at least one prior systemic therapy.	Dec 29 1999
bexarotene gel	Targretin	For the topical treatment of cutaneous manifestations of cutaneous T-cell lymphoma in patients who are refractory to at least one prior systemic therapy.	Jun 28 2000
bleomycin	Blenoxane	Sclerosing agent for the treatment of malignant pleural effusion (MPE) and prevention of recurrent pleural effusions.	Feb 20 1996
bortezomib	Velcade	Conversion to regular approval for treatment of multiple myeloma patients who have received as least one prior therapy	Mar 25 2005
busulfan intravenous	Busulfex	Use in combination with cyclophoshamide as conditioning regimen prior to allogeneic hematopoietic progenitor cell transplantation for chronic myelogenous leukemia.	Feb 04 1999
capecitabine	Xeloda	Conversion to regular approval for treatment in combination with docetaxel of patients with metastatic breast cancer after failure of prior anthracycline containing chemotherapy	Sep 07 2001

TABLE 6-2: SELECTED FDA-APPROVED ONCOLOGY DRUGS WITH INDICATIONS, JULY 2007 (2 OF 7)

Drug Generic Name	Drug Trade Name	Additional Information About Approved Use	Approval Date
capecitabine	Xeloda	Adjuvant treatment in patients with Dukes' C colon cancer who have undergone complete resection of the primary tumor when treatment with fluoropyrimidine therapy alone is preferred	Jun 15 2005
carboplatin	Paraplatin	Palliative treatment of patients with ovarian carcinoma recurrent after prior chemotherapy, including patients who have been previously treated with cisplatin.	Mar 03 1989
carboplatin	Paraplatin	Initial chemotherapy of advanced ovarian carcinoma in combination with other approved chemotherapeutic agents.	Jul 05 1991
carmustine	BCNU, BiCNU		Mar 07 1977
carmustine	Gliadel	Treatment of patients with malignant glioma undergoing primary surgical resection	Feb 25 2003
cetuximab	Erbitux	Accel. Approv. (clinical benefit not established) for treatment of EGFR-expressing metastatic colorectal carcinoma in patients who are refractory to irinotecan-based chemotherapy (in combination with irinotecan); as a single agent, treatment of EGFR-expressing metastatic colorectal carcinoma in patients who are intolerant to irinotecan-based chemotherapy	Feb 12 2004
cetuximab	Erbitux	For use in combination with radiation therapy (RT) for the treatment of locally or regionally advanced squamous cell carcinoma of the head and neck (SCCHN) or as a single agent for the treatment of patients with recurrent or metastatic SCCHN for whom prior platinum-based therapy has failed.	Mar 01 2006
chlorambucil	Leukeran		Mar 18 1957
cisplatin	Platinol	Metastatic testicular-in established combination therapy with other approved chemotherapeutic agents in patients with metastatic testicular tumors who have already received appropriate surgical and/or radiotherapeutic procedures. An established combination therapy consists of Platinol, Blenoxane and Velbam.	Dec 19 1978
cisplatin	Platinol	Metastatic ovarian tumors - in established combination therapy with other approved chemotherapeutic agents: Ovarian-in established combination therapy with other approved chemotherapeutic agents in patients with metastatic ovarian tumors who have already received appropriate surgical and/or radiotherapeutic procedures. An established combination consists of Platinol and Adriamycin. Platinol, as a single agent, is indicated as secondary therapy in patients with metastatic ovarian tumors refractory to standard chemotherapy who have not previously received Platinol therapy.	Dec 19 1978
cisplatin	Platinol	As a single agent for patients with transitional cell bladder cancer which is no longer amenable to local treatments such as surgery and/or radiotherapy.	Apr 22 1993
cladribine	Leustatin, 2-CdA	Treatment of active hairy cell leukemia.	Feb 26 1993
cyclophosphamide	Cytoxan, Neosar		Nov 16 1959
cytarabine	Cytosar-U		Jun 17 1969
dacarbazine	DTIC-Dome		May 27 1975
dactinomycin, actinomycin D	Cosmegen		Feb 04 1964
dasatinib	Sprycel	Chronic myelogenous leukemia	Jun 28 2006
daunorubicin, daunomycin	Daunorubicin	Leukemia/myelogenous/monocytic/erythroid of adults/remission induction in acute lymphocytic leukemia of children and adults.	Jan 30 1998

TABLE 6-2: SELECTED FDA-APPROVED ONCOLOGY DRUGS WITH INDICATIONS, JULY 2007 (3 OF 7)

Drug Generic Name	Drug Trade Name	Additional Information About Approved Use	Approval Date
daunorubicin, daunomycin	Cerubidine	In combination with approved anticancer drugs for induction of remission in adult ALL.	Mar 11 1987
docetaxel	Taxotere	Conversion to regular approval – treatment of locally advanced or metastatic breast cancer which has progressed during anthracycline-based treatment or relapsed during anthracycline-based adjuvant therapy.	Jun 22 1998
docetaxel	Taxotere	For use in combination with cisplatin for the treatment of patients with unresectable, locally advanced or metastatic non-small cell lung cancer who have not previously received chemotherapy for this condition cisplatin for the treatment of patients with unresectable, locally advanced or metastatic non-small cell lung cancer who have not previously received chemotherapy for this condition.	Nov 27 2002
docetaxel	Taxotere	For use in combination with prednisone as a treatment for patients with androgen independent (hormone refractory) metastatic prostate cancer	May 19 2004
docetaxel	Taxotere	For use in combination with doxorubicin and cyclophosphamide for the adjuvant treatment of patients with operable nodepositive breast cancer	Aug 18 2004
docetaxel	Taxotere	For use in combination with cisplatin and fluorouracil for the induction treatment of patients with inoperable, locally advanced squamous cell carcinoma of the head and neck.	Oct 17 2006
doxorubicin	Adriamycin PFS	For use in combination with cyclophosphamide as a component of adjuvant therapy in patients with evidence of axillary node tumor involvement following resection of primary breast cancer	May 08 2003
doxorubicin liposomal	Doxil	Conversion to regular approval for treatment of patients with ovarian cancer whose disease has progressed or recurred after platinum-based chemotherapy	Jan 28 2005
epirubicin liposomal	Ellence	A component of adjuvant therapy in patients with evidence of axillary node tumor involvement following resection of primary breast cancer.	Sep 15 1999
erlotinib	Tarceva	For use in combination with gemcitabine for the first-line treatment of patients with locally advanced, unresectable or metastatic pancreatic cancer	Nov 02 2005
etoposide phosphate	Etopophos	Management of refractory testicular tumors and small cell lung cancer.	Feb 27 1998
exemestane	Aromasin	For adjuvant treatment of postmenopausal women with estrogen-receptor positive early breast cancer who have received two to three years of tamoxifen and are switched to AROMASIN® for completion of a total of five consecutive years of adjuvant hormonal therapy	Oct 05 2005
exemestane	Aromasin	Treatment of advance breast cancer in postmenopausal women whose disease has progressed following tamoxifen therapy.	Oct 21 1999
gemcitabine	Gemzar	Treatment of patients with locally advanced (nonresectable stage II or III) or metastatic (stage IV) adenocarcinoma of the pancreas. Indicated for first-line treatment and for patients previously treated with a 5-fluorouracil-containing regimen.	May 15 1996
gemcitabine	Gemzar	For use in combination with cisplatin for the first-line treatment of patients with inoperable, locally advanced (Stage IIIA or IIIB) or metastatic (Stage IV) non-small cell lung cancer.	Aug 25 1998
gemcitabine hcl	Gemzar	Ovarian cancer	Jul 14 2006
gemicitabine	Gemzar	For use in combination with paclitaxel for the first-line treatment of patients with metastatic breast cancer after failure of prior anthracycline-containing adjuvant chemotherapy, unless anthracyclines were clinically contraindicated	May 19 2004

TABLE 6-2: SELECTED FDA-APPROVED ONCOLOGY DRUGS WITH INDICATIONS, JULY 2007 (4 OF 7)

Drug Generic Name	Drug Trade Name	Additional Information About Approved Use	Approval Date
imatinib mesylate	Gleevec	Accel. Approv. (clinical benefit not established) Treatment of pediatric patients with Ph+ chronic phase CML whose disease has recurred after stem cell transplant or who are resistant to interferon alpha therapy.	May 20 2003
imatinib mesylate	Gleevec	Conversion to regular approval for treatment of patients with Philadelphia chromosome positive chronic myeloid leukemia (CML) in blast crisis, accelerated phase, or in chronic phase after failure of interferon-alpha therapy	Dec 08 2003
imatinib mesylate	Gleevec	For the treatment of pediatric patients with newly diagnosed Philadelphia chromosome positive chronic myelogenous leukemia (Ph+ CML).	Sep 27 2006
imatinib mesylate	Gleevec	Single agent for the treatment of multiple indications	Oct 19 2006
interferon alfa 2a	Roferon A	Treatment of patients with hairy cell leukemia	Jun 04 1986
interferon alfa 2a	Roferon A	Chronic phase, Philadelphia chromosome positive chronic myelogenous leukemia (CML) patients who are minimally pretreated (within 1 year of diagnosis)	Oct 19 1995
Interferon alfa-2b	Intron A	Interferon alfa-2b, recombinant for Injection is indicated for the treatment of patients 18 years of age or older with hairy cell leukemia.	Jun 04 1986
Interferon alfa-2b	Intron A	Interferon alfa-2b, recombinant for injection is indicated for the treatment of selected patients 18 years of age or older with AIDS-related Kaposi's Sarcoma. The likelihood of response to INTRON A therapy is greater in patients who are without systemic symptoms, who have limited lymphadenopathy and who have a relatively intact immune system as indicated by total CD4 count.	Nov 21 1988
Interferon alfa-2b	Intron A	Interferon alfa-2b, recombinant for injection is indicated as adjuvant to surgical treatment in patients 18 years of age or older with malignant melanoma who are free of disease but at high risk for systemic recurrence within 56 days of surgery.	Dec 05 1995
Interferon alfa-2b	Intron A	Interferon alfa-2b, recombinant for Injection is indicated for the initial treatment of clinically aggressive follicular non-Hodgkin's Lymphoma in conjunction with anthracycline-containing combination chemotherapy in patients 18 years of age or older.	Nov 06 1997
irinotecan	Camptosar	Accel. Approv. (clinical benefit subsequently established) Treatment of patients with metastatic carcinoma of the colon or rectum whose disease has recurred or progressed following 5-FU-based therapy.	Jun 14 1996
irinotecan	Camptosar	Conversion to regular approval - treatment of metastatic carcinoma of the colon or rectum whose disease has recurred or progressed following 5-FU-based therapy.	Oct 22 1998
irinotecan	Camptosar	For first line treatment n combination with 5-FU/leucovorin of metastatic carcinoma of the colon or rectum.	Apr 20 2000
lapatinib ditosylate	Tykerb	For use in combination with capecitabine for the treatment of patients with advanced or metastatic breast cancer whose tumors overexpress HER2 (ErbB2) and who have received prior therapy including an anthracycline, a taxane, and trastuzumab.	Mar 13 2007
lenalidomide	Revlimid	Multiple myeloma	Jun 29 2006
letrozole	Femara	Treatment of advanced breast cancer in postmenopausal women.	Jul 25 1997
letrozole	Femara	First-line treatment of postmenopausal women with hormone receptor positive or hormone receptor unknown locally advanced or metastatic breast cancer.	Jan 10 2001
letrozole	Femara	Accel. Approv. (clinical benefit not established) for the extended adjuvant treatment of early breast cancer in postmenopausal women who have received five years of adjuvant tamoxifen therapy.	Oct 29 2004

TABLE 6-2: SELECTED FDA-APPROVED ONCOLOGY DRUGS WITH INDICATIONS, JULY 2007 (5 OF 7)

Drug Generic Name	Drug Trade Name	Additional Information About Approved Use	Approval Date
leucovorin	Leucovorin	In combination with fluorouracil to prolong survival in the palliative treatment of patients with advanced colorectal cancer.	Dec 12 1991
Leuprolide Acetate	Eligard	Palliative treatment of advanced prostate cancer.	Jan 23 2002
levamisole	Ergamisol	Adjuvant treatment in combination with 5-fluorouracil after surgical resection in patients with Dukes' Stage C colon cancer.	Jun 18 1990
lomustine, CCNU	CeeBU		Aug 04 1976
meclorethamine, nitrogen mustard	Mustargen		Mar 15 1949
megestrol acetate	Megace		Aug 18 1971
melphalan, L-PAM	Alkeran	Systemic administration for palliative treatment of patients with multiple myeloma for whom oral therapy is not appropriate.	Nov 18 1992
mercaptopurine, 6-MP	Purinethol		Sep 11 1953
methotrexate	Methotrexate		Dec 07 1953
mitomycin C	Mutamycin		May 28 1974
mitomycin C	Mitozytrex	Therapy of disseminated adenocarcinoma of the stomach or pancreas in proven combinations with other approved chemotherapeutic agents and as palliative treatment when other modalities have failed.	Nov 14 2002
mitoxantrone	Novantrone	For use in combination with corticosteroids as initial chemotherapy for the treatment of patients with pain related to advanced hormone-refractory prostate cancer.	Nov 13 1996
mitoxantrone	Novantrone	For use with other approved drugs in the initial therapy for acute nonlymphocytic leukemia (ANLL) in adults.	Dec 23 1987
nelarabine	Arranon	Accel. Approv. (clinical benefit not established) for the treatment of patients with T-cell acute lymphoblastic leukemia and T-cell lymphoblastic lymphoma whose disease has not responded to or has relapsed following treatment with at least two chemotherapy regimens	Oct 28 2005
oxaliplatin	Eloxatin	Accel. Approv. (clinical benefit not established) in combination with infusional 5-FU/LV, is indicated for the treatment of patients with metastatic carcinoma of the colon or rectum whose disease has recurred or progressed during or within 6 months of completion of first line therapy with the combination of bolus 5-FU/LV and irinotecan.	Aug 09 2002
oxaliplatin	Eloxatin	For use in combination with infusional 5-FU/LV, for the adjuvant treatment of stage III colon cancer patients who have undergone complete resection of the primary tumor	Nov 04 2004
paclitaxel	Taxol	For first-line therapy for the treatment of advanced carcinoma of the ovary in combination with cisplatin.	Apr 09 1998
paclitaxel	Taxol	For use in combination with cisplatin, for the first-line treatment of non-small cell lung cancer in patients who are not candidates for potentially curative surgery and/or radiation therapy.	Jun 30 1998
paclitaxel	Taxol	For the adjuvant treatment of node-positive breast cancer administered sequentially to standard doxorubicin-containing combination therapy.	Oct 25 1999
paclitaxel protein-bound particles	Abraxane	For the treatment of breast cancer after failure of combination chemotherapy for metastatic disease or relapse within 6 months of adjuvant chemotherapy. Prior therapy should have included an anthracyline unless clinically contraindicated	Jan 07 2005
pegaspargase	Oncaspar	Acute lymphocytic leukemia in L-asparaginase hypersensitive patients	Feb 01 1994
pegaspargase	Oncaspar	Acute lymphoblastic leukemia	Jul 24 2006

TABLE 6-2: SELECTED FDA-APPROVED ONCOLOGY DRUGS WITH INDICATIONS, JULY 2007 (6 OF 7)

Drug Generic Name	Drug Trade Name	Additional Information About Approved Use	Approval Date
pemetrexed disodium	Alimta	For use in the treatment of patients with malignant pleural mesothelioma whose disease is either unresectable or who are otherwise not candidates for curative surgery	Feb 04 2004
pemetrexed disodium	Alimta	Accel. Approv. (clinical benefit not established) as a single agent for the treatment of patients with locally advanced or metastatic non-small lung cancer after prior chemotherapy	Aug 19 2004
pentostatin	Nipent	Single-agent treatment for untreated hairy cell leukemia patients with active disease as defined by clinically significant anemia, neutropenia, thrombocytopenia, or disease-related symptoms. (Supplement for front-line therapy.)	Sep 29 1993
plicamycin, mithramycin	Mithracin		May 05 1970
procarbazine	Matulane		Jul 22 1969
rituximab	Rituxan	For the first-line treatment of patients with low grade or follicular, CD20-positive B-cell non-Hodgkin's lymphoma.	Sep 29 2006
Rituximab	Rituxan	Treatment of patients with relapsed or refractory low-grade or follicular B-cell non-Hodgkin' lymphoma	Nov 26 1997
Rituximab	Rituxan	Non-Hodgkin's lymphoma	Feb 10 2006
sargramostim	Leukine	Acceleration of myeloid recovery following autologous bone marrow transplant in patients with non-Hodgkin's lymphoma, acute lymphocytic leukemia, or Hodgkin's disease	Mar 05 1991
Sargramostim	Prokine		Nov 07 1996
sorafenib	Nexavar	For the treatment of patients with advanced renal cell carcinoma	Dec 20 2005
streptozocin	Zanosar	Antineoplastic agent.	May 07 1982
tamoxifen	Nolvadex	To reduce the incidence of breast cancer in women at high risk for breast cancer	Oct 29 1998
tamoxifen	Nolvadex	In women with DCIS, following breast surgery and radiation, Nolvadex is indicated to reduce the risk of invasive breast cancer.	Jun 29 2000
temozolomide	Temodar	Conversion to regular approval for the treatment of patients with newly diagnosed high grade gliomas concomitantly with radiotherapy and then as adjuvant treatment	Mar 15 2005
teniposide, VM-26	Vumon	In combination with other approved anticancer agents for induction therapy in patients with refractory childhood acute lymphoblastic leukemia (all).	Jul 14 1992
thalidomide	Thalomid	Multiple myeloma	May 26 2006
thioguanine, 6-TG	Thioguanine		Jan 18 1966
thiotepa	Thioplex		Mar 09 1959
topotecan	Hycamtin	Treatment of patients with metastatic carcinoma of the ovary after failure of initial or subsequent chemotherapy.	May 28 1996
topotecan	Hycamtin	Treatment of small cell lung cancer sensitive disease after failure of first-line chemotherapy. In clinical studies submitted to support approval, sensitive disease was defined as disease responding to chemotherapy but subsequently progressing at least 60 days (in the phase 3 study) or at least 90 days (in the phase 2 studies) after chemotherapy	Nov 30 1998
topotecan hcl	Hycamtin	Cervical carcinoma	Jun 14 2006
toremifene	Fareston	Treatment of advanced breast cancer in postmenopausal women.	May 29 1997

TABLE 6-2: SELECTED FDA-APPROVED ONCOLOGY DRUGS WITH INDICATIONS, JULY 2007 (7 OF 7)

Drug Generic Name	Drug Trade Name	Additional Information About Approved Use	Approval Date
Tositumomab/ I-131 tositumomab	Bexxar	Expand the indication to include patients with relapsed or refractory low grade follicular transformed CD20-positive non-Hodgkin's lymphoma who have not received rituximab	Dec 22 2004
trastuzumab	Herceptin	Early Stage Breast Cancer After Primary Therapy	Nov 16 2006
Trastuzumab	Herceptin	HERCEPTIN as a single agent is indicated for the treatment of patients with metastatic breast cancer whose tumors overexpress the HER2 protein and who have received one or more chemotherapy regimens for their metastatic disease.	Sep 25 1998
Trastuzumab	Herceptin	Herceptin in combination with paclitaxel is indicated for treatment of patients with metastatic breast cancer whose tumors overexpress the HER-2 protein and had not received chemotherapy for their metastatic disease	Feb 09 2000
vincristine	Oncovin		Jul 10 1963
vinorelbine	Navelbine	Navelbine is indicated as a single agent or in combination with cisplatin for the first-line treatment of ambulatory patients with unreseactable, advanced non-small cell lung cancer (NSCLC). In patients with Stage IV NSCLC, Navelbine is indicated as a single agent or in combination with cisplatin. In Stage III NSCLC, Navelbine is indicated in combination with cisplatin.	Nov 05 2002
vorinostat	Zolinza	for the treatment of cutaneous manifestations of cutaneous T-cell lymphoma (CTCL) in patients with progressive, persistent, or recurrent disease on or following two systemic therapies.	Oct 06 2006

Note. From List of Approved Oncology Drugs with Approved Indications, by U.S. Food and Drug Administration (FDA), 2006. Retrieved October 31, 2006, from http://www.fda.gov/cder/cancer/druglistframe.htm

to nanomedicine, which focuses on the development of a wide spectrum of nanoscale technologies for disease diagnosis, treatment, and prevention (Moghimi, Hunter, & Murray, 2005). Drug delivery and targeting using nanotechnology methods include development of nanoparticles—dedrimers, polymeric micelles, liposomes, nanospheres, aquasomes, and polyplexes/lipopolyplexes.

A current application in clinical practice is the nanosphere, a spherical synthetic or natural substance that is 10 to 100 nanometers. Nanosphere technology allows an agent to dissolve, be entrapped, or be encapsulated within the nanosphere and then released when given to the patient.

Chemotherapy agent examples based on nanotechnology include the liposomal-encapsulated doxorubicin (Doxil) and the nanoparticle albumin-bound paclitaxel (Taxol). The application of this technology allows selective delivery of the agent in high concentrations to tumor tissues and reduced

delivery to normal tissues. Therefore, dose density is possible with limited toxicity (ONS, 2005). Nanotechnology will continue to be introduced as a means to deliver chemotherapy agents more effectively.

CHEMOTHERAPY ADMINISTRATION

Dose Calculation

The dose of drug to be administered is generally based on the individual's body surface area (BSA), usually expressed in milligrams per square meter or milligrams per kilogram. BSA is traditionally determined by a height and weight nomogram (see Figure 6-3). These calculations are completed by using special BSA calculators. Then the chemotherapy doses (especially IV doses) are

FIGURE 6-3: NOMOGRAPH FOR CALCULATING THE BODY SURFACE AREA OF ADULTS

Body Surface of Adults

Nomogram for determination of body surface from height and mass[1]

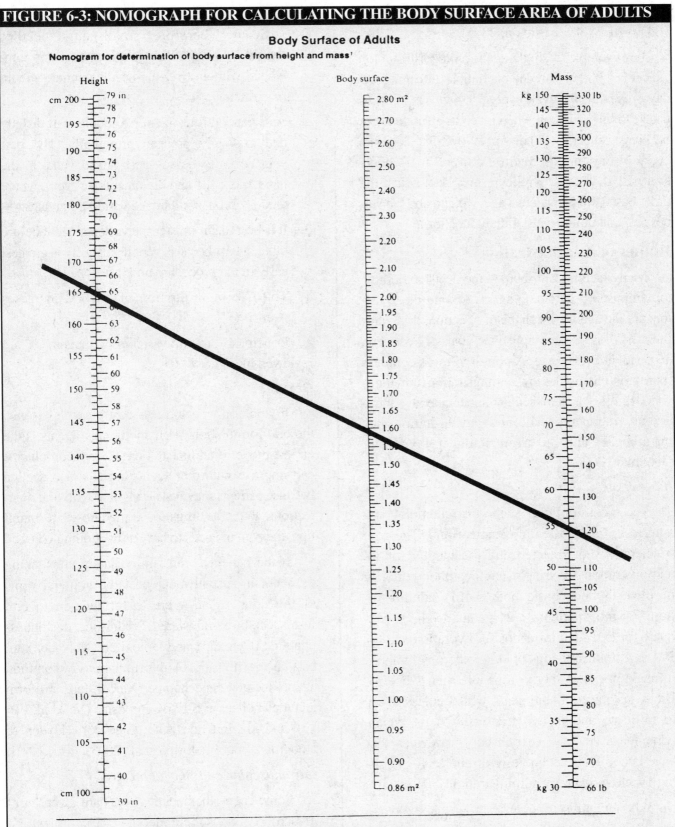

[1] From the formula of DU BOIS and DU BOIS, *Arch. intern. Med.*, 17, 863 (1916): $S = M^{0.425} \times H^{0.725} \times 71.84$, or $\log S = \log M \times 0.425 + \log H \times 0.725 + 1.8564$ (S: body surface in cm², M: mass in kg, H: height in cm).

Note. From "Nomographic charts for the calculation of the metabolic rate by the gasometer method," by W. Boothby & R. Sandiford, 1921. *Boston Med Surg Journal,* 185(12), 337. (Based on the formula of Duboise and Duboise: BSA in m² = [71.84] [kg$^{0.425}$] [cm$^{0.725}$] [10^{-4}].)

written as milligrams per square meter (mg/m²) (Ellsworth-Wolk & Maxon, 2005).

For example, a single agent protocol for colon cancer is 1,000 mg/m²/day continuous infusion for 5 days, repeating the cycle every 3 to 4 weeks. A paclitaxel (Taxol) protocol, when given as a single agent for breast cancer, is 250 mg/m² IV over 3 to 24 hours every 21 days or 175 mg/m² IV over 3 to 24 hours every 21 days. The physician may also adjust the order based on the patient's age, weight, and lab values (e.g., albumin levels, kidney function).

Routes of Administration

Many factors contribute to the decision on how to administer a cytotoxic agent. Among those factors are the agent's mechanism of action, drug half-life, best route to accomplish the goals of treatment, and patient preference. Among the most common routes of chemotherapy administration are intravenous, oral, intramuscular, subcutaneous, intra-arterial, intraperitoneal, intrapleural, intravesical, intrathecal, and intraventricular (Hayden & Goodman, 2006).

Intravenous

The most common method of chemotherapy administration is the intravenous route. The type of therapy should determine the method of IV administration. A simple angiocath or butterfly needle is the most basic method of IV administration. For most patients, a 21-gauge needle is adequate for extended infusions for hydration and for 3- and 4-hour infusions of chemotherapy. If an IV infusion needs to stay in for more than 1 hour, it is best to place an angiocath, which is less likely to infiltrate and is less traumatic to the veins. (Chapter 8 reviews venous access devices that have become the technology of choice for ongoing IV chemotherapy administration.)

When administering vesicant agents, the nurse should keep these points in mind (Ellsworth-Wolk & Maxon, 2005; Hayden & Goodman, 2006; Polovich et al., 2005):

1. A good blood return is crucial when giving a vesicant. Therefore, small-gauge needles should be avoided. An angiocath that is thin-walled with an over-the-needle cannula should be chosen.

2. As a general rule, the nurse should start distally and gradually proceed proximally. The best vein needs to be selected. Avoid veins in the hand and wrist and the antecubital vein, where tendon and nerve damage would be greatest.

3. It is best to administer the vesicant agent before other agents because venous integrity is greatest early in the procedure and infusion.

4. The risk of infiltration of any IV increases over time.

Principles of extravasation management are reviewed in Figure 8-2.

Oral

In addition to being less costly and less toxic, the oral formulation of chemotherapy agents is the easiest mode of administration. Patient compliance can improve with oral agents but can also decline because patients may be less vigilant with oral medications. For oral drugs to be the chosen formulation, the patient needs to have a functioning GI tract.

If the patient vomits immediately after taking the agent, it is usually not repeated. Parenteral forms of the drug, as an alternate formulation to oral forms, can be administered. Prednisone, cyclophosphamide (Cytoxan), and tamoxifen (Nolvadex) are best taken with food. Oral formulations of common agents include capecitabine (Xeloda [an oral form that metabolizes as 5-FU]), etoposide (VePesid, VP-16), and imatinib mesylate (Gleevec) (Hayden & Goodman, 2006; Polovich et al., 2005).

Intramuscular and Subcutaneous

Some chemotherapeutic agents are given intramuscularly or subcutaneously. Examples are methotrexate (Mexate), cytarabine (Cytosar-U), and L-asparaginase (Elspar). Biological agents, such as interferon, the interleukins, and colony-stimulating factors, have increased the number of agents given via these routes.

Intra-arterial

In intra-arterial drug administration, drugs are delivered directly through an arterial catheter to the tumor. This practice increases the drug concentration and decreases systemic drug spread, thus limiting side effects. A treatment for metastasis of colon cancer to the liver or hepatocellular carcinoma can be administered through the hepatic artery. Among the antineoplastic drugs used in these protocols are 5-FU, floxuridine, doxorubicin (Adriamycin), and mitomycin (Mutamycin).

Intra-arterial administration can include the use of an implanted pump. This can be a costly method of therapy and increases the risk of infection. More often, an ambulatory or a stationary infusion pump is used (Hayden & Goodman, 2006).

Intraperitoneal

For recurrent ovarian cancer, chemotherapy may be administered into the peritoneal space. This technique allows a high concentration of drug to be administered near the tumor but with lower drug concentrations in the bloodstream. Agents used include cisplatin (Platinol), paclitaxel (Taxel), carboplatin (Paraplatin), etoposide (VePesid), doxorubicin (Adriamycin), and cytarabine (Cytosar-U). Depending on the goals of therapy and its duration, intraperitoneal administration can involve a temporary indwelling catheter, an external catheter, or an implanted port (Hayden & Goodman, 2006).

Intrapleural

Care of the patient with a malignant pleural effusion involves insertion of chest tubes, drainage of the fluid, and sclerosis of the pleural space to prevent recurrence of the effusion. Among sclerosing agents are talc, minocycline (Minocin), doxycycline (Vibramycin), tetracycline (Achromycin), 5-FU, and bleomycin (Blenoxane).

Intravesical

An example of chemotherapy administered directly into a vessel is the treatment for bladder cancer. Intravesical agents include thiotepa (Thioplex), doxorubicin (Adriamycin), mitomycin (Mutamycin), and bacillus Calmette-Guerin.

Intrathecal or Intraventricular

Cancer cells can cross the blood-brain barrier and appear in the cerebrospinal fluid (CSF). Among malignant cells that cross the blood-brain barrier are leukemia (meningeal leukemia), breast cancer, lymphoma, and rhabdomyosarcoma (meningeal carcinomatosis).

To get around the barrier, chemotherapy is injected directly into the CSF via intrathecal or intraventricular administration. The antineoplastic agents used include methotrexate (Mexate), cytarabine (Cytosar-U), thiotepa (Thioplex), and interferon (Intron A). The device used for repeated intraventricular administration is called an *Ommaya reservoir* (Hayden & Goodman, 2006).

Safe Handling of Agents

Depending on the work setting, nurses may be responsible for both preparing and administering chemotherapeutic drugs. Procedures that ensure safe handling and disposal of antineoplastic drugs are based on professional guidelines (Polovich et al., 2005).

Areas of practice covered by these guidelines include preparation, handling, administration, storage, transport, disposal, and procedures for accidental spills or exposure (Polovich et al., 2005). Table 6-3 highlights some basic safe-handling principles that are included in most guidelines.

Despite well-established recommendations, many clinicians do not follow guidelines. Over the past two decades, studies have contributed to policies that underscore safety and personal protection of the clinician from the short- and long-term effects of antineoplastic exposure.

TABLE 6-3: SELECTED SAFE-HANDLING GUIDELINES FOR CHEMOTHERAPY DRUGS

Note: Follow the institution's policies, based on latest recommendations from OSHA, the Infusion Nurses Society (INS), and the Centers for Disease Control and Prevention.

Barriers
- Clothing: Chemotherapy administration–approved gown (covers body and arms)
- Gloves (without powder; sometimes double-gloving is recommended)
- Mask (in certain situations if risk of spray is high)

Technique
- Select site so that there is:
  – adequate vein size
  – stable site (avoid wrist and other areas of the body with risk of infiltration)
  – good venous blood return.
- Use extra vigilance when administering vesicant chemotherapies.
- Prime IV solutions with a compatible solution (not chemotherapy).
- Flush the line well between chemotherapy administrations.
- Do not clip or recap needles.

Disposal
- Dispose of all supplies—gowns, gloves, masks, IV tubing, syringes, needles, tubing attachments— in designated (and labeled) chemotherapy waste containers.
- Clean spills per protocol. (Spill kit contents listed in Table 6-4.)

(INS, 2006; OSHA, 1995; Polovich et al., 2005)

Studies support safe-handling guidelines for all clinicians. However, for pregnant employees, the hazards of exposure to antineoplastic agents (which have mutagenic, teratogenic, and carcinogenic properties) are not known. Therefore, the Occupational Safety and Health Administration (OSHA) recommends that pregnant employees be informed of potential risks and, if necessary, reassigned to other duties (Polovich et al., 2005). OSHA also recommends establishing minimum standards based on updated scientific information and policies and procedures. It also recommends ongoing monitoring to ensure compliance and continuous quality improvement.

Medication Errors

Despite extensive preventive measures, medication errors can occur. With chemotherapy administration, drug errors can be fatal. Therefore, a clear, steadfast adherence to safe drug dosing and administration policies is the best foundation for safe practice.

Most chemotherapy agents are strong medications with toxic effects on tumor cells and normal cells. Moreover, most protocols include multiple agents, each with their own toxicity profiles and complexities. Nurses in any clinical practice are challenged by the care of more patients, multiple tasks, and ongoing stress and pressure to complete their work efficiently. Still, attention to the principles of safe practice cannot be compromised. To maintain safe practices, the nurse can follow these safeguards:

- Provide ongoing education about chemotherapy agents, their side effects, and procedures that ensure their safe delivery. Special attention is given to vesicant agents, which can cause extravasation.

- Only experienced clinicians should write chemotherapy orders. They are familiar with the drug regimens and the patient.

- Drug name and doses should be clear and written in full (include dose in milligrams per square meter, dose to be given, the total daily dose, and number of days that dose is given). Abbreviations should be avoided when ordering and in documentation. The use of extraneous "0" decimals at the end of dosing should be avoided. For example, vincristine 1.0 mg should not be written since it could be misread as vincristine 10 mg.

- Special attention should be given to sound-alike, look-alike agents, such as cisplatin (Platinol) and carboplatin (Paraplatin), paclitaxel (Taxol) and docetaxel (Taxotere), mitomycin (Mutamycin) and mitoxantrone (Novantrone), vinblastine (Velban) and vinorelbine (Navelbine), and floxuridine (FUDR) and fluorouracil (5-FU).

- Whenever possible, typed or prewritten orders should be used.

- When transcribing physician's original drug order, the original form of the order should remain throughout the process of drug administration. Extra care is taken with investigational protocols.

- Systems should be in place to verify the order through pharmacy and nursing policies. Before administration, the nurse should double-check the order against the physician's order and with a nurse colleague. Specific guidelines for the verification of chemotherapeutics and the right patient should be in place. (Certification of nurses as chemotherapy-certified is highly recommended.)

- Drug-checking databases and technology need to be incorporated to avoid medication errors.

- Institutional policies and procedures should be in place to prevent errors and to report drug errors that allow systemic solutions and not individual blame. Those policies should be regularly reviewed.

- A chemotherapy spill kit should be created (see Table 6-4).

- Everyone responsible for chemotherapy drug preparation and administration is empowered to question the order (drug, dose, route, or schedule).

(Ellsworth-Wolk & Maxon, 2005; Fortenbaugh & Rummel, 2004; Polovich et al., 2005; Schulmeister, 2005, 2006).

SUMMARY

Considerations for choosing chemotherapy as a treatment involve the mechanism of the agent during the cell cycle, its pharmacokinetics and resistance profile related to the tumor cells, and its interaction with other chemotherapies in a chemotherapy regimen. By understanding how specific chemotherapies work, nurses can better care for patients and anticipate problems or side effects. Safe administration and handling of chemotherapy agents are crucial.

TABLE 6-4: CONTENTS OF A CHEMOTHERAPY SPILL KIT

Number	Item
1	Gown with cuffs and back closure (made of water nonpermeable fabric)
1 pair	Shoe covers
2 pair	Gloves
1 pair	Utility gloves
1 pair	Chemical splash goggles
1	Rebreather mask (National Institutes of Occupational Safety and Health approved)
1	Disposable dust pan (to collect any broken glass)
1	Plastic scraper (to scoop materials into dust pan)
2	Plastic-backed or absorbable towels
1 each	250 ml and 1 L spill-control pillows
2	Disposable sponges (one to clean up spill, one to clean up floor after removal of spill)
1	"Sharps" container
2	Large, heavy-duty waste disposal bags
1	Container of 70% alcohol for cleaning soiled area

Note. From "Controlling occupational exposure to hazardous drugs," by Occupational Safety and Health Administration (OSHA), 1995. (*OSHA Instruction CPL2-2.20B* [pp. 21-1 to 21-34]). Washington, DC: Author.

EXAM QUESTIONS

CHAPTER 6
Questions 21-25

Note: Choose the option that BEST answers each question.

21. The phase of the cell cycle when DNA replication occurs is

    a. S phase.

    b. G_1.

    c. G_2.

    d. M phase.

22. The action of an alkylating agent is

    a. specific during the cell cycle to G_1 phase.

    b. nonspecific or active during the entire cell cycle.

    c. specific during the cell cycle in M phase.

    d. specific during the cell cycle in S phase.

23. A hormone used to treat breast cancer is

    a. levothyroxine (Synthroid).

    b. anastrozole (Arimidex).

    c. cytarabine (Cytosar-U).

    d. vincristine (Oncovin).

24. A bisphosphonate used to treat bone metastasis is

    a. tamoxifen (Nolvadex).

    b. zolendronic acid (Zometa).

    c. allopurinol (Zyloprim).

    d. streptozocin (Zanosar).

25. One method that can be used to prevent extravasation of a vesicant chemotherapy is to

    a. maintain good blood return.

    b. hang an extra bag of blood.

    c. stop the infusion 2 minutes after it begins.

    d. administer the vesicant after all other chemotherapies.

REFERENCES

Adams, V., DeRemer, D., & Holdsworth, M. (2005). *Cancer chemotherapeutic regimens: 2005.* Available from http://www.oncologyse.com

Alley, E., & Haller, D. (2001). *Advances in chemotherapy for colo-rectal cancer.* Oncology special edition (4), 17-20. New York: McMahon.

Boothby W., & Sandiford, R (1921). Nomographic charts for the calculation of metabolic rate by the gasometer method. *Boston Med Surg Journal, 184*(12), 337.

Ellsworth-Wolk, J., & Maxon J. (2005). Principles of preparation, administration, and disposal of hazardous drugs. In J. K. Itano & K. N. Taoka (Eds.), *Core curriculum for oncology nursing* (4th ed., pp. 802–808). St. Louis: Elsevier.

Fortenbaugh, C., & Rummel, M. (2004). Chemotherapy safety. *Clinical Journal of Oncology Nursing, 8*(4), 424–425.

Gerken, P. (2004a). Cancer treatments: Letrozole (Femara). *Clinical Journal of Oncology Nursing, 8*(3), 314–315.

Gerken, P. (2004b). Cancer treatments: Toremifene citrate (Fareston). *Clinical Journal of Oncology Nursing, 8*(5), 529–530.

Hayden, B., & Goodman, M. (2006). Chemotherapy: Principles of administration. In C. Yarbro, M. Frogge, & M. Goodman (Eds.), *Cancer nursing: Principles and practice* (6th ed., pp. 351–382). Sudbury, MA: Jones & Bartlett.

Infusion Nurses Society. (2006). *Infusion Nursing Standards of Practice.* New York: Lippincott Williams & Wilkins.

Maltzman, J. (2004). Bone metastasis and the bisphosphonates. Available from http://www.oncolink.upenn.edu

Maxwell, C., & Viale, P. (2005). Cancer treatment-induced bone loss in patients with breast or prostate cancer. *Oncology Nursing Forum, 32*(3), 589–603.

Moghimi, S., Hunter, A., & Murray, J. (2005) Nanomedicine: Current status and future prospects. *Federation of American Societies for Experimental Biology Journal, 19*(3), 311–330.

National Cancer Institute. (2006). Newly approved cancer treatments. Available from http://www.cancer.gov/clinicaltrials/developments/newly-approved-treatments

Occupational Safety and Health Administration. (1995). *Controlling occupational exposure to hazardous drugs.* OSHA Instruction CPL2-2.20B (pp. 21-1 to 21-34). Washington, DC: Author.

Oncology Nursing Society. (2005, April). *Nanotechnology: New developments for breast cancer treatment.* Symposium: 4/30/05, ONS Congress, 2005.

Polovich, M., White, J.M., & Kelleher, L.O. (Eds.). (2005). *Chemotherapy and biotherapy guidelines and recommendations for practice* (2nd ed.). Pittsburgh, PA: Oncology Nursing Society.

Schulmeister, L. (2005). Ten simple strategies to prevent chemotherapy errors. *Clinical Journal of Oncology Nursing, 9*(2), 201–205.

Schulmeister, L. (2006). Look-alike, sound-alike oncology medications. *Clinical Journal of Oncology Nursing, 10*(1), 35–41.

Temple, S., & Poniatowski, B. (2005). Nursing implications of antineoplastic therapy. In J. K. Itano & K. N. Taoka (Eds.), *Core curriculum for oncology nursing* (4th ed., pp. 785–801). St. Louis: Elsevier.

U.S. Food and Drug Administration. (2006). *List of approved oncology drugs with approved indications.* Retrieved October 31, 2006, from http://www.fda.gov/cder/cancer/druglistframe.htm

Vachani, C. (2005). *Hormonal therapies in breast cancer.* Available from http://www.oncolink.upenn.edu

Viale, P. (2005). Aromatase inhibitor agents in breast cancer: Evolving practices in hormonal therapy treatment. *Oncology Nursing Forum, 32*(2), 343–353.

CHAPTER 7

TARGETED THERAPIES

CHAPTER OBJECTIVE

After completing this chapter, the reader will be able to recognize selected targeted therapies for selected malignancies and identify their mechanisms of action.

LEARNING OBJECTIVES

After studying this chapter, the reader will be able to

1. describe one clinical advantage of targeted therapies.

2. identify the mechanism of action of monoclonal antibodies.

3. identify one example of U.S. Food and Drug Administration approved monoclonal antibodies.

4. cite an approved indication for a tyrosine kinase inhibitor.

INTRODUCTION

An emerging treatment category for cancer is the so-called *targeted therapies*. These agents have been developed based on understanding the narrow and precise changes that occur on a cellular level and lead to tumor growth. Targeted therapies focus on signals, processes, and interactions on the surface of or within the internal mechanisms of a cell. By adjusting these communication pathways to halt tumor growth, targeted therapies can spare more serious adverse effects on surrounding healthy tissues. By sparing this damage to healthy cells and tissues, side effects from the therapies are less than those expected with conventional chemotherapy protocols.

In many cases, these agents are given in combination with chemotherapy to create a synergy of effect toward tumor cells.

PATHWAYS

An analogy for the cellular communication of targeted therapies is when a person receives commands from others (or stimuli) to perform such activities as eat, run, and answer the phone. The brain processes the information and then sends signals to the part of the body performing the action—mouth, legs, speech center, respectively.

Scientists believe that cellular communication behaves with a similar process of messages, creating a matrix or web of signals that stop and start—and ultimately affect tumor growth (CancerSource, 2005a, 2005b; Maltzman, 2004).

The language of this cellular communication includes terms such as *potentiate, stimulate, activate, transmission, translation,* and *defective genes* (CancerSource, 2005b; Viele, 2005). Figure 7-1 provides a schematic of the action of targeted therapies within the cell.

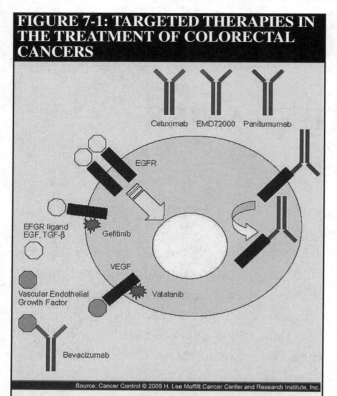

FIGURE 7-1: TARGETED THERAPIES IN THE TREATMENT OF COLORECTAL CANCERS

Source: Cancer Control © 2005 H. Lee Moffitt Cancer Center and Research Institute, Inc.

FIGURE 1. Monoclonal antibodies cetuximab (chimeric), EMD72000 (humanized), and panitumumab (fully human) bind cell surface epidermal growth factor receptor (EGFR) and inhibit binding of natural ligands epidermal growth factor (EGF) and transforming growth factor beta (TGF-ß), in addition to causing receptor internalization and proteosomal degradation. The humanized antibody bevacizumab binds circulating vascular endothelial growth factor (VEGF), preventing binding to receptor. Receptor tyrosine kinase inhibitors gefitinib and vatalanib work intracellularly to inhibit the EGFR and VEGF receptor (VEGFR), respectively.

Note. Reprinted by permission from Cancer Control: Journal of the Moffitt Cancer Center. *Targeted Therapies in the Treatment of Colorectal Cancers* by T. Alekshun & C. Garrett, 2005. Vol. 12 No 2.

MONOCLONAL ANTIBODIES

Antibodies are normal components of the immune system that help rid the body of foreign invaders or infectious agents such as bacteria. Antibodies are a type of protein that responds to an antigen (foreign substance). Each antibody can bind to only one specific antigen. The purpose of this binding is to help destroy the antigen.

Antibodies can work in several ways, depending on the nature of the antigen. Some antibodies destroy antigens directly. Antibodies can also trigger the body's immune response to an invader. Then they are programmed to remember the invaders so that they can effectively and quickly destroy the invaders if they return to attack the body again.

Monoclonal antibodies are produced in a laboratory. They work in a similar way to the body's natural antibodies. They locate and bind to antigens found on cancer cells and eliminate them from the body. Monoclonal antibodies can be used alone to stimulate an immune response, or they can be used to deliver drugs, toxins, or radioactive materials directly to a tumor. (See Table 7-1.)

One of the first targeted therapeutics developed to fight cancer is the monoclonal antibody rituximab (Rituxan). Rituximab is an antibody that targets a protein found on lymphocytes that are activated in lymphoma. Rituximab is used to treat B-cell non-Hodgkin's lymphomas that carry a protein called CD20. The CD20 protein is found in more than 90% of B-cell lymphomas (Maltzman, 2004; Marrs, 2004).

Another monoclonal antibody, trastuzumab (Herceptin), targets the gene that seems to be over-expressed in aggressive forms of breast cancer. This monoclonal antibody targets a protein on breast cancer cells called *human epidermal growth factor receptor-2* (HER-2). HER-2 is overproduced in about 25% to 30% of breast cancers. Trastuzumab is only effective against breast tumors that overproduce the HER-2 protein.

The monoclonal antibody gemtuzumab ozogamicin (Mylotarg) targets a protein only seen in leukemia cells. This antibody is linked to a powerful antibiotic. As the antibody finds and binds to its target, the antibiotic is released and helps to kill the target cell. This monoclonal antibody is a treatment for acute myelogenous leukemia (AML).

The monoclonal antibody alemtuzumab (Campath) works similarly to rituximab in certain lymphomas but targets a different cell surface protein.

Two more monoclonal antibodies are bevacizumab (Avastin) and cetuximab (Erbitux).

TABLE 7-1: MONOCLONAL ANTIBODIES, IMMUNOTHERAPY

- Monoclonal antibodies and immunotherapies bind to their targets (antigens on cell surfaces), not to interfere with growth signals but rather to *trigger* immune signals.

- This signalling leads to a series of antitumor immune reactions in the body, ultimately causing the tumor cells to die.

- When immunotherapy drugs are chemically attached to radioactive substances, tumor cells are attacked in two ways, taking advantage of both the antitumor immune response and the antitumor radiation reaction.

- Targeted immunotherapy drugs are essentially a collection of monoclonal antibodies with different targets.

- Antibodies are proteins that seek out and bind to specific antigens; every antibody has a particular antigen with which it "fits." Antibodies are named for the antigen to which they bind (e.g., the anti-CD20 antibody binds to the antigen CD20).

Brand Name	Generic Name	Lab Development Name
Rituxan	Rituximab	anti-CD20
Bexxar	Tositumomab	I-131-radiolabelled anti-CD20
Zevalin	Ibritumomab	Y-90-radiolabelled anti-CD20

(Vapiwala, 2005)

Bevacizumab has been approved by the U.S. Food and Drug Administration (FDA) as first-line treatment for metastatic colorectal cancer. Its mechanism targets angiogenesis, which is the formation of new blood vessels to the tumor (see Table 7-2). Bevacizumab selectively inhibits VEGF, thereby preventing VEGF activation of VEGFR-1 and VEGFR-2. Promising study results are being reported on the use of this agent for lung cancer.

Cetuximab has been approved for advanced colorectal cancer that has metastasized. It is thought to work by targeting the EGFR on the surface of cancer cells (see Figure 7-1). Studies are evaluating the use of this targeted therapy for lung cancer and head and neck cancers.

Adding to Monoclonal Antibodies

When tumor cells grow, they can form into a dense "ball" of cancer cells. When a radioactive isotope is added to an antibody like rituximab, the antibody binds to and kills the tumor cells and also releases radioactivity that kills the surrounding mass of dense cancerous cells. Using such a radioisotope actually makes sense when one considers how a mass of malignant cells grows.

The antibodies ibritumomab tiuxetan (Zevalin) and tositumomab (Bexxar) work in this way. Ibritumomab tiuxetan binds to the same CD20 target that rituximab does, so it is used to treat the same types of cancer as rituximab. However, ibritumomab tiuxetan carries an additional punch

TABLE 7-2: ANGIOGENESIS INHIBITORS

- Angiogenesis inhibitors thwart adequate blood supply so that tumor cells cannot perform vital cellular functions.

- Angiogenesis inhibitors interrupt blood supply for dividing tumors, which secrete special proteins (proangiogenic factors) that signal the surrounding area to sprout new blood vessels.

- The main proangiogenic factor is VEGF.

- Anti-VEGF leads to angiogenesis inhibition.

Brand Name	Generic Name	Lab Development Name
Avastin	Bevacizumab	anti-VEGF

(Ellis, 2005; Vapiwala, 2005)

because its monoclonal antibody is bound to a radioactive compound called yttrium-90 (y-90), which can kill cancer cells. By delivering this damaging compound directly to the tumor, ibritumomab tiuxetan allows larger and more-deadly doses of the radioactive agent to reach the tumor while minimizing its damage to healthy cells.

SMALL-MOLECULE COMPOUNDS

Small-molecule compounds are agents that either destroy cancer cells or stop their growth. Many of these agents can be taken by mouth.

Tyrosine Kinase Inhibitors (Table 7-3)

Imatinib (Gleevec) is a small molecule that can inhibit proteins called *tyrosine kinases,* the molecules involved in the cell signaling of the largest family of dominant oncogenes. It is used as a treatment against chronic myelogenous leukemia (CML) and some gastrointestinal stromal tumors. Imatinib targets and then inhibits an abnormal protein, programming the cell to die. This unique mechanism of action results in the death of all cancerous cells harboring the protein, without affecting normal or healthy cells.

CML is an unusual type of cancer in that only one molecular defect is needed to turn a normal cell into a cancerous one. The abnormality arises when two genes fuse together and, as a result, produce an abnormal protein. This protein sends a signal to the cell that tells it to grow in an uncontrolled manner. Imatinib controls the growth of CML tumors by preventing the abnormal protein from signaling the cancer cells to grow.

Gefitinib (Iressa), another tyrosine kinase inhibitor, targets malignant non-small-cell lung cancer (NSCLC). Preclinical studies suggested that gefitinib—a tyrosine kinase inhibitor of the EGFR—may have significant single-agent activity in colorectal cancer.

Erlotinib (Tarceva) is an EGFR inhibitor. It treats locally advanced NSCLC when other therapies have failed. Tarceva works by inhibiting EGFR. EGFR is present in excessive amounts in many tumors, such as those found in the lung, breast, and colon. Because additional molecular defects give rise to these cancers, more than just one drug is likely be needed to effectively control or destroy these tumors (CancerSource, 2005a, 2005b; Krozley, 2004).

OTHER TARGETED THERAPIES

In 2006, thalidomide (Thalomid), an immunomodulatory agent, was approved as a treatment for newly diagnosed multiple myeloma (in combination with dexamethasone). The precise mechanism of action of thalidomide is unknown. Thalidomide's mechanism of action against myeloma cells is based on several theories, theories of antiangiogenesis, stromal cell inhibition, and alteration of the activity of cytokines or stimulation of T cells (Multiple Myeloma Research Foundation, 2006).

VACCINES

Cancer vaccines attempt to treat cancer by stimulating the immune system to attack cancer cells. Genetically modified vaccines alter and reintroduce the patient's own cancer cells to stimulate an immune response.

As of 2006, most cancer vaccines as treatments were still in the experimental phase. Clinical trials have yet to show prolonged survival in patients receiving vaccines as treatment. The focus of cancer researchers is to use tumor-associated antigens in vaccines in ways that will activate the immune system to attack and stop tumor growth (Viele, 2005).

Vaccine approaches in trials include cell-based vaccines. In this approach, the patient's own (or

TABLE 7-3: SELECTED TYROSINE KINASE INHIBITORS

- A tyrosine kinase receptor is a molecular structure or site on the surface of a cell that binds with substances such as hormones, antigens, drugs, and neurotransmitters.

- When it binds with one of these triggering substances, the receptor performs a chemical reaction, which in turn triggers a series of reactions inside the cell.

- These reactions include cell multiplication, death, maturation, and migration. In tumor cells, all of these reactions are critical for the tumor to survive, thrive, and spread throughout the body.

- By blocking the receptor, the tyrosine kinase inhibitor prevents the cascade of reactions that enable tumor survival.

- One family of tyrosine kinase receptors is called the *human epidermal receptor* family, or the HER family:
  - HER-1 (also called EGFR)*
  - HER-2 (also called ErbB2 or HER2/*neu*)*
  - HER-3 (also called ErbB3)
  - HER-4 (also called ErbB4)

  *EGFR and HER2/*neu* are the two most extensively studied targets in oncology.

EGFR INHIBITORS

SMALL-MOLECULE INHIBITORS

Brand Name	Generic Name	Lab Development Name
Iressa	Gefitinib	ZD1839
Tarceva	Erlotinib	OSI 771
Gleevec	Imatinib	ST1571
Nexavar	Sorafenib	BAY 43-9006
Sprycel	Dasatinib	BMS-354825
Tykerb	Lapatinib	GW572016

SMALL-ANTIBODY INHIBITORS

Brand Name	Generic Name	Lab Development Name
Erbitux	Cetuximab	C225

HER2/*neu* INHIBITORS

Brand Name	Generic Name	Lab Development Name
Herceptin	Trastuzumab	NO 34

(FDA, 2007; Genentech BioOncology, 2005, n.d.; Vapiwala, 2005)

another patient's) tumor cells are inactivated in the laboratory and then injected back into the patient as vaccines. This approach is impractical because each patient requires a costly, unique vaccine. Also, these vaccines do not mobilize a strong immune response. To boost their effectiveness, adjuvants such as detoxified bacterial toxins or cytokines (interleukin-2 and granulocyte-macrophage colony-stimulating factor [Leukine]) are added.

Another approach in vaccine research is developing antigen-specific vaccines. Targeted antigens are administered, mobilizing an antitumor response.

In the next few years, more will be known about the effectiveness of vaccines. Initial clinical trials are focused on end-stage colorectal and metastatic lung cancer (CancerSource, 2005b; Maltzman 2004; Viele, 2005).

SUMMARY

Targeted therapies—including monoclonal antibodies, tyrosine kinase inhibitors, and angiogenesis inhibitors—show great promise in the treatment of selected malignancies. Among their advantages is their ability to target and destroy tumor cells with limited side effects on healthy adjacent tissue.

EXAM QUESTIONS

CHAPTER 7
Questions 26-29

Note: Choose the option that BEST answers each question.

26. An advantage of targeted therapies is that they

    a. can be used in any hematologic malignancy.
    b. spare normal tissue around the tumor site.
    c. are not used in combination with other treatment modalities.
    d. destroy the body's immune system.

27. Monoclonal antibodies work by

    a. providing one clone of a cell to replace the tumor cell.
    b. substituting for a cell antigen.
    c. locating and binding to antigens found on cancer cells and eliminating them from the body.
    d. eliminating the cell's blood supply.

28. An FDA-approved monoclonal antibody for cancer treatment is

    a. rituximab (Rituxan).
    b. tamoxifen (Nolvadex).
    c. mercaptopurine (Purinethol).
    d. prednisone (Deltasone).

29. Imatinib (Gleevec), a tyrosine kinase inhibitor, is an approved treatment for

    a. acute myelogenous leukemia.
    b. chronic myelogenous leukemia.
    c. human immunodeficiency virus.
    d. chronic lymphocytic leukemia.

REFERENCES

CancerSource. (2005a). *Biological therapy.* Retrieved April 17, 2007, from http://www.cancersource.com/CancerBasics/Cancer Treatment/BiologicalTherapy/45,NCIGenT2

CancerSource. (2005b). *Targeted therapies take aim at cancer.* Retrieved April 17, 2007, from http://www.cancersource.com/CancerBasics/CancerTreatment/TargetedTherapy/34,27737

Ellis, L. (2005). *How angiogenesis inhibition improves chemotherapy outcomes: An expert interview with Dr. Lee Ellis.* Retrieved April 17, 2007, from http://www.medscape.com/viewarticle/506591

Genentech BioOncology. (2005). *Innovative research: Attacking cancer from multiple angles.* Retrieved April 17, 2007, from http://www.biooncology.com/bioonc/pdf/BIO NP-25438_P01_Pathways.pdf

Genentech BioOncology. (n.d.). *Fundamentally transforming the way cancer is treated.* Retrieved April 17, 2007, from http://www.biooncology.com/bioonc/approach/index.m

H. Lee Moffitt Cancer Center and Research Institute, Inc. (2005). Targeted therapies in the treatment of colorectal cancer. *Cancer Control, 12*(2), 105–110.

Krozely, P. (2004). Epidermal growth factor receptor tyrosine kinase inhibitors: Evolving role in the treatment of solid tumors. *Clinical Journal of Oncology Nursing, 8*(2), 163–168.

Maltzman, J. (2004). *Targeted therapies: Navigating the "Other" web.* Available from http://www.oncolink.upenn.edu

Marrs, J. (2004). The use of monoclonal antibodies in oncology. *Clinical Journal of Oncology Nursing, 8*(3), 311–313, 315.

Multiple Myeloma Research Foundation. (2006). *Myeloma treatments.* Retrieved April 17, 2007, from http://www.multiplemyeloma.org/treatments/index.html

U.S. Food and Drug Administration. (2007). *List of approved oncology drugs with approved indications.* Available from http://www.fda.gov/cder/cancer/druglist-frame.htm

Viele, C. (2005). Keys to unlock cancer: Targeted therapy. *Oncology Nursing Forum, 32*(5), 935–940.

Vapiwala, N. (2005). *Introduction to targeted therapy.* Available from http://www.oncolink.upenn.edu

CHAPTER 8

TREATMENT ADMINISTRATION USING VENOUS ACCESS DEVICES

CHAPTER OBJECTIVE

After completing this chapter, the reader will be able to recognize common venous access devices, describe their care and maintenance, and identify ways to troubleshoot common problems associated with their use.

LEARNING OBJECTIVES

After studying this chapter, the reader will be able to

1. identify three types of vascular access devices (VADs).

2. list steps in maintaining the patency of VADs.

3. identify two complications associated with VADs.

4. list two methods to avoid infection related to VAD use.

INTRODUCTION

An important area of oncology nursing care and competence is the use of venous access devices (VADs) when administering IV chemotherapy, biotherapy, or targeted therapies. Before the insertion of a VAD, experienced oncology nurses can help advise physicians and the patient about choosing a device that is clinically appropriate and convenient for the patient. The nurse is also responsible for teaching the patient and family members about the device and its long-term care.

Selection of the appropriate VAD for a patient depends on many factors, including the type of therapy being administered; the duration of the therapy course; the patient's diagnosis, self-care ability, preference, and lifestyle; physician preference; and the risk of complications. This chapter provides an overview of commonly used VADs. Table 8-1 lists types of VADs. Figure 8-1 shows catheter landmarks for insertion.

TABLE 8-1: VENOUS ACCESS DEVICES
Peripheral VAD
• Angiocath
• Butterfly
Tunneled VAD
• Hickman
• Groshong
• Broviac
Subcutaneous VAD (implanted)
• Ports, single and double
Percutaneous VAD (nontunneled)
• Triple lumen central venous catheter (CVC)
• Small-gauge silastic CVC
Peripherally Inserted Central Catheter (PICC)
• PICC
• Midline
• Groshong PICC

FIGURE 8-1: CATHETER LANDMARKS

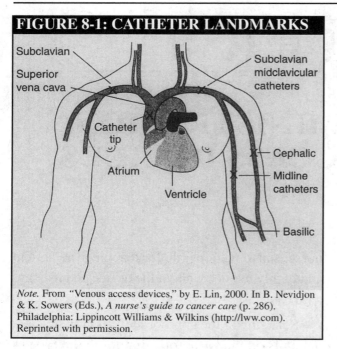

Note. From "Venous access devices," by E. Lin, 2000. In B. Nevidjon & K. Sowers (Eds.), *A nurse's guide to cancer care* (p. 286). Philadelphia: Lippincott Williams & Wilkins (http://lww.com). Reprinted with permission.

PERIPHERAL INTRAVENOUS CATHETERS

The most common type of VAD is the peripheral IV catheter. For nonvesicant agents, a nurse inserts this catheter into the patient's peripheral vein on the hand, wrist, or arm. If the catheter is inserted in an infant or a small child, one of the child's feet or head veins is used. The peripheral catheter provides patient access for short periods of time. To avoid inflammation and infection, a peripheral IV site is usually changed every 72 hours or per institutional protocol. Complications of peripheral IV catheters are infiltration, occlusion, phlebitis, catheter embolism, and hematoma. Some medications cause severe necrosis and pain if they are infused into the tissues instead of the vein. These agents are called *vesicants.* Pain or burning occurs when the agent infused extravasates into the vein and surrounding tissue. Standard care of an IV site includes careful assessment of the site before administering agents. With vesicant agents, that assessment is even more important (Schulmeister, 2005).

To prevent irritation and extravasation, the nurse should assess the site before medications are administered to clearly confirm adequate blood return and should frequently reassess the site during the infusion. Areas that are fragile or have low-flow veins and areas that are vulnerable (near tendons, previously inflamed or overused sites, or hands) should not be used as infusion sites for vesicants. After the infusion, the site should also be carefully assessed, with a focus on any postadministration signs or symptoms of infiltration.

Vesicants should be administered as boluses or slow infusions under the constant guidance of the nurse, not as continuous infusions. At a minimum, if daily vesicant infusions are ordered, the administration site should be changed daily. If infiltration of a vesicant occurs, follow facility procedures to manage the infiltration. (Figure 8-2 reviews the main strategies and steps to manage extravasation.)

CENTRAL VENOUS ACCESS DEVICES (CENTRAL LINES OR CATHETERS)

Central VADs provide the patient with many benefits. Among them are the elimination of needle sticks, more reliable and available venous access, and a ready means for special infusions (vesicant and continuous infusions) or scheduling of infusions, such as long-term total parenteral nutrition (TPN).

Central VADs differ in their characteristics: external or internal, tunneled or nontunneled, open or slit valve (Petree, 2005; Polovich, White, & Kelleher, 2005). They can also have multiple lumens (more than one lumen, or line).

External, Nontunneled, and Tunneled Central VADs

Externally accessed central catheters are either tunneled or nontunneled. An example of a nontunneled catheter is the subclavian catheter (percutaneously inserted catheter). It is typically indicated for short-term use (5 to 7 days) and is used to

FIGURE 8-2: STEPS TO ADDRESS SUSPECTED EXTRAVASATION

(Special concern with vesicant medications)

Below are general steps included in most protocols. Check with your institution's policy for specific steps.

Patient reports symptoms such as: warmth at injection site, stinging, redness, swelling

Peripheral

| Stop IV Infusion |
| Disconnect tubing, keeping cannula in place |
| (Follow institution policy) |
| Attach empty 10 to 20 cc syringe |

Central

| Stop IV Infusion |
| Assess for proper needle placement |
| Aspirate drug from the line |
| Notify physician |

If in tunneled section	If deep extravasation
	Notify plastic surgeon

| Attempt to aspirate drug and blood |
| If required by policy, administer antidote thru cannula or subcutaneously |
| Remove cannula |
| Apply direct, manual pressure |
| Mark and photograph site |
| Apply ice periodically on site for 24 to 48 hours |
| Notify physician |

Instruct patient (according to policy) to:

- Elevate extremity
- Gradually increase extremity normal activity
- Follow-up with physician for assessment two times during first week after incident
- Photograph site weekly
- Document observations and interventions
- Consider plastic surgeon referral if pain, redness, and ulceration do not stop

(Goolsby & Lombardo, 2006; Hayden & Goodman, 2006; Polovich et al., 2005)

monitor the patient, administer multiple medications (including TPN and blood products), and provide access for blood draws. Nontunneled catheters are inserted under sterile conditions in an X-ray suite, cardiac catheterization laboratory, or treatment room or at the patient's bedside (Petree, 2005).

Tunneled catheters have an entrance site distant from where the catheter enters the vascular system. These are "tunneled" through the skin and subcutaneous tissue to a great vein. These catheters stay in place because the patient's tissue forms around the catheter's Dacron cuff, stabilizing its placement and acting as a barrier to infection. The cuff design helps prevent bacteria from traveling up the catheter. Examples of these catheters include the Groshong catheter and the Hickman catheter (see Figure 8-3).

FIGURE 8-3: HICKMAN CATHETER

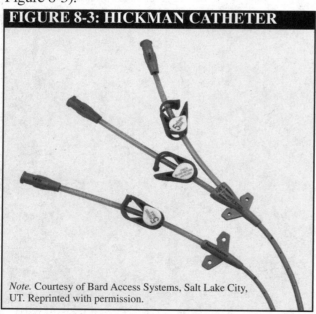

Note. Courtesy of Bard Access Systems, Salt Lake City, UT. Reprinted with permission.

Peripherally Inserted Central Catheters

A popular type of tunneled central VAD is a variation of surgically placed catheters. For patients needing intermediate-length therapy (i.e., 3 to 12 months), specially trained nurses can implant PICCs (see Figure 8-4). These catheters are appropriate for long-term antibiotic use, chemotherapy, TPN, blood products, and blood draws. They are available in single or multiple lumens. If the patient requires multiple

simultaneous infusions or large infusions, surgically placed central VADs are the best long-term access choice (Petree, 2005).

FIGURE 8-4: PERIPHERALLY INSERTED CENTRAL CATHETER

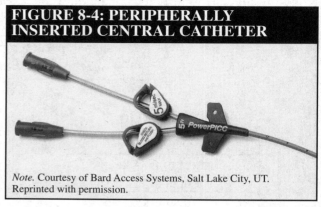

Note. Courtesy of Bard Access Systems, Salt Lake City, UT. Reprinted with permission.

To place a PICC line, the specially trained nurse (certified in PICC placement) creates sterile conditions at the patient's bedside. The catheter is then inserted into the cephalic or basilic vein. The catheter tip is then advanced into the superior vena cava or subclavian vein. (The superior vena cava is the recommended tip placement site.)

From the patient's viewpoint, the PICC is the least expensive and most easily inserted long-term central VAD, but it requires careful and vigilant self-care skills. The manufacturers of PICCs provide special recommendations for care and maintenance protocols.

Care and Maintenance of External Central VADs

Care and maintenance of external central VADs are necessary so that these devices can provide ongoing benefit. Depending on the catheter, manufacturers—in tandem with clinical sites—recommend various maintenance protocols; for care, there is no one standard recommendation. Included in any central catheter maintenance protocol are these elements:

1. Use recommended products and techniques (Luer-lock tips, appropriate adaptors, padded clamps). Establish a clean area to perform self-care.

2. Regularly flush the line, either with sterile normal saline solution or an anticoagulant (e.g., low-molecular-weight heparin). Depending on the catheter, the flushing schedule can vary between every few hours to every few days or weeks.

3. Avoid the use of sharps or scissors near catheters. Use needleless systems whenever possible.

4. Regularly monitor for complications, such as redness, rash, or blistering of the skin around the port. When these complications occur, the patient may be having an allergic reaction to the tape or dressing. In these cases, use an alternative type of tape, dressing, or skin-disinfecting agent.

5. Miscellaneous issues:

   • After central catheter placement, confirm placement and position with a chest X-ray.

   • Do not use blood pressure cuffs and tourniquets above the insertion site.

   • Clamp central catheters with an open port (i.e., Hickman) when the line is not used.

   • Groshong central catheters (also available as PICC and midline versions) each have a slit valve. They do not require heparin flushes.

   • Some patients are allergic to latex, betadine, plastic, or alcohol—materials or substances common to catheters or their care. To avoid problems, review and document the patient's allergies before catheter placement.

   • For blood infusions, use at least a 20-gauge needle. For ports, use larger needle gauges.

6. Regularly clean the exit site with recommended sterile dressings and supplies. Usually, catheter protocols require a scheduled change of the catheter cap (if the product has one). Studies evaluating the use of transparent and gauze dressings show that either dressing type can be used.

(Hayden & Goodman, 2006; Petree, 2005; Polovich et al., 2005)

OTHER LONG-TERM ACCESS DEVICES

Implanted Ports

Implanted ports, also called Portacaths, are another central VAD for long-term access. A port is a hollow housing of stainless steel, titanium, or plastic that contains a compressed latex septum over a portal chamber. It is connected via a small tube to a silicone or polyurethane catheter that is inserted into a blood vessel. The port is placed subcutaneously, and the nurse accesses the port percutaneously using a special noncoring needle. The implanted catheter is attached to a plastic or metal reservoir, which is surgically implanted on the chest wall. The implanted port provides access for long-term intermittent therapy or cyclic therapy.

Implanted ports can also provide the patient with a way to preserve body image because they have no external catheters. Figure 8-5 shows a portacath.

FIGURE 8-5: IMPLANTED PORT

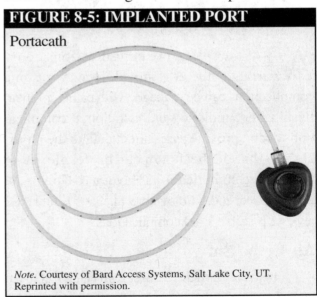

Portacath

Note. Courtesy of Bard Access Systems, Salt Lake City, UT. Reprinted with permission.

A port should have a brisk blood return and allow easy flow of fluids. Watch for edema, redness, or pain in the tissues surrounding the port.

Long-Arm Catheters

Another venous access option is the long-arm catheter (LAC), also called the *midline catheter* (see Figure 8-6). A LAC is a central VAD-like device, although when threaded, it does not end in the superior vena cava. The LAC is a variation of the PICC line. The tip of this catheter lies in the midclavicle, providing venous access through a larger vein than peripheral lines placed more distally on the lower arm. Although not a central line, maintenance care of the LAC is similar to a PICC.

FIGURE 8-6: MIDLINE CATHETER

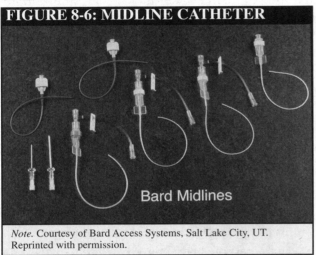

Bard Midlines

Note. Courtesy of Bard Access Systems, Salt Lake City, UT. Reprinted with permission.

COMPLICATIONS OF CENTRAL CATHETERS

Any of the following complications could warrant catheter removal. However, some complications can be managed with catheter repair, flushing, or antibiotic administration. If complications occur, provide assessment data to the physician so that the best plan can be developed to address the complication (Hayden & Goodman, 2006; Petree, 2005; Polovich et al., 2005). Table 8-2 reviews possible VAD complications.

Air Embolism

A bolus of air in the bloodstream can travel to the lungs, heart, or brain, disrupting blood flow or causing brain damage or death. Clinical signs of an air embolism present as respiratory distress. On examination, the patient has unequal breath sounds, weak pulses, decreased blood pressure, and a decreased level of consciousness. Air embolism is a risk when a central VAD is inserted or removed during tubing or cap changes. The risk increases when the patient's

TABLE 8-2: VENOUS ACCESS DEVICE COMPLICATIONS

Obstruction
* Tip placement, catheter migration
* Development of fibrin sheath or thrombi
* Development of drug precipitate
* Catheter fracture

Air Embolism

Extravasation
* Dislodged catheter or needle
* Catheter fracture or defect
* Catheter migration

intrathoracic pressure changes—for example, during coughing, sneezing, crying, or laughing. To prevent air embolism, clamp central lines (exception: Groshong) when the catheter is open to air, such as when changing tubing or adaptors.

If an air embolism is suspected, fold the catheter back on itself and clamp it at the proximal end (if clamping is allowed). Otherwise, reconnect the IV tubing (if it is disconnected) or cap the catheter. Next, turn the patient onto his or her left side. If possible, the patient should be placed head down so that the air collects in the right atrium. Administer oxygen.

To reduce the risk of air embolism during catheter insertion and removal, ask the patient to perform the Valsalva maneuver to increase intrathoracic pressure. After catheter removal, cover the insertion site and surrounding area with a gel-based ointment, such as petroleum jelly gauze or ointment. Cover the area with a dressing. Inspect the insertion site every 24 hours. Once a scab has formed, the site is effectively sealed (Petree, 2005; Polovich et al., 2005).

Venous Thrombosis

A thrombus may develop in the vein holding the catheter. Signs of venous thrombosis include edema at the puncture site, erythema, and ipsilateral swelling of the arm, neck, and face. The patient may complain of pain along the vein, fever, malaise, and tachycardia. When the inner layer of a vein wall is injured, platelets and fibrin collect at the injury site and an intravascular thrombus can form. The results are a clot or a fibrin sheath.

Thrombi occurring in the upper superior vena cava result from an improperly placed central VAD tip (in the upper portion of the superior vena cava instead of the midproximal third) that irritates the vessel. The patient can develop swelling on the affected side within 96 hours of catheter insertion.

Thrombi in the subclavian vein are usually related to improper insertion technique, during which the vessel wall is injured (rather than improper tip placement). Early indications of this complication are when the IV solution does not infuse by gravity or when the pump signals an occlusion. If the thrombosis is not treated, this swelling progresses up the arm and into the patient's chest and neck. In extreme cases, the mammary veins on the affected side become engorged.

If a patient shows signs of a thrombosis, stop the infusion and contact the physician. The patient will need anticoagulants and may need thrombolytic therapy. Treatment, based on clinical signs, can include leaving the central VAD in place until a venogram shows complete resolution of the thrombus or removing the central VAD entirely (Petree, 2005; Polovich et al., 2005).

For some patients, physicians order a protocol of low-dose warfarin therapy to prevent thrombosis.

Pneumothorax

Pneumothorax, hemothorax, and hydrothorax can occur during insertion. With these complications, the patient suddenly complains of chest pain and dyspnea and has decreased breath sounds. The patient may also become cyanotic. While waiting for physician assistance, the nurse should clamp the catheter (exception: Groshong) and provide the patient with oxygen (Petree, 2005).

Occlusion

If fluids cannot infuse and the catheter is not clamped, the line may be occluded. Before attempting to administer medications, most catheters need to be checked for blood return. Some institutions allow the administration of anti-thrombolytic medications to clear an occlusion. The institution's protocol needs to be followed. In any case, avoid forcing fluids because doing so puts the patient at risk for embolism.

Sepsis

Patients who are immunosuppressed or leukopenic cannot mount a strong immune response to infection (Hayden & Goodman, 2006). A typical response to infection is fever and redness, warmth, tenderness, or purulent exudate at the catheter site. In immunocompromised patients with developing infections, the signs and symptoms are more subtle.

Catheter-related sepsis is the most common life-threatening complication of central VADs. In fact, catheter-related devices account for 2.7% to 60% of patient infections (Hayden & Goodman, 2006). In most cases, microorganisms invade the bloodstream through the catheter insertion site, either by migration along the catheter's external surface or through contamination that enters the internal port. With an environment for bacterial entry, the maintenance of sterile technique during catheter procedures and manipulation is even more important.

Signs of a systemic infection include fever, chills, an increased white blood cell (WBC) count, nausea and vomiting, malaise, and increased urine glucose. (Exception: Patients who are neutropenic do not have elevated WBC counts.) If an infection is suspected, the catheter tip is cultured. In some cases, catheter-based infections are treated with antibiotics. In other cases, the catheter—as the source of the infection—is pulled (Petree, 2005; Polovich et al., 2005).

These factors can increase a patient's risk of catheter-related sepsis:

- Poor insertion technique— Failing to maintain a sterile field or prepare the skin properly may be the leading factor contributing to catheter-related sepsis.

- Multilumen catheters— Because a larger-gauge introducer is needed to insert a multilumen catheter, trauma is created at the insertion site. Also, these catheters may be handled more often, increasing the opportunity for microorganisms to enter the line.

- Use of stopcocks— This increases handling of the catheter and the access area.

- A jugular or femoral insertion site— A jugular site is difficult to keep immobilized and to keep adequately dressed. Both sites are close to areas with large numbers of microorganisms (the mouth and the groin).

- Catheter material— Most catheters are made of polyurethane, polyvinyl chloride, or silicone. When the catheter is inserted into the vein, the body responds to the foreign object by encapsulating it in a fibrin sheath. Bacteria can adhere to this sheath and multiply.

- Long-term catheterization— The length of therapy should be a factor in catheter selection. Access should be discontinued at the end of therapy. Risk is considered cumulative and therefore increases with time, so the need for central access should be frequently reevaluated.

- Frequent manipulation of the dressing— Extra care should be taken when the patient is in declining health or has an acute illness, including critical illness, immunosuppression, diabetes, and hypercoagulability.

SUMMARY

The use of VADs in administering IV chemotherapy, biotherapy, or targeted therapies is a mainstay of oncology nursing practice. The type of VAD chosen for the patient depends on the treatment being administered, the duration of the treatment or course of treatment, and patient and physician preferences. Proper VAD maintenance includes careful technique, adhering to protocols that address sterility of the site, regular dressing changes, and proper flushing schedules. VAD complications that nurses should know how to manage include extravasation, catheter occlusions, air embolism, thrombosis, and sepsis.

EXAM QUESTIONS

CHAPTER 8
Questions 30-33

Note: Choose the option that BEST answers each question.

30. One type of VAD is the

    a. time-release capsule.
    b. Foley catheter.
    c. PICC line.
    d. arterial line.

31. To maintain the patency of VADs, the nurse should

    a. regularly flush the line.
    b. clamp off the line every hour.
    c. use a blood pressure cuff above the insertion site.
    d. avoid cleaning the exit site.

32. A complication associated with VADs is

    a. infection.
    b. absorption.
    c. disintegration.
    d. portability.

33. The best way to avoid infection related to VAD use is to

    a. change the tubing every 2 weeks.
    b. apply warm compresses to the site every hour.
    c. frequently manipulate the dressing.
    d. maintain a sterile field during insertion.

REFERENCES

Goolsby, T., & Lombardo, F. (2006). Extravasation of chemotherapeutic agents: Prevention and treatment. *Seminars in Oncology, 33*(1), 139-43.

Hayden, B., & Goodman, M. (2006). Chemotherapy: Principles of administration. In C. Yarbro, M. Frogge, & M. Goodman (Eds.), *Cancer nursing: Principles and practice* (6th ed., pp. 351-382). Sudbury, MA: Jones & Bartlett.

Lin, E. (2000). Venous access devices. In B. Nevidjon & K. Sowers (Eds.), *A nurse's guide to cancer care* (p. 284-294). Philadelphia: Lippincott Williams & Wilkins.

Petree, J. (2005). Supportive care: Supportive therapies and procedures; Vascular access: Venous, arterial, and peritoneal devices. In J. K. Itano & K. N. Taoka (Eds.), *Core curriculum for oncology nursing* (4th ed., pp. 149-160). St. Louis: Elsevier.

Polovich, M., White, J.M., & Kelleher, L. (Eds.). (2005). *Chemotherapy and biotherapy guidelines and recommendations for practice* (2nd ed.). Pittsburgh, PA: Oncology Nursing Press, Inc.

CHAPTER 9

BONE MARROW AND PERIPHERAL STEM CELL TRANSPLANT

CHAPTER OBJECTIVE

After completing this chapter, the reader will be able to recognize bone marrow and peripheral stem cell transplants as treatments for selected cancers and describe the processes of transplantation and donor matching.

LEARNING OBJECTIVES

After studying this chapter, the reader will be able to

1. identify factors that allow an allogenic match, donor to recipient.

2. list supportive therapies during the engraftment period.

3. identify symptoms of graft-versus-host disease.

4. recognize the benefits of cord transplants.

INTRODUCTION

Bone marrow transplants (BMTs) and peripheral stem cell transplants (PSCTs) have become the standard of care for selected hematologic malignancies, such as leukemias and lymphoproliferative disorders (see Table 9-1). The goal of the transplant process is to first kill as many of the cancer cells as possible with very high doses of chemotherapy and radiation and then rescue the body with new noncancerous stem or bone marrow cells. Because of improvements in transplant procedures and effective supportive therapies, transplants have become an effective—albeit complicated—cancer treatment.

Stem Cell Lines

Pluripotent stem cells are immature body cells that can make identical copies of themselves. Depending on the body's needs, stem cells can provide the early cells to replace aging or damaged cells. Once stem cells mature, they cannot duplicate.

Blood stem cells, known as *hematopoietic stem cells,* are in the bone's marrow. Hematopoietic stem cells supply three types of blood cells: erythrocytes (commonly known as *red blood cells* [RBCs]); platelets (also called *blood-clotting cells*); and leukocytes, the white blood cells (WCBs) of the immune system. The constant process of replacing red or white cells or platelets by moving the stem cells from the bone marrow to the bloodstream is called *hematopoiesis*. (See Figure 9-1.)

Immune cells—also called WBCs or lymphocytes—leave the bone marrow while still immature, maturing until they become T or B cells in the immune system. Other blood components, like RBCs, completely mature in the bone marrow and go directly into the bloodstream. For every blood stem cell in the bloodstream, there are approximately 100 stem cells in the bone marrow. The timing and rate of release of those cells into the

TABLE 9-1: COMMON DISEASES TREATED WITH BONE MARROW OR STEM CELL TRANSPLANTS

	BMT	PSCT
Leukemias		
Acute myelogenous leukemia	X	X
Acute lymphoblastic leukemia	X	X
Chronic myelogenous leukemia	X	X
Myelodysplastic syndromes	X	
Lymphoproliferative Disorders		
Hodgkin's disease	X	X
Non-Hodgkin's disease	X	X
Multiple myeloma	X	X
Chronic lymphocytic leukemia	X	X
Lymphoproliferative Disorders		
B-thalassemia	X	
Sickle cell anemia	X	

(Baltic & Bakitas, 2006; Shapiro, 2005)

FIGURE 9-1: HEMATOPOIESIS CHART

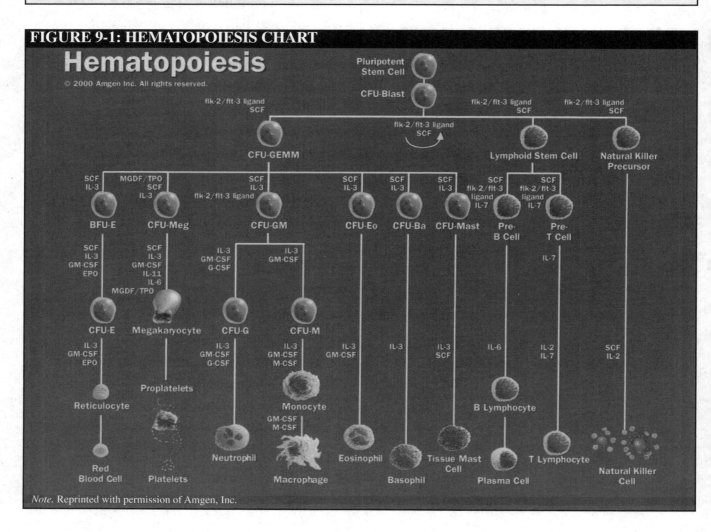

Note. Reprinted with permission of Amgen, Inc.

bloodstream is not clearly understood (National Cancer Institute [NCI]), 2006a, 2006b).

TRANSPLANTS AS TREATMENT

Blood stem cell transplants are classified into two types: BMTs or PSCTs. Either type of transplant can restore normal hematopoiesis. With BMT, the new or replaced bone marrow is a source for disease-free hematopoietic cell lines. Before aggressive chemotherapy or radiation treatments begin, circulating stem cells are collected and cryopreserved (frozen in liquid nitrogen). To step up the production of stem cells harvested from peripheral blood, patients receive growth factors to move blood stem cells from the marrow into the bloodstream. Growth factors can increase the blood stem cell concentration 10- to 100-fold in the blood.

The process of harvesting blood stem cells from a donor's peripheral blood is called *apheresis* and can take several hours. This process involves removal of whole blood from the donor and separation of component blood types via centrifuge.

The blood itself, minus the stem cells, is returned to the donor (NCI, 2006b; Shapiro, 2005).

After harvesting the patient's cells, high-dose treatments begin. This stage of the treatment is called the *conditioning regimen for myeloablation.* As soon as possible after conditioning treatment, clinicians return the bone marrow or stem cells to the patient for engraftment (production of new healthy blood cells.) Engraftment generally starts to occur within 2 weeks after PSCT. For BMT, the start of engraftment can take as long as 5 weeks after transplant (NCI, 2006a; Vachani, 2005a).

The best strategy for transplant is based on the patient's disease, clinical data, treatment plan, and histocompatibility of cell matches. When transplanted cells come from a compatible donor, the transplant is an allogenic transplant. (Figure 9-2 illustrates the process of allogenic transplant.) When cells are taken from the patient and later returned to the patient, the transplant is an autologous transplant. (Figure 9-3 illustrates the steps in an autologous transplant.)

Currently more common than BMTs are PSCTs, which focus on peripheral stem cell harvests rather than bone marrow harvests. Stem cells can be

FIGURE 9-2: SCHEME OF BONE MARROW TRANSPLANTATION FROM AN ALLOGENIC DONOR

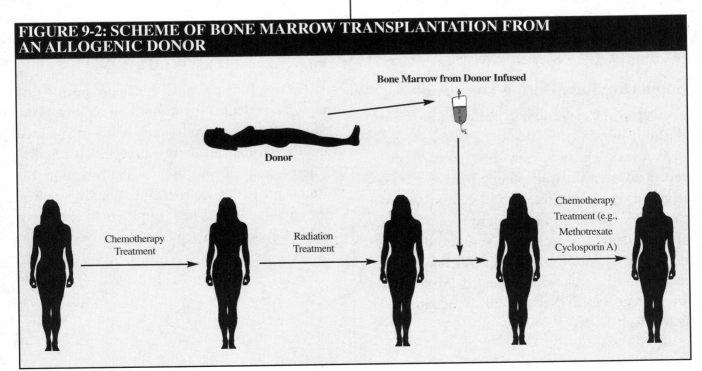

FIGURE 9-3: SCHEME OF AUTOLOGOUS BONE MARROW OR STEM CELL TRANSPLANTATION

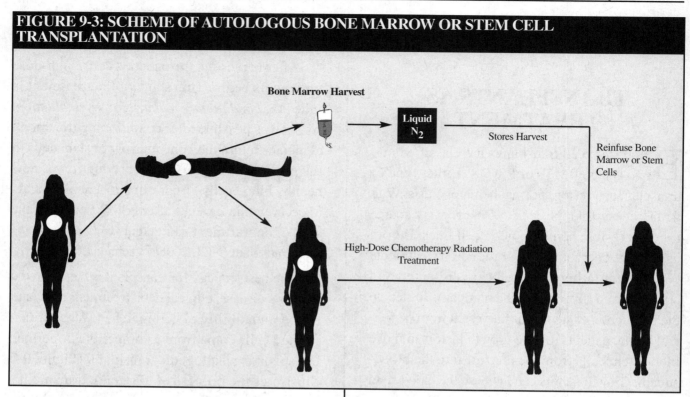

harvested from a patient in an outpatient setting through a peripheral IV or central venous catheter site. The process of PSCT is less traumatic to the patient, is more cost-effective (more outpatient procedures, shorter hospital stays), and typically offers a posttransplant course equivalent to that of the more complicated BMT. Both transplant procedures benefit from effective supportive therapy, which contributes to better transplant courses and outcomes (Papayannopoulou, 2004; Shapiro, 2005).

Supportive Care During Transplant

During the conditioning phase of transplant, the body normally would not be able to handle high doses of chemotherapy and radiation. Thus, recent advances in transplant effectiveness are largely due to developments in effective supportive therapies. These therapies fight off infection, anemia, thrombocytopenia, immune disorders, and the possible toxic effects of chemotherapy agents themselves (e.g., nausea, vomiting, diarrhea, stomatitis, fatigue, pain) (Vachani, 2005a, 2005b; West & Mitchell, 2004).

One of the main purposes of supportive therapies is to provide agents that boost or quicken the returned bone marrow's functioning once stem cells are reinfused. Growth factors such as granulocyte macrophage colony-stimulating factor (sargramostine [Leukine]), granulocyte-colony stimulating factor (pegfilgrasim [Neulasta]), and erythropoietin (epoetin alfa [Procrit]) are a few of the available supportive therapies that help increase the success rate of BMTs and PSCTs.

Transplant patients can have periods of multiple, serious complications. In addition to the various physical challenges that patients face before, during, and after treatment, they can also suffer from profound fatigue and depression (El-Banna et al., 2004). Therefore, nursing care of transplant patients needs to include extensive emotional and psychological support.

POSTTRANSPLANT COURSE

When stem cells repopulate the bloodstream with normal RBCs and immune cells, the stem cells "rescue" the patient. To determine if a stem cell transplant has been effective, the interaction of certain markers that are found on the surface of all body cells is evaluated. The markers—or antigens—recognize self and nonself cells.

Antigens can mobilize powerful immune reactions when they are first introduced to a new, nonself environment. The adverse reaction of antigens from a donor source responding to the patient or host and determining an unmatch can trigger the patient's immune cells to attack the donated (transplanted) cells, which are referred to as *graft cells.* When this occurs after a transplant, the disconnect means that the transplant is being rejected. Another term for this dire situation is graft-versus-host disease (GVHD).

Graft-Versus-Host Disease

Graft rejection can occur if immune system cells are left in the patient after the preparative regimen. These "native" cells attack the donor cells because they recognize them as being foreign to the body.

GVHD can be prevented most of the time by making sure the preparative regimen is sufficiently strong to kill any native immune cells. Table 9-2 highlights the focus of nursing care when the patient has GVHD.

Acute GVHD generally occurs during the first 2 months after transplant. Chronic GVHD starts at least 2 to 3 months after transplant. Almost all allogeneic transplant patients have some degree of this complication, which can range from very mild to very severe.

Treatments for GVHD include immunosuppressive medications, including steroids and

TABLE 9-2: FOCUS OF NURSING CARE: GRAFT VERSUS HOST DISEASE (GVHD)
Signs of GVHD
• Skin (rash)
• Intestinal tract (diarrhea)
• Liver (elevated liver blood tests and decreased liver function)
• Pulmonary complications are generally caused by pneumonia
Especially with allogeneic transplants:
• Pulmonary complications
• Liver problems (veno-occlusive disease of the liver)
– Jaundice
– Enlarged liver
– Swelling of the abdomen
– Liver failure

antithymocyte globulin (Atgam) (Shapiro, 2005; Wilson & Sylvanus, 2005).

Transfusion of irradiated blood products can decrease the GVHD in susceptible recipients (those with a limited immune systems). Irradiated blood products are exposed to approximately 2500 rads of gamma radiation to destroy the lymphocytes' ability to divide. Irradiation destroys the ability of transfused lymphocytes to respond to host foreign antigens. Patients with functional immune systems naturally destroy foreign lymphocytes, making irradiation of blood and blood components unnecessary.

Engraftment

Graft failure occurs when the donor's cells fail to start working (producing new blood cells). Physicians usually consider a diagnosis of graft failure if engraftment has not occurred by 42 days after transplant. This complication is rare, occurring in only about 5% of patients. The only treatment for graft failure is to receive another transplant (NCI, 2006a, 2006b).

Engrafting directly from the bone marrow takes longer—up to 5 weeks. For patients to have completely restored immune function, autologous transplants take several months; allogenic transplants can take 1 to 2 years (Bevans & Shelburne, 2004; NCI, 2006a; Shapiro, 2005).

MATCHING DONOR CELLS TO THEIR HOST

The goal of transplanting stem cells is to find a compatible match of the antigens on the donor cells and tissues with those on the patient's cells. The two sources of cells can be different, but not too different. Closely matched donors are usually relatives, but donor-to-patient transplants do not necessarily need to be related. They only need to be reasonably compatible.

To determine compatibility, the patient's and donor's blood are tested in a process called *tissue typing*. One method to find a better match for a patient is to have the patient donate stem cells to himself or herself. This is called an *autologous transplant*. When an identical twin donates to his or her twin, it is called a *syngeneic transplant*. When donated cells come from a nonself donor, the transplant is allogeneic.

Individuals have a unique "self" set of antigens, which are major histocompatibility complex (MHC) proteins. When these MHC proteins mark the surface of immune cells (leukocytes), the antigens are referred to as *human leukocyte antigens* (HLAs). Leukocytes are the cells used for tissue typing. The HLAs determine if a reasonable match is possible for a patient. To establish a match, a donor's leukocytes are removed from a blood sample and then evaluated for HLA markers.

HLA Markers

Six important genes for HLAs are contributed by each parent. Therefore, an individual inherits a double set of six major genes that produce six major corresponding antigens: HLA-A, HLA-B, HLA-C, HLA-DP, HLA-DQ, and HLA-DR. Because as many as 20 varieties exist for each of these HLA-producing genes in different individuals, the number of possible HLAs that can mark "self" and trigger an immune response can approach 10,000 (NCI, 2006a; Shapiro, 2005).

Studies have identified that the three most important antigens to match when choosing nonself donors for a transplant are HLA-A, HLA-B, and HLA-DR. An ideal 6:6 antigen match, known as a *clinical match,* means that both sets of the three "most important" inherited HLAs in the donor match perfectly with those of the body (and immune) cells in the patient. As the number of HLA matches decreases among donors and recipients, the chances of finding a donor decrease (Shapiro, 2005).

Approximately 35% of matches can be made with siblings (Baltic & Bakitas, 2006). More than 90% of patients can find a haplo-identical donor if they are willing to accept a three-antigen match. This threshold is determined as acceptable for severely ill patients who cannot wait several months to find a four-, five-, or six-antigen match donor. Patients who undergo these transplants are at increased risk for GVHD and rejection of the transplant (NCI, 2006a, 2006b).

Graft-Versus-Tumor Effect

Haplo-identical transplants can provide a possible benefit to the donor as well. With these transplants, the process may enable an attack on malignant cells. A graft-versus-tumor effect occurs when a donor's mature immune cells join with the transplanted stem cells to recognize and attack "foreign" cancer cells. When this occurs, some patients can avoid a relapse; sometimes this process even creates a cure. To capitalize on the graft-versus-tumor effect, patients may be infused with the donor's stem cells and WBCs.

The downside of the graft-versus-tumor effect is that the donor's mature immune cells (T cells) can interfere with the stem cell graft; as a result, the patient's tissues are attacked. To minimize this risk, T cells may be depleted from the transplant, leaving stem cells only. When T cells are removed from the donated community of cells, the ability for T cells to join the attack on cancer cells is eliminated.

Probability of Clinical Match

Matched transplants between unrelated individuals can be challenging because the donor pool is large. For example, Japanese patients come from a confined gene pool due to island geography. Thus, in this geography population, the chances increase for a clinical match compared to a match based on a larger, more heterogenous gene pool. (Some estimate the chance of a clinical match is 99% [NCI, 2006a, 2006b]).

African American and Asian American patients are part of a large gene pool but are underrepresented in the donor pool. They have less than 50% probability of finding a 6:6 clinical match. The chance for a clinical match in the North American Caucasian population is 93% (NCI, 2006a, 2006b).

CORD BLOOD TRANSPLANTS

Cord blood transplants—from the rich supply of immature stem cells in the umbilical cord—were first performed in 1989 to help children with leukemia. Now cord transplants have been shown to help adults, as well. Stem cells from umbilical cords are capable of rebuilding all three types of blood cells in the body (RCBs, immune cells, and platelets).

Umbilical cord blood is now a readily available, easy-to-store alternative to the standard process of stem cell transplants. This option has been welcomed by those patients who are waiting to be matched to a suitable donor and those unable to find a donor. Even with a one- or two-antigen mismatch, cord-blood transplants succeed in a greater percentage of cases than those for equally mismatched BMTs. Cord transplants also expand the availability of transplant as an option to patients in under represented minority groups. Moreover, cord transplants decrease the risk of transferring cytomegalovirus, which is a problem in about 10% of marrow donations (NCI, 2006b).

Cord transplants are not without risk. Maternal cells or genetic disease from the child donating the cord can be transferred during transplant. Also, cord transplants on average include only one-tenth of the number of cells that can be harvested during a BMT. Cord transplants also may have a delayed period before engrafting, therefore leaving the patient open to complications, such as the risk of infection.

THE NATIONAL MARROW DONOR PROGRAM

The National Marrow Donor Program is the coordinating center for unrelated donors. Based in Minneapolis, MN, its data lists more than 3 million donors (more than 1 million are fully typed). During the initial search, potential matches are found in about 70% of cases (NCI, 2006b). The program's website is http://www.marrow.org.

Those interested in donating blood stem cells and mothers willing to donate cord blood are instructed to provide a blood sample at a local collection site, so that they are entered into the database. Further tissue typing occurs later if a potential match is anticipated (NCI, 2006a, 2006b).

SUMMARY

Because of improvements in transplant procedures and effective supportive therapies, bone marrow and stem cell transplants have become a standard treatment for selected hematologic malignancies. The process involves HLA matching of donor to recipient (for nonautologous transplants), aggressive pretransplant chemotherapy or radiation therapy regimens, and the return of transplanted cells to the patient. If the patient's allogenic transplant is rejected, GVHD can become a life-threatening complication. Cord blood transplants have emerged as an option for patients who cannot establish a safe clinical match, donor to host.

EXAM QUESTIONS

CHAPTER 9
Questions 34-37

Note: Choose the option that BEST answers each question.

34. Supportive therapy to boost bone marrow functioning during the engraftment period includes

    a. antibiotics.
    b. steroids.
    c. growth factors.
    d. antifungals.

35. A symptom of GVHD is

    a. depression.
    b. delerium.
    c. diarrhea.
    d. constipation.

36. An allogenic match, donor to recipient, is possible when

    a. HLA matching includes three of the main HLA markers.
    b. an autologous transplant is ruled out.
    c. both donor and recipient have type O blood.
    d. both donor and recipient live close to one another.

37. A benefit of cord transplants is that

    a. they are an option for difficult-to-match transplant recipients.
    b. they are convenient for the transplant recipient.
    c. they are low in cost.
    d. they provide an overabundance of cells to harvest during a bone marrow transplant.

REFERENCES

Baltic, T., & Bakitas, M. (2006). Principles of bone marrow and hematopoietic cell transplantation. In C. Yarbro, M. Frogge, & M. Goodman (Eds.), *Cancer nursing: Principles and practice* (6th ed., pp. 458–477). Sudbury, MA: Jones & Bartlett.

Bevans, M., & Shelburne, N. (2004). Hematopoietic stem cell transplantation. *Clinical Journal of Oncology Nursing, 8*(5), 541–543.

El-Banna, M., Berger, A., Farr, L., Foxall, M., Friesth, B., & Schreiner, E. (2004). Fatigue and depression in patients with lymphoma undergoing autologous peripheral blood stem cell transplantation. *Oncology Nursing Forum, 31*(5), 937–944.

National Cancer Institute. (2006a). *Bone marrow transplantation and peripheral blood stem cell transplantation: Questions and answers.* Available from http://cancer.gov/cancertopics/factsheet

National Cancer Institute. (2006b). *Understanding cancer series: Blood stem cell transplants.* Retrieved October 31, 2006, from http://www icic.nci.nih.gov/cancertopics/understanding cancer/stemcells

Papayannopoulou, T. (2004). Current mechanistic scenarios in hematopoietic stem/progenitor cell mobilization. *Blood, 103*(5), 1580–1585.

Shapiro, T. (2005). Nursing implications of hematopoietic stem cell transplantation. In J.K. Itano & K.N. Taoka (Eds.), *Core curriculum for oncology nursing* (4th ed., pp. 809–827). St. Louis: Elsevier.

Vachani, C. (2005a). *Autologous stem cell transplant or bone marrow transplant.* Available from http://www.oncolink.upenn.edu

Vachani, C. (2005b). *Allogeneic transplant (bone marrow & stem cell).* Available from http://www.oncolink.upenn.edu

West, F., & Mitchell, S. (2004). Evidence-based guidelines for the management of neutropenia following outpatient hematopoietic stem cell transplantation. *Clinical Journal of Oncology Nursing, 8*(6), 601–613.

Wilson, C., & Sylvanus, T. (2005). Graft failure following allogeneic blood and marrow transplant: Evidence-based nursing case study review. *Clinical Journal of Oncology Nursing, 9*(2), 151–159.

CHAPTER 10

CLINICAL TRIALS

CHAPTER OBJECTIVE

After completing this chapter, the reader will be able to describe the process for enrolling patients in clinical trials and define the role of the nurse in clinical trials.

LEARNING OBJECTIVES

After studying this chapter, the reader will be able to

1. recognize the phases of clinical trials.

2. identify web-based databases about clinical trials.

3. list two questions that patients may have about enrolling in clinical trials.

4. recognize two nursing interventions related to caring for patients enrolled in clinical trials.

INTRODUCTION

Patients considering enrollment in clinical trials require a special nursing focus. Among the patient education issues are the phases of a clinical trial, informed consent, enrollment processes, data gathering, and coverage outside of the patient's insurance plan. This chapter reviews these areas that impact the care of patients enrolled in clinical trials.

OVERVIEW

Six predominant types of clinical trials exist: prevention, screening, diagnostic, treatment, supportive care, and genetic studies (National Institutes of Health, 2006). In cancer care and treatment, of special focus are clinical trials that evaluate the merit of new drugs and determine appropriate drug doses, acceptable toxicities, and prevention and treatment strategies. Based on the data generated from clinical trials, effective cancer prevention agents and treatments continue to be developed (CancerSource, 2005; Harris, 2006).

National and local study groups, university-based research programs, and pharmaceutical manufacturers sponsor clinical trials. The effort is huge, both in the public and private sectors. The National Cancer Institute [NCI] and pharmaceutical manufacturers are the major sources of therapy research and development. The NCI coordinates the screening of more than 10,000 compounds each year in an effort to find new and potentially useful drugs for treating cancer. Less than 1% of screened compounds proceed to clinical trials (CancerSource, 2005). Figure 10-1 highlights where pharmaceutical manufacturers are targeting their developmental dollars.

FIGURE 10-1: MEDICINES IN DEVELOPMENT FOR CANCER*

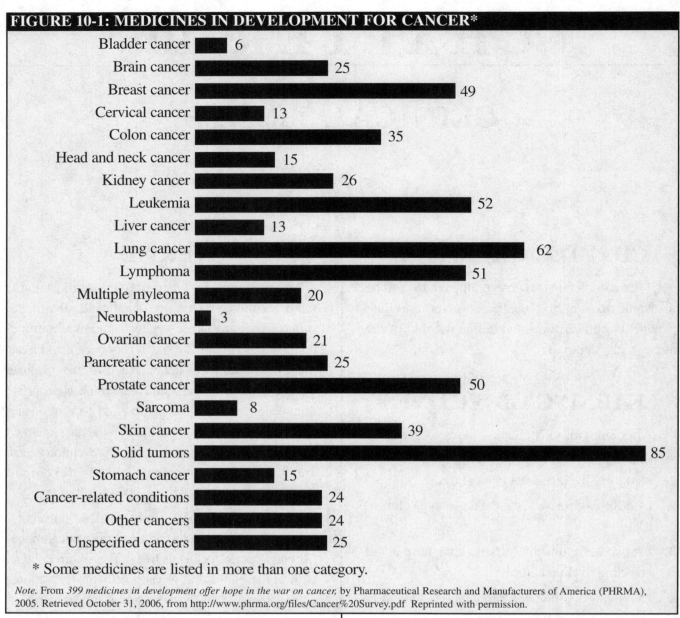

Bladder cancer 6
Brain cancer 25
Breast cancer 49
Cervical cancer 13
Colon cancer 35
Head and neck cancer 15
Kidney cancer 26
Leukemia 52
Liver cancer 13
Lung cancer 62
Lymphoma 51
Multiple myleoma 20
Neuroblastoma 3
Ovarian cancer 21
Pancreatic cancer 25
Prostate cancer 50
Sarcoma 8
Skin cancer 39
Solid tumors 85
Stomach cancer 15
Cancer-related conditions 24
Other cancers 24
Unspecified cancers 25

* Some medicines are listed in more than one category.

Note. From *399 medicines in development offer hope in the war on cancer,* by Pharmaceutical Research and Manufacturers of America (PHRMA), 2005. Retrieved October 31, 2006, from http://www.phrma.org/files/Cancer%20Survey.pdf Reprinted with permission.

PHASES OF CLINICAL TRIALS

Before clinical trials begin on humans in the United States, new compounds are tested on animals. Once enough human data are sufficiently compiled, the findings are submitted to the U.S. Food and Drug Administration (FDA) for approval. As clinical trials proceed, the process is lengthy and expensive. Some estimates report that the average time and cost to bring a drug to market is 10 to 12 years and $40 to $80 million. The phases of clinical trial development are listed in Table 10-1.

Trials bring to market compounds that are based on cumulative knowledge about the malignancy, the pharmacological properties of the compounds, and the ever-expanding knowledge about anticancer mechanisms of action.

ENROLLMENT IN CLINICAL TRIALS

Annually, only 3% of patients participate in clinical trials (Lara et al., 2006). The Internet has revolutionized the process for health care professionals and patients by making it easier to find out more about clin-

TABLE 10-1: PHASES OF CANCER CLINICAL TRIALS

PHASE I

Goals in new agents not approved by the FDA

Primary goal:	Establishes the maximum tolerated dose (MTD) by selecting a starting dose, then sequentially escalating the dose in groups of three or more patients until the MDT is reached.
Secondary goal:	Defines toxicities and quantifies the degree of their severity.

In agents already approved by the FDA

Primary goal:	May be a dose-finding study for a single agent or may be defining a dose when used in combination or in a new patient population.
Patient Population:	Usually conducted in a small number of patients (≤ 50) in a few centers.
Comments:	Pharmacokinetics are drawn at timed intervals to gather information on the drug's absorption, distribution, metabolism, and elimination.

PHASE II

Primary goal:	Performed to test the effectiveness of a drug in a specific tumor type.
Patient Population:	Performed in a larger number of patients and at several sites simultaneously. Patients must have measurable disease and adequate anticipated life expectancy to permit enough data collection for analysis of results.
Comments:	Pharmacokinetics collection may continue. Safety information continues to be collected. Must involve enough subjects to produce statistically significant conclusions about the activity of the agent in the population being studied.

PHASE III

Primary goal:	Compares a new drug/treatment to current drugs/treatments to prove that the new drug/treatment is at least as effective as the standard drug.
Patient population:	Conducted in a large number of patients, usually in multiple centers.
Comments:	May contain a quality-of-life component. Trial design is often randomized and blinded.

PHASE IV

Primary goal:	Continues collection of safety and efficacy data after the drug is approved for marketing and use.
Secondary goal:	Expands the "off-label" use.
Patient population:	Same as Phase III.
Comments:	These trials may continue for several years after the drug has been FDA-approved.

(Delaney, 2006)

ical trials. In the United States, the NCI has a well-established web site (http://www.cancer.gov/clinical trials) that allows access to its database about clinical trials and provides comprehensive information on open clinical trials. In 2005, approximately 10,000 clinical trials were listed, with almost 300 of those trials targeted to cancer care and treatment (Lee, 2005).

In addition to the NCI, other databases provide listings of clinical trials. They include:

- Center Watch Clinical Trials Listing Service (http://www.centerwatch.com) provides information about 41,000 active industry- and government-sponsored clinical trials in the United States and is designed for patients and research professionals. Of those trials, approximately 130 were cancer care trials in 2005.

- PDQ (http://wwwicic.nci.nih.gov/cancertopics/pdq/cancerdatabase#clinical_trial) holds about 2,000 trials in its international registry and is maintained by the NCI. In 2005, this database had approximately 2,000 cancer trials listed.

- Trial Check (http://www.cancertrialshelp.org) provides information about 350 trials and is available to members of the Coalition of Cancer Cooperative Groups.

(Lee, 2005)

Although some clinical trials are coordinated in the community, most originate and are managed at comprehensive cancer centers and university hospitals. Trials can also originate from community hospitals and physician groups.

Matching the patient to the trial's eligibility requirements is key to receiving treatment through a clinical trial (e.g., sex, age range, type of cancer, previous treatments, state of disease, comorbidi-

ties). Table 10-2 provides answers to common questions that patients have when considering enrollment in a clinical trial.

The constant stream of clinical trial data in the press can make it difficult to sift through what is important or promising. Data from each trial protocol present various benefits and challenges to the patient. Nurses caring for patients who contemplate joining a clinical trial must serve as patient educators and advocates. Table 10-3 reviews nursing interventions for patients enrolled in clinical trials.

When discussing trials with patients, an emphasis is needed on how the proposed treatment—through a clinical trial—is not compromising patient care. Physicians, especially those in the community, need to be informed of available protocols.

TABLE 10-2: TEN THINGS TO KNOW ABOUT CANCER TREATMENT TRIALS

1. Each clinical trial tries to answer scientific questions and to find better ways to prevent, diagnose, or treat cancer in people.

2. In cancer research, a clinical trial is designed to show how a particular anticancer strategy—a promising drug, a gene therapy treatment, a new diagnostic test, or a possible way to prevent cancer—affects the people who receive it.

3. A clinical trial is one of the stages of a long and careful cancer research process. Getting promising results from testing a new drug on mice, for example, is a preliminary step to human research studies. Treatments that work well in mice do not always work well in people.

4. In treatment trials, participants receive high-quality cancer care and are among the first to benefit if a new approach is proven to work.

5. Each clinical trial has its own guidelines for who can participate. Generally, participants are alike in key ways, such as the type and stage of cancer, age, gender, and other factors.

6. New treatments under study are not always better than—or even as good as—standard care. They may also have unexpected side effects. Through a process called *informed consent,* potential participants learn about a study's treatments and tests and their possible benefits and risks before deciding whether to participate.

7. In treatment trials involving people who have cancer, placebos are very rarely used.

8. Many treatment trials are designed to compare a new treatment with a standard treatment. In these studies, patients are randomly assigned to one group or another.

9. Clinical trials enroll patients all over the country—in cancer centers, other major medical centers, community hospitals and clinics, physicians' offices, and veterans' and military hospitals in numerous cities and towns.

10. Health plans and managed care providers do not always cover all patient care costs in a study. What they cover varies by plan and by study. The research costs, such as data management, are covered by the study sponsor.

(CancerSource, 2005; NCI, 2006)

TABLE 10-3: NURSING CONSIDERATIONS: PREPARING PATIENTS TO ENROLL IN A CLINICAL TRIAL

Adhere to the ethical principle of beneficence (i.e., patient safety and freedom from harm)

- Identify patients' understanding of and participation in their health care decisions.

- Provide unbiased information when offering a clinical trial and be aware of conflicting agendas and patient misconceptions.

- Provide patients with the information necessary to make informed decisions. (Many patients with cancer are not aware of nonstandard treatments, the unproven nature of the drug or treatment being investigated, and the uncertainty of possible risks and benefits.)

- Educate the patient to the best of his or her knowledge and report these findings to the research nurse or principal investigator.

- Assess the educational and psychosocial needs of patients on a continual basis, including understanding of the response to current and prospective treatment options.

- Provide needed reassurance to patients that clinical trial enrollment does not mean that the patient will be abandoned during the clinical trial period.

(CancerSource, 2005; NCI, 2006)

In a 2004 study, respondents asked about clinical trial recruitment reported that the most effective strategy for increasing public awareness of clinical trials was to highlight participants in past trials. They also stressed the value of increasing the visibility of clinical trials through campaigns sponsored by nonprofit organizations (Connolly, Schneider, & Hill, 2004).

Just in the informed consent process alone, nurses can be pivotal sources of support and clarity. Table 10-4 reviews elements to include in the patient's informed consent.

COVERAGE OF CLINICAL TRIALS

In 2000, Medicare began covering beneficiaries' patient care costs in clinical trials. Up-to-date information about what Medicare covers can be found on the website of the Centers for Medicare & Medicaid Services (formerly the Health Care Financing Administration; http://www.cms.hhs.gov).

Many states have now passed legislation or created special arrangements for patients' health

TABLE 10-4: SELECTED ELEMENTS OF INFORMED CONSENT

Treatment/Therapy
- Appropriate (understandable) explanation of the treatment or therapy and goal of therapy
- Known treatment benefits
- Expected outcome from the therapy or treatment
- Length of recovery from treatment
- Expected outcome if the patient's decision is to not pursue the therapy or treatment
- Possible complications and risks
- Other treatment options
- Circumstances when the physician or investigator may choose to stop treatment

Patient Rights
- Voluntary consent
- Right to refuse consent
- Right to withdraw consent—process of orderly termination
- Anticipated circumstances if treatment stops
- Confidentiality of records

Miscellaneous Elements
- Compensation if patient is injured or harmed during treatment
- Contact information regarding treatment, research (if study), patient rights, and compensation if patient is injured
- Additional costs to the patient (if applicable)

plans to provide coverage for care associated with clinical trials that is not covered by the plan's standard care coverage. Figure 10-2 identifies states with clinical trials provisions, as of March 2007. These laws and agreements do not cover the research costs associated with conduct of the trial, such as tests performed purely for research purposes.

SUMMARY

Nurses caring for patients enrolled in clinical trials should be aware of the phases of clinical trials, questions that patients may have about clinical trials, principles of informed consent, and out-of-insurance-plan coverage for a particular clinical trial. Using the networking and information-sharing capabilities of the Internet for clinical trials has significantly improved the processes of enrollment, data gathering, and data sharing.

FIGURE 10-2: STATES WITH PROVISIONS TO COVER SOME COSTS OF CARE ASSOCIATED WITH CLINICAL TRIALS

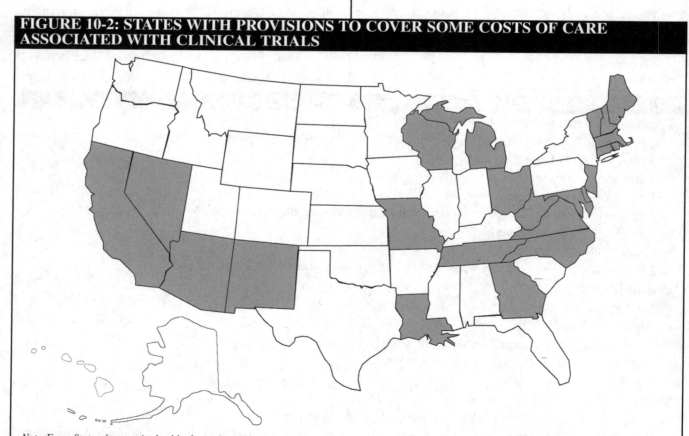

Note. From *States that require health plans to cover patient care costs in clinical trials* by National Cancer Institute, 2007. Retrieved May 29, 2007, from http://www.cancer.gov/clinicaltrials/learnign/laws-about-clinical-trial-costs

EXAM QUESTIONS

CHAPTER 10
Questions 38-41

Note: Choose the option that BEST answers each question.

38. Phase III clinical trials focus on

    a. the optimal dose.

    b. the optimal schedule.

    c. the treatment's effectiveness compared with standard therapies.

    d. the treatment's effectiveness for new indications.

39. One web-based database about clinical trials is available on the Internet at

    a. http://www.centerwatch.com

    b. http://www.cancer.org

    c. http://www.cms.hhs.gov

    d. http://www.cancer.com

40. A patient may be concerned about enrolling in a clinical trial because of the

    a. benefits.

    b. risks.

    c. pain.

    d. certainty.

41. When caring for a patient enrolled in clinical trials, one of the roles of the nurse is to

    a. address questions about the trial.

    b. offer the best randomized arm of the trial.

    c. provide decisions.

    d. provide comfort care.

REFERENCES

CancerSource. (2005). *Clinical trials.* Available from http://www.cancersource.com/clinicaltrials/

Connolly, N., Schneider, D., & Hill, A. (2004). Improving enrollment in cancer clinical trials. *Oncology Nursing Forum, 31*(3), 610–614.

Delaney, P. (2006). *Understanding clinical trials from the patient's perspective.* Retrieved May 30, 2007, from http://www.fda.gov/oashi/cancer/pdart.html

Harris, G. (2006, March 6). New drugs hit the market, but promised trials go undone. *The New York Times,* p. 8.

Lara, P., Jr., Paterniti, D., Chiechi, C., Turrell, C., Morain, C., Horan, N., et al. (2006). Evaluation of factors affecting awareness of and willingness to participate in cancer clinical trials. *Journal of Clinical Oncology, 23*(36), 9282–9289.

Lee, C. (2005). Clinical trails in cancer. Part 1. Biomedical, complementary, and alternative medicine: Finding active trials and results of closed trials. *Clinical Journal of Oncology Nursing, 8*(5), 531–535.

National Cancer Institute. (2006). *Ten things to know about cancer treatment trials.* Retrieved October 31, 2006, from http://www.cancer.gov/clinicaltrials/learning/things-to-know-treatment-trials

National Cancer Institute. (2007). *States that require health plans to cover patient care costs in clinical trials.* Retrieved May 29, 2007, from http://www.cancer.gov/clinicaltrials/learnign/laws-about-clinical-trial-costs

National Institutes of Health. (2006). *An introduction to clinical trials.* Available from http://clinicaltrials.gov

Pharmaceutical Research and Manufacturers of America. (2005). *399 medicines in development offer hope in the war on cancer.* Retrieved October 31, 2006, from http://www.phrma.org/files/Cancer%20Survey.pdf

CHAPTER 11

SIDE EFFECTS OF CANCER TREATMENT

CHAPTER OBJECTIVE

After completing this chapter, the reader will be able to recognize the most common side effects associated with cancer treatment and identify appropriate nursing interventions.

LEARNING OBJECTIVES

After studying this chapter, the reader will be able to

1. recognize interventions to manage the effects of myelosuppression.

2. identify strategies to minimize constipation.

3. indicate strategies to help patients gain weight.

4. list patient-focused teaching points about sun exposure.

5. cite two interventions to help relieve fatigue.

INTRODUCTION

Patients undergoing treatments for malignancies can experience side effects or complications from their disease. They also can experience side effects from treatments, due to scheduling, dosing, or tumor response to the treatment.

Side effects frequently are the unfortunate by-products of treatment because the treatment targeting the malignancy also affects normal cells. Moreover, the intensity and aggressiveness of treat-ment—and the combination of treatment modalities used—usually affect the severity of the patient's experience of side effects. Treatment primarily affects the fastest growing cells—those in the bone marrow, gastrointestinal (GI) tract, mucous membranes, hair follicles, and reproductive cells.

In managing side effects, nurses can call on an extensive body of knowledge and interventional strategies, based on evidence-based practice guidelines and years of health care professionals' experience in caring for patients. The nurse's role in managing side effects includes anticipating, preventing, and assessing side effects; intervening as appropriate; and educating patients and their families about side effects. The nurse, as the patient's guide before and during the experience of these side effects, is an important contributor to patient compliance with therapy. If side effects are unmanaged, the patient's compliance with therapy can decline (Krumwiede et al., 2004; West & Mitchell, 2004; Wickham, 2004).

The following review of selected side effects provides basic information about each side effect and suggested nursing interventions. (Table 11-1 provides a broad list of cancer treatment side effects.)

Included in this chapter are sections on the most commonly experienced symptoms and side effects, which include myelosuppression, GI effects (nausea and vomiting, diarrhea, constipation, mucositis, and stomatitis), alterations in nutrition, cutaneous changes (skin and hair), fatigue, and miscellaneous

TABLE 11-1: MISCELLANEOUS SIDE EFFECTS OF CANCER TREATMENT

- Alopecia (hair loss)
- Anemia
- Anxiety
- Appetite loss
- Bladder incontinence
- Bone issues
- Chemo brain
- Constipation
- Depression
- Diarrhea
- Dry mouth
- Fatigue
- Fluid imbalance
- Hot flashes
- Hypersensitivity
- Infection
- Lymphedema
- Mouth sores/mucositis
- Nausea and vomiting
- Neurological disturbances
- Neutropenia
- Pain
- Peripheral neuropathy
- Radiation therapy skin changes
- Sexual issues
- Shortness of breath
- Sleep-wake issues
- Problems with swallowing
- Thrombocytopenia
- Wound care

side effects from treatment (hemorrhagic cystitis, neurotoxicity, cardiac toxicity, hot flashes, cognitive dysfunction, and nephrotoxicity). Pain is reviewed in Chapter 22. When caring for individual patients, the nurse should always consult cancer therapy references, the drug protocol, and other reliable sources of information to best manage side effects.

MYELOSUPPRESSION

Many cytotoxic agents and biologic therapies can affect the patient's hematopoietic system, the bone marrow's ability to produce blood cells. All blood cells develop from immature cells known as *stem cells*. The majority of stem cells are found within the bone marrow. Most of these stem cells mature in the bone marrow and are then released into the bloodstream (see Figure 11-1). Stem cells are the precursors of white blood cells (WBCs), red blood cells (RBCs), and platelets (Eggenberger, Krumwiede, Meiers, Bliesmer, & Earle, 2004). When patients experience myelosuppression (a condition in which bone marrow activity decreases), they can experience neutropenia, anemia, and thrombocytopenia (Eggenberger et al., 2004).

Neutropenia

WBCs are responsible for fighting infection. Leukopenia is a decrease in the number of WBCs. (WBCs are also called *leukocytes*). Neutrophils or granulocytes, a subset of WBCs, are the body's first line of defense against infection, launching an allergic or inflammatory response. In a normal person, 60% of WBCs are neutrophils.

Neutropenia is a decrease in neutrophils. (Neutropenia can occur with and without the presence of infection.) It is potentially the most serious complication of myelosuppression. Patients with hematopoietic malignancies, such as leukemia, have abnormal WBC (and neutrophil) counts. Patients receiving radiation therapy (RT) or chemotherapy for their tumors can become neutropenic because their therapies affect the hematopoietic system, destroying the rapidly dividing hematopoietic cells (Larson & Nirenberg, 2004).

The normal range for a neutrophil count is 2,000 to 6,000 cells/mm^3. Once the number of neutrophils falls below 1,500 cells/mm^3, the patient is considered neutropenic and is susceptible to infection.

Table 11-2 shows how to calculate absolute neutrophil count (ANC). ANC is an important ongoing measurement of the patient's neutrophils and thus the patient's ability to fight infection. ANC indicates how

FIGURE 11-1: HEMATOPOIESIS CHART

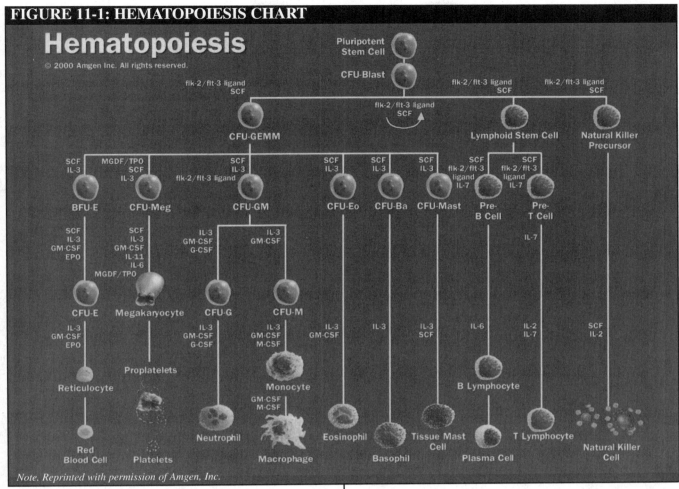

Note. Reprinted with permission of Amgen, Inc.

well the patient is doing with treatment. Therefore, monitoring ANC is important.

Alkylating chemotherapy agents can produce prolonged periods of myelosuppression or failure of bone marrow recovery (Krumwiede et al., 2004), which can require patient hospitalization. The development of hematopoietic growth factors (e.g., granulocyte-macrophage colony-stimulating factor and granulocyte colony-stimulating factor) boosts the return of functioning neutrophils, thus accelerating the return of a functioning immune system. Growth factors have decreased the risk of febrile neutropenia and acute infection (Amgen, 2006; Cappozzo, 2004; West & Mitchell, 2004). Side effects of colony-stimulating factors can include bone pain and signs of an allergic reaction.

By far, the most important way to prevent infection is hand washing—by the patient, staff, and caregivers. Other neutropenia precautions are listed in

Table 11-3. Because some patients can take these suggestions to the extreme, nurses should provide practical advice for following the precautions so that patients can still enjoy life and keep healthy (West & Mitchell, 2004).

Other WBCs types are also monitored when patients are diagnosed with hematologic malignancies or during chemotherapy or targeted therapy treatments—to determine the effects of treatment:

- **Lymphocytes** are in the blood as well as in the lymph nodes, spleen, and thymus. As part of the immune system, they interact in complex ways to produce specific antibodies. When the body produces antibodies, those antibodies attack "foreign" substances in the body. Antibodies and other cells and processes regulate the immune system.

- **Monocytes** move into tissues and develop into macrophages. They play a role in phagocytosis, the cleaning up of cells from the body.

TABLE 11-2: CALCULATING ABSOLUTE NEUTROPHIL COUNT

1. From laboratory results, determine WBC count. (This is the percentage of segmented neutrophils and bands.)

2. Use this formula to determine ANC:

$$ANC = \frac{(\% \text{ segments} + \% \text{ bands}) \times WBC}{100}$$

Example: $ANC = \dfrac{(22 + 3) \times 4000}{100}$

Results: $ANC = 1,000/mm^3$

Normal Ranges

Cell type	Relative value (%)	Absolute value (cells/mm^3)
Neutrophils	60–70	3,000–7,000
Eosinophils	1–4	50–400
Basophils	0.5–1.0	25–100
Lymphocytes	20–30	1,500–4,000
Monocytes	2–6	100–500

Infection Risk

ANC = 1500–2000	Not significant
ANC = 1000–1500	Minimal risk
ANC = 500–1000	Moderate risk
ANC = < 500	Severe risk

- **Eosinophils** play an important role in phagocytosis, an inflammatory process that clears debris such as bacteria, fungi, and viruses, from the body.

- **Basophils** play a significant role in allergic reactions.

Anemia

Anemia is when RBC count falls below a normal, functioning range. RBCs are also called *erythrocytes*.

RBCs have two important functions: They carry oxygen from the lungs to cells throughout the body, and they carry carbon dioxide and other cellular waste products out of the circulation. The life span of an RBC is approximately 120 days.

Anemia may cause weakness, fatigue, shortness of breath, and palpitations or an irregular heartbeat. Anemia associated with cancer therapy is not usu-

ally a severe problem. For patients on certain regimens, however, the risk of anemia increases.

Transfusion of RBCs or use of the growth factor erythropoietin (Epogen, Procrit) can diminish the degree of anemia. Patient fatigue may be correlated with the degree of anemia as well as with other factors.

Patients at risk for anemia should be instructed in ways to decrease fatigue. Methods to address fatigue include getting sufficient rest, eating protein-rich foods and, in some cases, adding nutritional supplements to the diet (Nail, 2004). Fatigue is further reviewed later in this chapter.

The growth factor erythropoietin stimulates and accelerates RBC production. Side effects of erythropoietin include hypertension, skin rashes, and blood clots.

Thrombocytopenia

Thrombocytopenia occurs when platelet levels fall. It can be a complication of both the underlying cancerous condition and of the chemotherapy used to treat malignancies. Platelets, or thrombocytes, help to prevent bleeding by mobilizing clot formation at the site of injury.

A normal platelet range is 150,000 to 400,000/mm^3. The risk of thrombocytopenia increases when platelet count is in the range of 40,000 to 60,000/mm^3. The risk of spontaneous bleeding occurs when the count is less than 20,000/mm^3 and can be fatal at less than 10,000/mm^3.

Indications of thrombocytopenia include petechiae, easy bruising, oozing from gums or other tissues, and frank bleeding (especially from the GI tract). Patients should be advised to avoid potentially traumatic activities, especially falls. Trauma to the head, particularly when platelet count is low (< 5,000/mm^3), can be serious. A low platelet count should be correlated with a possible intracranial bleed or subdural hematoma. Patients should also avoid activities in which cuts or bruises can occur, such as using a straight razor or a hard toothbrush. Table 11-4 lists bleeding precautions.

When thrombocytopenia is severe, patients receive platelet transfusions. The growth factor oprelvekin (Neumega) and thrombopoietin are agents that can stimulate more-rapid production of platelets (Friend & Pruett, 2004).

TABLE 11-3: NEUTROPENIA PRECAUTIONS FOR PATIENTS AND VISITORS

- **Wash your hands**. *Hand washing is the single most important and effective way to prevent infection.*
- If you are a visitor, you should wash your hands before and after any direct contact with a patient.
    - All visitors should be required to wash all surfaces of their hands for a minimum of 15 seconds prior to entering a patient's room.
    - Wash all surfaces of the hands with antibacterial soap for at least 15 seconds; then thoroughly rinse with water. Any time you wash your hands, use disposable paper towels to dry them and use that paper towel to turn off the faucet.
- Avoid fresh fruits, vegetables, flowers, dried flowers, and live plants.
- Avoid people recently vaccinated with live organisms or viruses (e.g., polio) for 48 to 72 hours.
- Avoid pet excreta (e.g., litter boxes, fish tanks and aquariums, turtle bowls).
- Avoid people who have a transmissible illness (e.g., chicken pox, herpes zoster, influenza, common cold).
- Use good personal hygiene: hand washing, daily bathing, mouth care after meals and at bedtime (per oral care protocol), and perineal care after voiding and bowel movements.
- Once therapy begins (e.g., chemotherapy, immunosuppressant therapy, RT), wear a face mask when you are outside of your room or home.
- Use high-efficiency particulate air (HEPA) filters to specially clean room air. These filters are used in rooms for all allogenic transplant recipients. For the filter to be effective, keep the door of a HEPA filter room closed at all times. The filter should be in the center of the room, with enough space around it so that air can circulate.
- Prevent trauma to the skin and mucous membranes:
    - Do not use enemas, rectal thermometers, or tampons.
    - Prevent constipation by exercising and increasing fluid and fiber intake. Notify the transplant physician or nurse if you have not had a bowel movement in the past 3 days.
    - Prevent pressure sores by exercising frequently and changing positions, such as getting out of bed and sitting up in chair.
    - Use only an electric razor to shave unwanted body hair.
    - Promote healing of all wounds by cleansing and dressing them as directed.
- Use a water soluble lubricant during intercourse and practice good postcoital hygiene. Avoid intercourse during periods of neutropenia.
- Maintain optimal function of the respiratory system:
    - Exercise daily (e.g., walking, riding stationary bike).
    - Do coughing and deep-breathing exercises to decrease the risk of pneumonia.
    - When activity is low, use an incentive spirometer as directed by the transplant nurse.
- Report:
    - temperature higher than 100.4° F (38° C)
    - shaking chills
    - pain when urinating
    - pain when breathing
    - respiratory congestion or the appearance of sputum
    - pain.

(Eggenberger et al., 2004; Krumwiede et al., 2004; West & Mitchell, 2004)

TABLE 11-4: BLEEDING PRECAUTIONS (< 20,000 cells/mm³ platelet count)

Use
- Lotions and creams on the skin
- Only an electric razor
- Soft-bristled toothbrush
- Alcohol-free mouthwash
- Stool softeners
- Shoes when walking

Avoid
- Dental toothpicks
- Aspirin or aspirin-containing medications
- Invasive procedures, as much as possible (enemas, rectal temperatures, suppositories, bladder catheterization, venipunctures, fingersticks, subcutaneous or intramuscular injections)
- Overinflation of blood pressure cuff

Other Considerations
- Apply pressure to puncture sites for at least 5 minutes; use icepacks—when appropriate—to decrease bleeding.
- Support methods to avoid forceful coughing, nose blowing, sneezing, and vomiting.
- Remove items from the environment that have the potential to cause trauma (pad side rails, rearrange furniture to eliminate sharp corners).

(Camp-Sorrell, 2005; Gobel, 2006)

FATIGUE

Fatigue can be one of the most disturbing and frequently reported side effects of cancer treatment. Almost all cancer patients report that they experience fatigue.

Fatigue for patients with cancer is a weariness that cannot be relieved with sleep or enough rest. Cancer-related fatigue is usually not linked to activity. It can be caused by physiologic deficits (e.g., anemia, hypoxia), emotional fatigue (e.g., grief, anxiety), or treatments (e.g., steroids, various chemotherapies, RT) (Nail, 2004; Stricker, Drake, Hoyer, & Mock, 2004).

The nurse should assess fatigue using tools similar to those used with pain assessment (i.e., 0-to-10 scales). Fatigue is what the patient says it is; appearance, activity, and affect of the patient are not valid indicators of the quality or intensity of fatigue.

Energy-sparing behaviors help minimize the problems associated with fatigue. Approaches to address fatigue are listed in Table 11-5.

TABLE 11-5: WAYS TO REDUCE CANCER-RELATED FATIGUE

- Address anemia by dealing with its root cause.
- Boost hemoglobin with transfusions or erythropoietin.
- Conserve energy by organizing tasks and managing activities of the day with a focus on simple, limited priorities.
- If possible, promote exercise or mild physical activity.
- Allow enough sleep and effective rest periods.
- Encourage the patient to eat balanced, nutritious foods and supplement meals with vitamins or minerals (based on physician or dietician guidance).

(Nail, 2004; Porock, Beshears, Hinton, & Anderson, 2005)

GASTROINTESTINAL EFFECTS

GI side effects can occur with many cancer treatments. GI effects include nausea and vomiting, diarrhea, constipation, and inflammation of the mucous membrane and GI tract (mucositis and stomatitis). In most cases, these side effects can be effectively managed. As part of management, the nurse anticipates these side effects so that they are not an inevitable part of cancer treatment.

Nausea and Vomiting

Cancer patients can experience nausea, vomiting, and retching during the course of their disease and its treatment. Nausea is an unpleasant sensation experienced when a person feels as if he or she must vomit. Vomiting is an involuntary reflex that results in the forceful expulsion of gastric contents. Retching occurs when the stomach contains no gastric contents to expel (Viale, 2005).

Those at risk for nausea and vomiting include patients:

- receiving high-emetic-potential treatment regimens, such as cyclophosphamide (Cytoxan), cisplatin (ciplatinum, Platinol), and selected biotherapies, especially interleukin-2 (Proleukin)

- undergoing RT to treatment fields involving the brain, large portions of the abdomen, the pelvic area, the epigastrium, or the whole body

- with metastases to the central nervous system or liver

- who have intestinal inflammatory disease

- who have fluid and electrolyte imbalances (e.g., hypercalcemia), intestinal obstruction (e.g., ileus), infections, sepsis, or uremia

- receiving antibiotics, narcotic analgesics, or long-acting bronchodilators.

(Rittenberg & Cunningham, 2005)

Pathophysiology

In general, nausea precedes vomiting. Physiologic changes accompanying nausea include an increase in respirations, increased heart rate, dilated pupils, and pallor. Patients may also have decreased gastric motility. The feeling of nausea may persist even after the patient vomits, although many patients feel relief after vomiting (Rittenberg & Cunningham, 2005; Wickham, 2004).

Vomiting can be caused by many factors:

- The vomiting center, located in the medulla, is stimulated by input from a variety of pathways via neurotransmitters, such as acetylcholine, dopamine, histamine, serotonin, and norepinephrine. The vomiting center includes the chemoreceptor trigger zone in the fourth ventricle and the true vomiting center.

- Stimuli in the GI tract can trigger a response from the body's vomiting center.

- The patient's cerebral cortex can trigger a nausea and vomiting response when affected by noxious stimuli, such as odors and tastes.

When nausea and vomiting are severe and protracted, other complications can arise. Prolonged vomiting can lead to anorexia, dehydration, malnutrition, metabolic imbalances, depression, and poor compliance with treatment (Rittenberg & Cunningham, 2005; Wickham, 2004).

Perceptions

The perception that all patients on chemotherapy experience nausea and vomiting stems from the early history of chemotherapy treatment. Those memories make some people assume that all chemotherapy causes severe nausea and vomiting. Fortunately, nausea and vomiting are no longer inevitable side effects of treatment thanks to the appropriate choice and schedule of antiemetic drugs and a plan to manage nausea early in the patient's experience (Viale, 2005).

In addition, each patient has his or her own threshold for the development of nausea and vomiting. That threshold is influenced by the disease process and treatment regimen.

Types

Nausea and vomiting can be acute, delayed, or anticipatory. Acute (and breakthrough) nausea and vomiting generally begin a few hours after treatment and last for approximately 24 hours.

The cancer treatment—its route of administration, dose, frequency and, for RT, the treatment field irradiated—influences the nausea and vomiting experience. Selected cytotoxic agents can cause a predictable nausea and vomiting response (Rittenberg & Cunningham, 2005; Wickham, 2004). (See Chapter 6.)

Delayed nausea and vomiting follow treatment, usually about a day later. The peak of their severity can last 48 to 72 hours. If nausea and vomiting continue, they usually pass after 7 days.

Anticipatory nausea and vomiting, a learned or conditioned response, begins before treatment starts, sometimes as early as the day before. Patients with poor emesis control are at greatest risk for anticipatory nausea and vomiting. Patients who achieve effective emesis control during the first 24 hours after treatment are less likely to experience this type of nausea and vomiting for subsequent courses of therapy. Treatment for anticipatory nausea and vomiting may include administration of lorazepam (Ativan) to decrease anxiety and methods to relax, which provide a sense of control (Wickham, 2004).

Interventions

Nursing care includes assessment, support, and education as well as administration of antiemetics. Care includes monitoring for fluid and electrolyte imbalances and anorexia by checking lab values. Other interventions include:

- placing an emesis basin within easy reach of the patient

- offering the patient mouth rinses to cleanse after each vomiting episode

- teaching the patient to avoid stimuli that can begin an anticipatory nausea and vomiting response, such as sights, sounds, smells, or simply the thought of chemotherapy.

    As part of an overall antiemetic management plan, consider adding or substituting amnesiacs, tranquilizers, or psychotropic medications. (An effective antiemetic regimen generally incorporates more than one agent and involves combining agents with different actions and side effects.) (Viale, 2005; Wickham, 2004).

Table 11-6 lists some common nonpharmacologic interventions for managing nausea and vomiting. Antiemetics are generally administered 30 to 60 minutes before the treatment and, depending on the emetogenic potential of the treatment, may be administered around the clock for up to 24 hours after treatment (Rittenberg, 2004). (See Table 11-7 for a list of commonly used aniemetic agents.)

Patients younger than age 30 are more susceptible to developing dystonic reactions from antiemet-

---

TABLE 11-6: NONPHARMACOLOGIC INTERVENTIONS FOR NAUSEA AND VOMITING

Behavioral
- Biofeedback, deconditioning or desensitization, distraction or diversion, guided imagery, hypnosis, and relaxation

Dietary
- Eating small, frequent meals and easily digested foods (e.g., toast, crackers, rice)

- Avoiding fatty and spicy foods

- Avoiding eating or drinking favorite foods (some patients develop aversions to foods they associate with periods of nausea and vomiting)

- Maintaining fluid intake to prevent dehydration. (Begin by drinking clear liquids and then, if these are tolerated, try soups and broths as tolerated; flat carbonated beverages, popsicles, and gelatin are also often well-tolerated.)

Environment
- Creating a conducive environment, avoiding food odors that enhance the potential for nausea and vomiting, and avoiding unpleasant sights and smells (e.g., perfumes, hair spray)

(Rittenberg & Cunningham, 2005; Wickham, 2004)

---

ics, such as butyrophenones (droperidol) and phenothiazines (prochlorperazine). Studies show that patients who have a history of alcohol abuse or chronic heavy alcohol use are less likely to experience problems with nausea and vomiting. Patients who have a history of motion sickness are more likely to have problems with nausea and vomiting (Wickham, 2004).

In the majority of cases, the nurse has the knowledge and methods at hand to manage the risk and occurrence of nausea and vomiting (Rittenberg & Cunningham, 2005; Wickham, 2004).

Diarrhea

Those at risk for diarrhea are patients:
- with cancers affecting the GI tract

TABLE 11-7: ANTIEMETIC AGENTS USED TO PREVENT OR TREAT NAUSEA AND VOMITING

Agent	Proprietary Name	Classification of agent
droperidol	Droperidol	Dopamine receptor antagonist
prochlorperazine	Compazine	Phenothiazine
ondansetron	Zofran	Serotonin antagonist
granisetron	Kytril	Serotonin antagonist
dolasetron	Anzemet	Serotonin antagonist
chlorpromazine	Thorazine	Phenothiazine
lorazepam	Ativan	Benzodiazepine
dexamethasone	Decadron	Corticosteroid
metoclopramide	Reglan	Dopamine receptor antagonist
aprepitant	Emend	Neurokinin receptor antagonist
dronabinol	Marinol	Cannabinoid

- with fecal impaction causing obstruction
- with pancreatic tumors
- undergoing allogenic bone marrow transplantation from the effects of graft-versus-host disease on the gut
- undergoing cancer treatments, including selected biotherapies, 5-fluorouracil (5-FU), capecitabine (Xeloda), cytarabine (Ara-C, cytosine arabinoside), 5-azacytidine, hydroxyurea (Hydrea), plicamycin (mithramycin, Mithracin), irinotecan (Camptosar), mitotane (Lysodren), and methotrexate (Trexall Rheumatrex)
- undergoing RT to the abdomen or pelvis (diarrhea usually begins after cumulative doses of 2000 cGy)
- with resections of the GI tract, causing dumping syndrome or malabsorption
- with bowel infections (e.g., *Clostridium difficile* infection) and malabsorption
- receiving antibiotics or supplemental feedings
- with high levels of stress or anxiety.

(Bush, 2005; Engelking, 2004)

Pathophysiology

Diarrhea is the frequent passage of soft or liquid stools with or without discomfort. Normal bowel function varies from person to person. The normal bowel pattern may range from as much as three times per day to as infrequently as three times per week.

Food digestion, absorption of nutrients, and the passage of stool through the colon constantly damage the mucosal layer of the GI tract. Because the tract is lined with rapidly dividing cells, the mucosa is continually renewed. However, when cancer or cancer treatments interrupt the normal process of renewal, inflammation and edema can occur. As a result, the production of mucus may increase, which increases the motility of stool through the intestines. With this increased motility, there is insufficient time for absorption of nutrients, electrolytes, and water (Bush, 2005; Engelking, 2004).

Many factors affect the severity of diarrhea. It can be severe enough to require therapy to stop peristalsis and allow bowel recovery. It can be a dose-limiting toxic effect of therapy.

Profound diarrhea often leaves patients feeling weak and exhausted. Skin integrity may become compromised, and the perianal area may become painful. Patients may express feelings of embarrassment. Their quality of life is disrupted (Bush, 2005; Engelking, 2004).

Signs and Symptoms

The signs and symptoms of diarrhea are loose, watery stools; hyperactive bowel sounds; cramping; and bloating; flatus; and pain.

Interventions

Nursing interventions are designed to promote healing and comfort (see Table 11-8). Interventions are based on assessment information. Loss of elec-trolytes through severe and chronic diarrhea should be carefully monitored in order to assess for other metabolic or functional changes, such as alteration in heart rhythms. Table 11-9 lists antidiarrheal agents.

Constipation

Constipation may be caused by chemotherapy, opioids, lack of exercise, or insufficient nutrition; or it may be a complication of the disease process.

TABLE 11-8: INTERVENTIONS FOR DIARRHEA

- Monitor intake and output.
- Monitor electrolyte levels.
- Weigh the patient.
- Maintain an accurate record of episodes of diarrhea.
- Test the stool for occult blood.
- Send stool samples for culture as ordered.
- Gently cleanse the patient's rectal area. Use warm water, rinse well, and pat dry.
- Apply barrier-type creams, ointments, or skin sealants (e.g., A & D Ointment, Soothe and Cool, Bard Protective Barrier) to protect skin and mucous membranes and promote healing.
- Administer total parenteral nutrition or fluids for hydration as necessary for treatment of severe and per-sistent diarrhea.
- Apply local anesthetics (e.g., Tucks®) as needed.
- Administer systemic medications for pain relief as needed.
- Administer antidiarrheals as ordered. Antidiarrheals are usually given every 4 to 6 hours around the clock or after each liquid bowel movement. The medication should be discontinued within 12 hours once the diarrhea subsides. Examples of antidiarrheals are opium derivatives (e.g., paregoric, tincture of opium), diphenoxylate hydrochloride (Lomotil), and loperamide hydrochloride (Imodium).
- To increase bulk, administer a fiber supplement (e.g., Metamucil).
- Support the patient psychologically.
- Patients should be encouraged to take these measures:
  – Eliminate foods that irritate or stimulate the GI tract.
  – Eat small, frequent meals.
  – Eat slowly and chew thoroughly.
  – Eat a low-residue diet, which increases absorption and decreases bowel irritation. Low-residue foods include bananas, applesauce, white rice, noodles, broth, bouillon, consomme, gelatin, and white bread. A nutritionist can provide a list of additional low-residue foods and beverages.
  – Avoid milk and milk products.
  – Avoid foods that are too hot or too cold. Extreme temperatures may stimulate GI activity or aggravate diarrhea.
  – Drink at least 3,000 ml of fluid each day. Gatorade; weak, tepid tea; gelatin; caffeine-free drinks; and flat, carbonated beverages are usually well tolerated. If diarrhea is severe, clear liquids may be neces-sary until the diarrhea resolves.
  – Apply heat to the abdomen to relieve cramping.
  – Take sitz baths.
  – Wear loose-fitting clothes that allow the rectal area to be exposed to air.
  – Schedule and use rest periods.
  – Decrease stress, because stress increases GI motility.

TABLE 11-9: AGENTS TO TREAT DIARRHEA
Absorbents
Charcoal
Kaolin + pectin (generic or branded [e.g., Kaopectate])
Anticholinergics
Atropine
Belladonna
Scopolamine
Antisecretory agents
Bismuth subsalicylate (e.g., Pepto-Bismol)
Octreotide acetate (Sandostatin)
Prednisone
Sulfasalazine
Opioids
Tincture of opium
Diphenoxylate

Those at risk for constipation are patients:

- receiving opioids for pain or therapy

- receiving neurotoxic chemotherapeutic agents, antidepressants, tranquilizers, or muscle relaxants

- taking antinausea medications in the category of 5HT-3 antagonists (e.g., ondansetron [Zofran])

- with intestinal obstruction or ileus (in these cases, intervention and discontinuation of the drug are necessary).

(Davison, 2006; Massey, Haylock, Curtiss, 2004)

Pathophysiology

Constipation occurs when bowel peristalsis becomes static. Its origin can be from the disease process or from opioids, which slow down GI motility.

Patients who are at risk for constipation may have been treated with chemotherapeutic drugs with potential neurotoxic effects, such as vinblastine (Velban), vincristine (Oncovin), docetaxel (Taxotere), paclitaxel (Taxol), cisplatin (Platinol), and vinorelbine (Navelbine). Constipation may be a sign of paralytic ileus from severe neurotoxic side effects of chemotherapy treatment.

Interventions

Based on a thorough assessment, nursing care for constipation includes prevention and management measures. Strategies include:

- support of a regular bowel management program: schedule for toileting, privacy, comfort, regular exercise

- increase in dietary bulk, fluids, and exercise, as tolerated

- administration of prescribed laxatives.

(Davison, 2006; Massey et al., 2004)

MUCOSITIS

Mucositis is a general term used to describe inflammation of the mucosa, which lines the body passages and cavities. The term *stomatitis* refers to oral mucositis, which is an inflammation of tissue in the mouth and salivary glands (Eilers, 2004).

The terms *mucositis* and *stomatitis* are often used interchangeably. Mucositis can progress to ulcerations, which can cause alterations in nutrition, sleep disturbance, and diminished quality of life.

Those at risk include patients:

- with head and neck cancer

- receiving RT or concurrent RT and chemotherapy (RT involving head, neck, and total-body irradiation can cause mucositis and stomatitis. Factors affecting the degree of mucositis or stomatitis include type of radiation, fraction per dose, total dose, time between fractions, type of tissues irradiated, size of the treatment field, and the anatomic structures exposed to radiation. Signs and symptoms usually resolve within 3 weeks after the end of therapy)

- who have had surgery of the head and neck for treatment of cancer

- receiving multimodality therapy, such as RT therapy and chemotherapy

- with hematologic tumors, such as leukemia

(immunosuppression and myelosuppression increase the risk of complications associated with stomatitis, such as infections and bleeding; stomatitis usually resolves when WBC count returns to normal)

- receiving chemotherapy, including antitumor antibiotics (e.g., doxorubicin [Adriamycin], bleomycin [Blenoxane], antimetabolites [e.g., 5-FU], methotrexate [Mexate], cytarabine [cytosine arabinoside; Ara-C], mercaptopurine [6-MP]) or biotherapy, such as interleukin-2 (aldesleukin)

- who have altered nutritional status (malnutrition, cachexia, anorexia, nutritional deficiencies)

- with poor oral hygiene (e.g., preexisting periodontal disease) or irritating dentures

- who use alcohol or tobacco.

(Eilers, 2004)

Pathophysiology

Because the mucous membranes are constantly being renewed, they are vulnerable to the effects of cancer, cancer treatments, and the side effects of treatments. The cells of the epithelial layer of the mucous membranes are generally replaced every 7 to 14 days. Mucosal thinning and ulcerations occur when the rate of cell loss (by sloughing off) is greater than the rate of cell renewal.

Because mucous membranes are barriers to microorganisms, any alteration in their integrity is an opening for organisms and increases the risk of infection (Cawley & Benson, 2005).

Signs and Symptoms

Signs and symptoms of oral mucositis include dry, rough, cracked, ulcerated, and bleeding lips. Drying of the mucosa, edema, erythema, swelling, and ulceration may occur in the oral cavity. Saliva may be profuse and watery in the early stages, then become thick and ropy, and finally be lacking. Because of mucositis, the patient can become more susceptible to bacterial and fungal infections. Patients may experience tenderness, a burning sen-

sation, pain, increased sensitivity to acidic and spicy substances, difficulty swallowing, and a decrease in oral intake. Maintaining a patent airway may be difficult if stomatitis is severe. In extreme cases, intubation may be necessary to protect the airway until the mucosal lining returns.

Stomatitis can begin 3 to 5 days after chemotherapy treatment, peak around 7 to 10 days, and begin to resolve over the next week with proper management (Cawley & Benson, 2005).

Interventions

Prevention of mucositis is key; using ice can be an effective prophylactic strategy. Nurses, in partnership with patients, can prevent mucositis or at least minimize its effects. Frequent assessment is essential. Table 11-10 lists strategies to manage stomatitis.

ALTERATIONS IN NUTRITION

Patients do not eat for many reasons. Among them are:

- fear of vomiting
- stomatitis
- changes in the ability to ingest and digest food
- anemia
- constipation
- fatigue
- infection
- inactivity and immobility
- physical discomfort and pain
- anxiety, depression, and discouragement.

Anorexia

A number of factors related to cancer contribute to alterations in the patient's nutritional status. Anorexia, or a loss of appetite, is often an initial indication of cancer and may be a sign of cancer recurrence or advanced or metastatic disease.

TABLE 11-10: MANAGING STOMATITIS (1 OF 2)

Assessment Components

- Recommending examination by a dentist before treatment of cancer begins.

- Checking the oral cavity at least twice a day; appearance of the mucosa, the quality of the voice, and the ability to swallow should be determined. Use consistent assessment criteria and grading systems to communicate with colleagues.

- Monitoring the patient's oral hygiene practices, ability to control secretions and maintain a patent airway, and hydration and nutritional status.

- Monitoring complete blood cell count.

Oral Care Recommendations

- Encourage a meticulous oral care program that is simple and easy for patients to follow. The frequency and consistency of oral care are more important than the actual products used. The optimum frequency depends on the severity of the stomatitis:
  - For mild stomatitis, every 4 hours while awake
  - For moderate stomatitis, every 2 hours while awake and every 4 hours during the night
  - For severe stomatitis, every 2 hours while awake and every 2 to 4 hours during the night
  - For no stomatitis or mild stomatitis, after meals and at bedtime.

- Promote rigorous use of mouth rinses that decrease or control stomatitis. Counsel patients to avoid using commercial mouthwashes, which often contain alcohol. Apply lip lubricants and avoid irritants to the oral cavity (tobacco, alcohol, poorly fitting dentures). Choices for mouth rinses include:
  - 1/2 tsp salt and sodium bicarbonate in 8 oz of warm water
  - Normal saline solution
  - 1 tsp of sodium bicarbonate in 8 oz of water
  - Sterile water
  - Hydrogen peroxide* diluted 1:1 with water or normal saline solution
    (*Use only when necessary to debride thick saliva or to clean teeth. Do not use longer than 48 hours. Chronic use impairs healing.)

- Use local antifungals as prescribed (prescribed prophylactically for patients at risk). Patients should not eat or drink anything for 30 minutes after using an oral antifungal. Choices include:
  - Clotrimazole, which is administered as a troche five times per day. To be effective, the troche must be dissolved completely in the mouth, a requirement that can make this agent inappropriate for patients with severe stomatitis.
  - Nystatin suspension is swished and swallowed; for patients unable to swallow, it can be swished and spit.
  - Intravenous antifungals such as fluconazole or amphotericin are used for more severe cases or when systemic infection is suspected.

- Use antivirals as prescribed. Patients receiving bone marrow transplants may take acyclovir prophylactically.

- Support dietary changes during periods of stomatitis. Encourage the patient to:
  - Eat bland, soft foods.
  - Eat cool foods (e.g., yogurt, ice cream), which may be soothing.
  - Avoid very hot foods.
  - Avoid acidic foods and beverages.

- Encourage oral intake and administer enteral or parenteral nutrition as ordered.

TABLE 11-10: MANAGING STOMATITIS (2 OF 2)

- Support the patient's comfort:
  - Offer ice chips and popsicles, which may be soothing.
  - Use topical anesthetics as indicated.
  - Administer systemic opioids in conjunction with topical anesthetics or when topical anesthetics are ineffective.
  - Apply antifibrolytics and administer platelets as ordered to control bleeding.
  - When needed, acquire samples for cultures.

(Cawley & Benson, 2005; Eilers, 2004)

Patients at risk for anorexia include:

- any cancer patient experiencing metabolic changes related to the tumor and wastes from tumor cell breakdown
- those with GI obstruction
- those diagnosed with head and neck cancer.

(Hartmuller & Desmond, 2004; Whitman, 2004)

Signs and Symptoms

Signs and symptoms of anorexia include malaise, pallor, weakness, and weight loss.

Cachexia is the most severe form of malnutrition in cancer patients. It is characterized by progressive loss of body weight and fat and lean muscle mass, anorexia, anemia, edema, hypoalbuminemia, hypoglycemia and glucose intolerance, and lactic acidosis. Patients with cachexia may also have mouth lesions, muscle and tissue wasting, dull sunken eyes, sparse and thinning hair, weight loss, and temporal wasting. Progressive weight loss is associated with a poor prognosis.

Most cancer patients experience anorexia, cachexia, or both at some time during the course of their disease. The prevalence and severity of cachexia increase as cancer progresses; cachexia can be a major contributor to the decline of patients with advanced stages of cancer.

Loss of Taste

Not wanting to eat can be due to loss of taste perception. Chemotherapeutic agents such as cisplatin, cyclophosphamide (Cytoxan), dactinomycin (Actinomycin D), 5-FU, methotrexate (Mexate), and mechlorethamine (nitrogen mustard) can affect the patient's sense of taste. Deficiencies in copper, nickel, niacin, vitamin A, and zinc are also associated with changes in taste.

RT to the head and neck destroys taste buds and the cells responsible for production of saliva. Surgery of the oral cavity, tongue, nasal area, olfactory nerve, and inner ear may also alter taste perception. Taste buds can regenerate, so the effects are generally temporary; however, permanent changes can occur.

Some patients report a decreased tolerance for bitter foods; these foods include meats, which can have high protein content. Patients also often have difficulty tasting sweet foods unless the foods are overly sweet.

For some, changes in taste can be temporary; taste may return to normal when the tumor responds to treatment. However, some report a lack of taste that extends indefinitely (Hartmuller & Desmond, 2004).

Interventions to Address Alterations in Nutrition

Interventions, based on assessment and a diet history, attempt to address the patient's disinterest in eating or inability to eat.

Finding high-protein, nutritious options can be challenging. Dieticians can offer their expertise and suggestions. If regular meals cannot address a patient's nutritional needs, enteral and parenteral nutrition may supplement or complete nutritional needs. Table 11-11 offers tips to address nutrition challenges and help patients gain weight. Patients' appetites may also be stimulated when patients are given megestrol acetate (Megace), dronabinol (Marinol), or low-dose steroids (Hartmuller & Desmond, 2004).

TABLE 11-11: STRATEGIES FOR PATIENTS TO GAIN WEIGHT
• Use smaller plates.
• Eat small, frequent meals (six to eight per day).
• Eat favorite foods.
• Eat protein and foods high in calories (e.g., cheese, peanut butter).
• Drink high-protein shakes and supplements; eat high-calorie snacks (e.g., ice cream).
• Experiment with new recipes.
• Avoid drinking fluids before and during meals. Fluids are filling and can create a feeling of satiety.
• Avoid fatty foods.
• Increase activity level, which may stimulate appetite.
• Drink a glass of wine, if permitted, to stimulate appetite.
• Monitor and record weight.
• Count calories.
• Use nutritional supplements.
• Marinate meats (e.g., in teriyaki sauce, soy sauce, or sweet marinades).
• Experiment with seasonings and different foods.
• Eat foods that are cold or at room temperature; they may be more palatable than hot foods.
• Eat acidic foods, pickled foods, citrus foods, citrus drinks, and lemon to stimulate taste buds.
• Experiment with spices.
• Consider zinc supplementation to stimulate taste and smell.
• Create a positive environment for eating.
• Eat with family and friends.
• Change settings for mealtime. For example, eat at a friend's house or at a restaurant.

CUTANEOUS CHANGES

Skin

The skin serves as the body's primary barrier against infection. Skin folds are particularly vulnerable to breakdown, allowing the development of infection. Highly vulnerable areas include the axillae, tissue under the breast, the groin, and the gluteal folds. Changes in the skin can range from mild (dryness, slight erythema) to severe (complete breakdown, sloughing that results in localized pain). Additionally, rashes or pruritus may develop (Goodman, 2004).

At Risk

The patient's underlying disease, treatment regimen, age, and nutritional status affect the type and severity of skin changes. Treatments can cause:

- **Hyperpigmentation.** Mechlorethamine, bleomycin, and 5-FU can cause the veins to darken. Nails can also become hyperpigmented, and their growth may be retarded.

- **Photosensitivity.** Treatments cause an increased sensitivity to sunlight. Among the chemotherapy agents that increase photosensitivity are dacarbazine, 5-FU, methotrexate, and vinblastine.

- **Radiation recall.** Several weeks after RT, some radiation patients experience radiation recall. Radiation recall is confined to the skin and tissue of the area (treatment field) that was irradiated. It often begins as erythema and can develop into blisters. It can progress to wet desquamation. Hyperpigmentation of skin can follow and can be permanent. Chemotherapeutic agent administration, such as doxorubicin, daunorubicin, or dactinomycin, can lead to radiation recall.

Most RT regimens are designed to minimize the risk of radiation recall. For patients treated with RT for spinal cord compression, the physician may delay for several weeks administration of chemotherapeutic agents associated with radiation recall (Nystedt et al., 2005; Wickline, 2004).

Interventions

Interventions and management strategies for skin changes are included in Table 11-12.

TABLE 11-12: MANAGING SKIN CHANGES

1. Complete frequent skin assessments. Include the onset of changes, the pattern and location of changes, and the severity of change. Examine the skin daily—especially the perineum and intravascular access sites—for breakdown and other reactions, such as rashes, bruising, and petechiae.

2. To maintain skin integrity, the nurse (and patient) should inspect and clean daily areas where the skin is changing or at risk for breakdown. To promote healing:
    *   Use mild hypoallergenic soaps (e.g., Aveeno, Dove, Neutrogena). Rinse the skin thoroughly. Pat dry. Avoid hot baths and showers.
    *   Use lotion to moisturize the skin. Avoid skin care products and lotions that contain alcohol or perfumes because they can dry the skin.
    *   Use water-soluble lotions (e.g., Lubriderm, Aquaphor, Soothe and Cool lotion). Patients receiving RT must remove all lotions before daily treatment.
    *   Avoid scratching the skin. Hydrocortisone 1% cream may be helpful for pruritus.
    *   Avoid exposure to sunlight, especially between 10 a.m. and 2 p.m. Wear protective clothing (e.g., long-sleeved shirts, hats) when exposed to sunlight. Apply sunscreen p-aminobenzoic acid–free and at least sun protection factor [SPF] of 15) to all exposed areas, especially the face, neck, and ears.

3. Have the patient undergoing RT avoid temperature extremes (e.g., hot, cold). Do not use perfumed lotions on the skin, and do not use tape over the treatment area. Patients who have severe skin reactions while receiving RT usually have their treatments temporarily stopped.

4. *Note:* Hyperpigmentation treatments do not exist; the condition is usually permanent. Dark-skinned patients who receive RT generally have more hyperpigmentation than lighter-skinned patients. (Dark-skinned patients have a greater amount of melanin in their skin.)

(Goodman, 2004; Wickline, 2004)

Hair

Alopecia, the loss of hair anywhere on the body, can have a profound impact on a patient's body image. Alopecia occurs because the hair follicles are rapidly dividing cells. Cancer treatments atrophy the hair bulb and can constrict the hair shaft, causing breaks.

The degree of hair loss with chemotherapy varies from thinning to complete loss, depending on the chemotherapy agent. In general, alopecia is temporary with selected chemotherapy agents; however, in some cases, it may be permanent.

Hair can grow back after the end of therapy, but the new hair may be fragile and break off easily. Many patients report that, when their hair returns, it is also a different color (lighter or darker) and has a different texture (Reeves, 2004).

At Risk

Only patients receiving certain chemotherapy agents experience thinning hair or lose their hair completely. Factors affecting the type and degree of hair loss are the chemotherapeutic agents and the dosage and intensity of the therapy. Hair loss can also include the eyebrows, eyelashes, and hair on the extremities and genitals.

For patients who receive RT, temporary alopecia may develop in the treatment area only. High doses of radiation (> 4500 to 6000 cGy), such as those used to treat brain tumors, may cause permanent alopecia (Reeves, 2004).

Interventions

Patients need support. Included in that support is teaching—about why and when they will lose their hair and information to prepare for their hair loss. This information can cover wigs, wig fittings, head covering options such as hats and scarves, scalp care, and make-up application. Support should boost self-esteem and encourage coping.

Once alopecia begins, patients should be instructed on how to care for their scalp and how to care for new hair once it appears. When caring for patients with anticipated or current alopecia, nurses need to encourage patients to:

- use gentle shampoos
- use soft brushes and combs with wide teeth
- avoid items that damage the hair, such as curling irons, hair dryers, electric curlers, permanents, and hair coloring
- minimize trauma to the hair and scalp and avoid items that place tension on the hair, such as hair bows, ponytail holders, and hair clips
- protect the scalp from sunburn. (apply sunscreen and wear protective covering [e.g., hat] when out in the sun)
- minimize heat loss from the scalp in cold weather by wearing a protective covering, such as a scarf or cap
- encourage expression of concern and feelings related to changes in body image (Reeves, 2004)
- seek support to help them feel better about their changed appearance. Programs, such as the American Cancer Society's "Look Good, Feel Better" program can provide that support.

CHEMOTHERAPY-RELATED TOXICITIES

Hemorrhagic Cystitis

Patients who receive cyclophosphamide (Cytoxan) are at risk for developing hemorrhagic cystitis (2% to 40%). Hemorrhagic cystitis can appear as slight hematuria or frank bleeding. The best way to manage cystitis is for the patient to continue to intake fluids and promote frequent voiding.

For example, ifosfamide (IFEX) can cause hemorrhagic cystitis; mesna taken with ifosfamide protects again cystitis (Berry, 2004).

Neurotoxicity

Neurotoxic side effects of treatment affect nerve endings and normal nerve function. With myalgias and arthralgias, pain occurs in the large joints.

Paresthesia—a tingling and numb feeling in the hands and feet—is a neurotoxic side effect of some chemotherapies. As a form of neurotoxicity, patients describe paresthesia and numbness distributed like a "glove and stocking."

Drugs that can cause neurotoxicity are vinblastine, vincristine, docetaxel, paclitaxel, cisplatin, and vinorelbine. If patients experience temporary neurotoxicity, the agent's dose is reduced; in some cases, dose limits do not eliminate permanent effects of neurotoxic agents, especially if the chemotherapy was given in high doses.

Medication administration, such as the tricylic antidepressant amitriptyline, which offers central nervous system (CNS) agent properties, can help alleviate neuropathic pain. Other pharmacologic interventions include nonsteroidal analgesics or opioids (Wilkes, 2004).

Administration of folic acid (B4) and amifostine (Ethyol) have shown some promise in treating neurotoxicities associated with oxaliplatin (Eloxatin) protocols for colorectal cancer (Grothey, 2005).

Cardiac Toxicity

Some chemotherapy agents, as well as RT to the chest, can cause abnormal conduction and function of the heart muscle. For example, anthracycline agents (e.g., doxorubicin, daunorubicin) can cause progressive cardiomyopathy, affecting cardiac tissue's contractility. Therefore, prevention of cardiomyopathy is the goal, by limiting the cumulative lifetime dose of the agent. For doxorubin, the maximum lifetime dose is 550 mg/m². For daunorubicin, the maximum lifetime dose is 600 mg/m² (Story, 2005).

Trastuzumab (Herceptin) is also known to contribute to the development of cardiomyopathy in patients receiving treatment. The pathogenesis of cardiotoxicity for patients receiving trastuzumab is not clearly understood. Researchers suggest that the agent may exacerbate damage to cardiac cells, either directly or by joining with other anthracycline chemotherapy agents. Some patients may also have a genetic susceptibility that contributes to cardiac toxicity when they receive certain agents (Bush & Griffin-Sobel, 2004).

Risk factors for developing cardiotoxicity from such agents are not clear, although age has been an associated factor. Obesity and hypertension are known risk factors for cardiac dysfunction with these chemotherapy agents (Bush & Griffin-Sobel, 2004).

Monitoring of cardiac function is the focus of nursing care for patients who develop cardiomyopathy from chemotherapy treatment. Patients who ultimately develop congestive heart failure (CHF) are treated with beta blockers and follow CHF protocols (Bush & Griffin-Sobel, 2004; Simpson, Herr, & Courville; 2004).

Hot Flashes

Hot flashes have been described as transient episodes of flushing, sweating, and heat, sometimes accompanied by palpitations, anxiety, and chills. They typically occur in healthy, postmenopausal women and breast cancer patients receiving therapy. Hot flashes are categorized as mild, moderate, and severe.

For those diagnosed with cancer, hot flashes usually are reported among women going through estrogen withdrawal, including those discontinuing hormone replacement therapy for chemoprevention or treatment (e.g., estrogen receptor modulators, aromatase inhibitors) of hormonally dependent cancers; those receiving chemotherapy; those undergoing oophorectomy; and those with radiation-induced ovarian damage. It is estimated that 50% to 75% of women in treatment for breast cancer experience hot flashes (Carpenter, 2005a).

For men, the most common risk factors include (a) endocrine therapies used for neoadjuvant or adjuvant treatment of prostate cancer and (b) orchiectomy for the treatment of advanced or metastatic prostate cancer. Hot flashes are also reported in women and men who are diagnosed with carcinoid tumors, medullary thyroid cancer, pancreatic cancer, or renal cell carcinoma. The cause of hot flashes is tumor secretion of various compounds (Carpenter, 2005a).

Studies continue to determine the best ways to alleviate hot flashes. To date, pharmacologic management of hot flashes includes prescribing selective serotonin reuptake inhibitors, antidepressants, anticonvulsants, and anti-adronergics. Nonpharmacologic treatment strategies include relaxation techniques (Carpenter, 2005b). Soy and black cohosh have been reported to relieve hot flashes, although they are contraindicated in women diagnosed with breast cancer (Lee, 2005; Montbriand, 2004).

More evidence-based studies are needed to establish effective treatments for hot flashes (Carpenter, 2005b).

Cognitive Dysfunction

Certain chemotherapy agents are associated with what is called "chemo brain," or impairments in cognitive function. These impairments can include changes in attention, concentration, and functioning (ability to plan, categorize, respond to changing stimuli, solve problems, achieve goals, be creative, be adaptive, or be flexible) as well as information processing, language, motor function, learning, and memory (Jansen, Miaskowski, Dodd, Dowling, & Kramer, 2005; Armstrong, Almadrones, & Gilbert, 2005).

The mechanisms for chemotherapy-induced impairments in cognitive function most likely are multifactorial. Although chemotherapy agents associated with cognitive dysfunction do not cross the blood-brain barrier, studies show that patients can have various cognitive impairments with certain chemotherapy administrations (Jansen et al., 2005).

Agents that have been associated with patients' experience of cognitive dysfunction include cyclophosphamide, doxorubicin, 5-FU, methotrexate, and paclitaxel. Cognitive dysfunction may be caused by processes triggered by chemotherapy in the system, which involve leukoencephalopathy (structural change in white matter, especially myelin), cytokine-induced inflammatory response, chemotherapy-induced anemia, chemotherapy-induced menopause, stress, and fatigue (Jansen et al., 2005).

Nurses need to be aware of this potential effect of chemotherapy and conduct ongoing assessments of patients. Although no valid and reliable clinical tools exist to assess for chemotherapy-induced cognitive impairments, nurses can evaluate patients for changes in attention and concentration or in the ability to perform routine cognitive tasks, such as balancing a checkbook (Jansen et al., 2005).

Observational assessment is the most sensitive and appropriate method to screen for cognitive dysfunction (Staat & Segatore, 2005). In the absence of clear and proven effective treatments for chemo brain, interventions are borrowed from strategies used for patients with brain injuries or cognitive impairment. No pharmacologic interventions have yet been proven as effective treatments (Armstrong et al., 2005; Staat & Segatore, 2005).

Nephrotoxicity

Nephrotoxicity can occur with administration of certain chemotherapy agents, such as cisplatin and ifosfamide, high-dose methotrexate, and mitomycin (Camp-Sorrell, 2006). To protect against nephrotoxicity, aggressive hydration accompanies the administration of these agents. The agent doses are also limited if the patient's renal function is compromised, based on increased serum creatinine levels, creatinine clearance, and other electrolyte levels. Chemoprotective agents, such as amifostine and dimesna, may be included as part of chemotherapy protocols to guard against nephrotoxicity and normal renal cell kill in an environment of tumor cell kill (Camp-Sorrell, 2006).

In addition to careful monitoring of laboratory values, nursing care to prevent nephrotoxicity also includes the careful monitoring of diuresis and urine output, which should accompany aggressive hydration.

SUMMARY

Various side effects from cancer treatment can be anticipated and managed. Among those discussed in this chapter were the effects of myelosuppression, GI disturbance, weight loss, skin and hair changes, fatigue, and chemotherapy-associated toxicities. Table 11-13 provides a summary of chemotherapy agents and their potential side effects. Nurses can call on well-known interventions to help patients avoid or minimize these side effects.

TABLE 11-13: SELECTED CHEMOTHERAPY AND TARGETED THERAPIES WITH SELECTED SIDE EFFECTS (1 OF 3)

(For a complete profile of toxicities and side effects, check recent drug references and agent web sites.)

Agent	Trade Name	Agent Class	Alopecia	Anemia	Constipation	Diarrhea	Mouth Sores	Nausea and Vomiting	Neutropenia	Peripheral Neuropathy	Pain (Joint or Bone) or Headache	Thrombocytopenia	Other Side Effects
alemtuzumab	Campath	MA			X		X	X	X	X	Headaches	X	
altretamine	Hexalen	AA							X		X		
anastrozole	Arimidex	H										X	Hot flashes
asparaginase	Elspar	E							X			X	
bevacizumab	Avastin	MA						X		X			Allergic reactions, proteinuria
bleomycin	Blenoxane	AAA	X				X	X					Fever, pulmonary fibrosis
busulfan	Myleran, Busulfex	AA			X					X			Hyperpigmentation, pulmonary fibrosis
capecitabine	Xeloda	AM			X		X			X			Fatigue, hand-and-foot syndrome
carboplatin	Paraplatin	AA	X		X				X	X	X	X	Ototoxicity, nephrotoxicity
carmustine, BCNU	BiCNU	N	X		X				X	X		X	Pulmonary fibrosis, elevated liver function tests (LFTs)
cetuximab	Erbitux	MA				X	X		X				Dermatologic toxicities
chlorambucil	Leukeran	AA			X				X		X		Decreased LFTs, pulmonary fibrosis
cisplatin	Platinol	AA			X	X			X		X		Ototoxicity, renal toxicity
cladribine, 2-CdA	Leustatin	AM							X	X	Headaches	X	Fever, rash
cyclophosphamide	Cytoxan, Neosar	AA	X		X				X	X		X	Hemorrhagic cystitis
cytarabine	Cytosar-U	AM			X		X	X	X	X		X	Skin rashes, ocular toxicities
dacarbazine	DTIC-Dome	AA			X			X	X	X		X	Hepatotoxicity
dactinomycin, actinomycin D	Cosmegen	AnA	X		X		X	X	X	X		X	
daunorubicin, daunomycin	Cerubidine	AAA	X		X			X	X	X		X	Hyperpigmentation, cardiac toxicity
docetaxel	Taxotere	PA	X		X					X		X	Fluid retention
doxorubicin	Adriamycin PFS	AAA	X		X			X		X		X	Cardiac toxicity, nail bed changes
doxorubicin liposomal	Doxil	AAA	X		X			X		X		X	Allergic reactions, hand-and-foot syndrome, cardiac toxicity
epirubicin	Ellence	AAA	X		X				X	X		X	Cardiac toxicity
etoposide, VP-16	VePesid	PA	X		X				X	X		X	
exemestane	Aromasin	H							X				Hot flashes
floxuridine (intra-arterial)	FUDR	AM	X		X				X	X			Weight loss, skin changes
fludarabine	Fludara	AM			X					X		X	
fluorouracil, 5-FU	Adrucil	AM					X	X	X		Headaches	X	Skin and nail bed changes

TABLE 11-13: SELECTED CHEMOTHERAPY AND TARGETED THERAPIES WITH SELECTED SIDE EFFECTS (2 OF 3)

(For a complete profile of toxicities and side effects, check recent drug references and agent web sites.)

Agent	Trade Name	Agent Class	Alopecia	Anemia	Constipation	Diarrhea	Mouth Sores	Nausea and Vomiting	Neutropenia	Peripheral Neuropathy	Pain (Joint or Bone) or Headache	Thrombocytopenia	Other Side Effects
fulvestrant	Faslodex	H				X	X		X			X	
gefitinib	Iressa	TKI					X		X				Rash
gemcitabine	Gemzar	AM	X						X	X		X	Flu-like syndrome
gemtuzumab	Mylotarg	MA			X				X			X	Veno-occlusive disease
hydroxyurea	Hydrea	MA			X		X		X	X		X	Dermatitis, dysuria
ibritumomab	Zevalin	MA			X				X			X	
idarubicin	Idamycin	AAA	X				X	X	X			X	Pink urine
ifosfamide	IFEX	AA	X	X					X			X	Urinary toxicity
imatinib	Gleevec	TKI					X		X			X	Fluid retention, muscle cramps
interferon alfa-2a	Roferon A	B						X	X			X	Flu-like syndrome
interferon alfa-2b	Intron A	B						X	X			X	Flu-like syndrome
interleukin-2, aldesleuken	Proleukin												Flu-like syndrome, CNS effects, renal dysfunction
irinotecan	Camptosar	TI			X		X		X	X		X	
L-asparaginase	Elspar	MA							X			X	Allergic reactions, rash
letrozole	Femara	H										X	Hot flashes, swelling, weight gain
leucovorin	Wellcovorin,	MA	X				X	X	X	X			
leuprolide acetate	Lupon	H										X	Numbness, dysuria
levamisole	Ergamisol	B					X		X				Metallic taste
lomustine, CCNU	CeeNU	N	X					X	X	X		X	
megestrol acetate	Megace	H									Headaches		Trouble sleeping
melphalan, L-PAM	Alkeran	AA			X				X	X			
mercaptopurine, 6-MP	Purinethol	AM						X					Fatigue, yellow eyes and skin
methotrexate	Trexall, Rheumatrex	AM			X			X	X	X		X	
mitomycin C	Mutamycin	AAA		A					X			X	
mitoxantrone	Novantrone	AAA	X	X	X		X	X	X	X		X	
oxaliplatin	Eloxatin	AA					X		X	X		X	
paclitaxel	Taxol	PA	X	X	X			X	X	X		X	
paclitaxel protein-bound particles	Abraxane	PA	X	X	X			X	X	X		X	
plicamycin, mithramycin	Mithracin	AAA							X			X	
procarbazine	Matulane	MA			X			X	X	X		X	
rituximab	Rituxan	MA										X	Allergic reactions
sorafenib	Nexavar	TKI											Hypertension, allergic reactions
streptozocin	Zanosar	N								X		X	Allergic reactions, nephrotoxicity

TABLE 11-13: SELECTED CHEMOTHERAPY AND TARGETED THERAPIES WITH SELECTED SIDE EFFECTS (3 OF 3)

(For a complete profile of toxicities and side effects, check recent drug references and agent web sites.)

Agent	Trade Name	Agent Class	Alopecia	Anemia	Constipation	Diarrhea	Mouth Sores	Nausea and Vomiting	Neutropenia	Peripheral Neuropathy	Pain (Joint or Bone)	Thrombocytopenia	Other Side Effects
tamoxifen	Nolvadex	H										X	Hot flashes, swelling
temozolomide	Temodar	AA							X		Headaches	X	Allergic reactions
teniposide, VM-26	Vumon	PA	X		X				X			X	
thalidomide	Thalomid	IA				X			X	X			Rash, fatigue
thioguanine, 6-TG	Thioguanine	AM					X	X				X	Hepatotoxicity
thiotepa	Thioplex	AA						X	X	X		X	
topotecan	Hycamtin	TI	X	X		X			X	X	X	X	Flu-like syndrome
toremifene	Fareston	H											Tumor flare, hot flashes, hypercalcemia
tositumomab	Bexxar	MA		X				X	X	X		X	Fever, urticaria, rash
trastuzumab	Herceptin	MA		X					X	X	X		Cardiomyopathy
vinblastine	Velban	PA	X			X			X		X	X	Rash
vincristine	Oncovin	PA			X						X		
vinorelbine	Navelbine	PA	X	X	X				X		X	X	Weight loss

Legend

AA = Alkylating agent
AAA = Anthracycline antitumor antibiotics
AM = Antimetabolite
AnA = Antitumor Antibiotic
B = Biotherapy
E = Enzyme
H = Hormone

IA = Immunomodulating agent
M = Miscellaneous agent
MA = Monoclonal antibody
N = Nitrosourea
PA = Plant alkaloid
TI = Topoisomerase inhibitor
TKI = Tyrosine kinase inhibitor

EXAM QUESTIONS

CHAPTER 11
Questions 42-46

Note: Choose the option that BEST answers each question.

42. The single most effective way to prevent infections in a patient with neutropenia is to

    a. apply hot packs frequently.
    b. promote hand washing.
    c. encourage a protein-rich diet.
    d. increase bed rest.

43. One way to minimize constipation is

    a. administering antiemetics.
    b. decreasing dietary bulk.
    c. increasing dietary bulk, fluids, and exercise.
    d. administering narcotics.

44. A method to help patients gain weight is to encourage the patient to

    a. eat small, frequent meals.
    b. eat three large meals daily.
    c. only eat in the evening.
    d. include spicy foods in the diet.

45. When teaching a patient about the risks of sun exposure, recommend

    a. limiting exposure to sunlight, especially between 10 a.m. and 2 p.m.
    b. using a sunscreen with an SPF of at least 8.
    c. staying inside.
    d. wearing sunglasses.

46. An intervention to help relieve fatigue is

    a. engaging in mild exercise.
    b. consuming frequent meals.
    c. sleeping more than 10 hours per night.
    d. using a personal trainer.

REFERENCES

Amgen. (2006). *Facts about neutropenia.* Retrieved October 31, 2006, from http://www.neulasta.com/professional/about_neulasta/facts_neutropenia.jsp

Armstrong, T., Almadrones, L., & Gilbert, M. (2005). Chemotherapy-induced peripheral neuropathy. *Oncology Nursing Forum, 32*(2), 305–311.

Berry, D. (2004). Bladder disturbances. In C. Yarbro, M. Frogge, & M. Goodman (Eds.), *Cancer symptom management* (3rd ed., pp. 493–511). Sudbury, MA: Jones & Bartlett.

Bush, N. (2005). Clinical Challenges: Chemotherapy-induced diarrhea. *Oncology Nursing Forum, 31*(5), 889–892.

Bush, J., & Griffin-Sobel, J. (2004). Clinical challenges: Chemotherapy-induced cardiomyopathy. *Oncology Nursing Forum, 31*(2), 185–188.

Camp-Sorrell, D. (2005). Myelosuppression. In J. K. Itano & K. N. Taoka (Eds.), *Core curriculum for oncology nursing* (4th ed., pp. 259–274). St. Louis: Elsevier.

Camp-Sorrell, D. (2006). Chemotherapy toxicities and management. In C. Yarbro, M. Frogge, & M. Goodman (Eds.), *Cancer symptom management* (3rd ed., pp. 412–457). Sudbury, MA: Jones & Bartlett.

Cappozzo, C. (2004). Optimal use of granulocyte-colony-stimulating factor in patients with cancer who are at risk for chemotherapy-induced neutropenia. *Oncology Nursing Forum, 31*(3), 569–576.

Carpenter, J. (2005a). State of the science: Hot flashes and cancer, Part 1: Definition, scope, impact, physiology, and measurement. *Oncology Nursing Forum, 32*(5), 959–968.

Carpenter, J. (2005b). State of the science: Hot flashes and cancer, Part 2: Management and future directions. *Oncology Nursing Forum, 32*(5), 969–978.

Cawley, M., & Benson, L. (2005). Current trends in managing oral mucositis. *Clinical Journal of Oncology Nursing, 9*(5), 584–592.

Davison, D. (2006). Constipation. *Clinical Journal of Oncology Nursing, 10*(1), 112–113.

Eggenberger, S., Krumwiede, N., Meiers, S., Bliesmer, M., & Earle, P. (2004). Family caring strategies in neutropenia. *Clinical Journal of Oncology Nursing, 8*(6), 617–621.

Eilers, J. (2004). Nursing interventions and supportive care for the prevention and treatment of oral mucositis associated with cancer treatment. *Oncology Nursing Forum, 31*(4 Suppl.), 13–23.

Engelking, C. (2004). Diarrhea. In C. Yarbro, M. Frogge, & M. Goodman (Eds.), *Cancer symptom management* (3rd ed., pp. 528–558). Sudbury, MA: Jones & Bartlett.

Friend, P., & Pruett, J. (2004). Bleeding and thrombotic complications. In C. Yarbro, M. Frogge, & M. Goodman (Eds.), *Cancer symptom management* (3rd ed., pp. 231–251). Sudbury, MA: Jones & Bartlett.

Gobel, B. (2006). Bleeding. In C. Yarbro, M. Frogge, & M. Goodman (Eds.), *Cancer symptom management* (3rd ed., pp. 723–740). Sudbury, MA: Jones & Bartlett.

Goodman, J. (2004). Skin and nail bed changes. In C. Yarbro, M. Frogge, & M. Goodman (Eds.), *Cancer symptom management* (3rd ed., pp. 319–330). Sudbury, MA: Jones & Bartlett.

Grothey, A. (2005). Clinical management of oxaliplatin-associated neurotoxicity. *Clinical Colorectal Cancer,* 5 Suppl.(1), S38–46.

Hartmuller, V., & Desmond, S. (2004). Professional and patient perspectives on nutritional needs of patients with cancer. *Oncology Nursing Forum, 31*(5), 989–996.

Jansen, C., Miaskowski, C., Dodd, M., Dowling, G., & Kramer, J. (2005). Potential mechanisms for chemotherapy-induced impairments in cognitive function. *Oncology Nursing Forum, 32*(6), 1151–1163.

Krumwiede, H., Meiers, S., Eggenberger, S., Murray, S., Bliesmer, M., Earle, P., et al. (2004). Turbulent waiting: Rural families experiencing chemotherapy-induced neutropenia. *Oncology Nursing Forum, 31*(6), 1145–1152.

Larson, E., & Nirenberg, A. (2004). Evidence-based nursing practice to prevent infection in hospitalized neutropenic patients with cancer. *Oncology Nursing Forum, 31*(4), 717–725.

Lee, C. (2005). Complementary and alternative medicine patients are talking about: Black cohosh. *Clinical Journal of Oncology Nursing, 9*(5), 628–629.

Massey, R., Haylock, P., & Curtiss, C. (2004). Constipation. In C. Yarbro, M. Frogge, & M. Goodman (Eds.), *Cancer symptom management* (3rd ed., pp. 512–527). Sudbury, MA: Jones & Bartlett.

Montbriand, M. (2004). Herbs or natural products that increase cancer growth: Part two of a four-part series. *Oncology Nursing Forum, 31*(5), E99–115.

Nail, L. (2004). Fatigue. In C. Yarbro, M. Frogge, & M. Goodman (Eds.), *Cancer symptom management* (3rd ed., pp. 47–60). Sudbury, MA: Jones & Bartlett.

Nystedt, K., Hill, J., Mitchell, A., Goodwin, F., Rowe, L., Wong, F., et al. (2005). The standardization of radiation skin care in British Columbia: A collaborative approach. *Oncology Nursing Forum, 32*(6), 1199–1205.

Porock, D., Beshears, B., Hinton, P., & Anderson, C. (2005). Nutritional, functional, and emotional characteristics related to fatigue in patients during and after biochemotherapy. *Oncology Nursing Forum, 32*(3), 661–667.

Reeves, D. (2004). Alopecia. In C. Yarbro, M. Frogge, & M. Goodman (Eds.), *Cancer symptom management* (3rd ed., pp. 561–570). Sudbury, MA: Jones & Bartlett.

Rittenberg, C. (2004). The next generation of chemotherapy-induced nausea and vomiting prevention and control: A new 5-HT3 antagonist arrives. *Clinical Journal of Oncology Nursing, 8*(3), 307–308, 310.

Rittenberg, C., & Cunningham, R. (2005). Chemotherapy-induced nausea and vomiting. *Clinical Journal of Oncology Nursing, 9*(2), 257–260.

Simpson, C., Herr, H., & Courville, K. (2004). Current therapies that protect against doxorubicin-induced cardiomyopathy. *Clinical Journal of Oncology Nursing, 8*(5), 497–501.

Staat, K., & Segatore, M. (2005). The phenomenon of chemo brain. *Clinical Journal of Oncology Nursing, 9*(6), 713–721.

Story, K. (2005). Alterations in circulation. In J. K. Itano & K. N. Taoka (Eds.), *Core curriculum for oncology nursing* (4th ed., pp. 364–379). St. Louis: Elsevier.

Stricker, C., Drake, D., Hoyer, K., & Mock, V. (2004). Evidence-based practice for fatigue management in adults with cancer: Exercise as an intervention. *Oncology Nursing Forum, 31*(5), 963–976.

Viale, P. (2005). Integrating aprepitant and palonosetron into clinical practice: A role for the new antiemetics. *Clinical Journal of Oncology Nursing, 9*(1), 77–84.

West, F., & Mitchell, S. (2004). Evidence-based guidelines for the management of neutropenia following outpatient hematopoietic stem cell transplantation. *Clinical Journal of Oncology Nursing, 8*(6), 601–613.

Whitman, M. (2004). Nutrition and surgery in patients with cancer. *Clinical Journal of Oncology Nursing, 8*(2), 217–219.

Wickham, R. (2004). Nausea and vomiting. In C. Yarbro, M. Frogge, & M. Goodman (Eds.), *Cancer symptom management* (3rd ed., pp. 187–214). Sudbury, MA: Jones & Bartlett.

Wickline, M. (2004). Prevention and treatment of acute radiation dermatitis: A literature review. *Oncology Nursing Forum, 31*(2), 237–47.

Wilkes, G. (2004). Peripheral neuropathy. In C. Yarbro, M. Frogge, & M. Goodman (Eds.), *Cancer symptom management* (3rd ed., pp. 338–358). Sudbury, MA: Jones & Bartlett.

CHAPTER 12

ONCOLOGY EMERGENCIES

CHAPTER OBJECTIVE

After completing this chapter, the reader will be able to recognize the signs and symptoms of the most common oncology emergencies and indicate interventions for each emergency.

LEARNING OBJECTIVES

After studying this chapter, the reader will be able to

1. identify tumors associated with hypercalcemia.

2. recognize the signs of superior vena cava syndrome.

3. identify the signs of spinal cord compression.

4. recognize the symptoms of sepsis.

5. cite the interventions for tumor lysis syndrome.

INTRODUCTION

Oncology emergencies are specific acute situations for cancer patients that require immediate or urgent medical intervention. These emergencies can occur because of the malignancy or, in some cases, are complications of treatments.

Oncology emergencies often can be anticipated because of the patient's diagnosis or the course of the disease or treatment. Therefore, the nurse caring for the patient—equipped with knowledge about these emergencies—is the first step in addressing the emer-

gency. The nurse can identify the condition, mobilize a response, and integrate treatment for that emergency in the scope of the patient's total care plan.

In many instances, treatment of the underlying tumor adequately addresses the presenting or impending oncology emergency. In some situations, however, the oncology emergency requires a focus of treatment for the emergency itself, although treatment of the underlying disease continues.

Oncology emergencies reviewed in this chapter include hypercalcemia, superior vena cava syndrome (SVCS), cardiac tamponade, spinal cord compression (SCC), brain metastasis, disseminated intravascular coagulation (DIC), sepsis, syndrome of inappropriate antidiuretic hormone (SIADH), tumor lysis syndrome (TLS), pleural effusion, and bone metastasis.

HYPERCALCEMIA

Hypercalcemia is the most common metabolic oncology emergency. Among hospitalized cancer patients, a malignant tumor is the primary cause of hypercalcemia, although abnormally high calcium levels can occur with other metabolic conditions, such as renal dysfunction and hyperparathyroidism (Shuey, 2004).

At Risk

Patients at risk for hypercalcemia include those who have a) renal or kidney cancer, b) malignant tumors of the breast, lung (squamous cell), head and neck, prostate, or thyroid, or c) lymphoma or multiple myeloma (Richerson, 2004). Also, patients are at risk for hypercalcemia when their malignancies spread as bony metastases. The extent of metastasis does not correlate with the level of hypercalcemia. Hypercalcemia occurs in 10% to 40% of patients with cancer (Shuey, 2004).

Pathophysiology

Calcium regulation is a function of three hormonal regulatory mechanisms: the parathyroid glands, calcitonin produced by the thyroid, and vitamin D.

Normally, the parathyroid glands regulate calcium levels by producing hormones that promote calcium release from the bones into the circulation (via renal resorption). This release is triggered when extracellular levels of calcium are low, accompanied by an increase of renal excretion of calcium when levels are abnormally high (Richerson, 2004). Calcitonin, which is produced by the thyroid, offsets the action of the parathyroid, decreasing renal resorption of calcium and inhibiting bone resorption.

Vitamin D increases the absorption of calcium in the gastrointestinal (GI) tract. It also increases the amount of calcium available, promoting bone mineralization. Dietary intake of calcium does not affect hypercalcemia (Shuey, 2004).

Kidney and renal cancer and other conditions that affect the kidneys' ability to excrete calcium also cause serum levels of calcium to increase. Normal range for calcium is 9 to 11 mg/dl (Shuey, 2004). With hypercalcemia, the levels are greater than the high-normal levels (> 11 mg/dl).

Bone metastases may directly or indirectly cause tumor-induced osteoclasts to become activated. Bone metastasis also may cause increased bone resorption due to the release of calcium. The dysfunctional cycle of osteoclastic activity leads to bone destruction, which leads to elevated calcium levels and more cycles of bone destruction.

Another origin of hypercalcemia is humoral hypercalcemia. In this condition, the patient's high calcium level is a result of the interaction of ectopic parathyroid hormone-like factors, prostaglandin release by the tumor cells, and osteoclast-activating factors (substances released by tumors, such as tumor necrosis factor, interleukin-2, and lymphotoxins) (Richerson, 2004).

In women with breast cancer metastatic to bone, use of hormonal therapy may cause increased bone resorption and production of osteolytic prostaglandin by breast cancer cells. Bone pain and serum calcium levels may increase temporarily. (This is called a "flare.") Prognostically, this increased calcium level effect is an indication that the patient may have a good response from hormonal manipulation as treatment. Head and neck and lung cancers may cause a pseudostate of hyperparathyroidism that, in turn, leads to deregulation of calcium levels (Gobel, 2005).

Diagnosis

The early signs and symptoms of hypercalcemia are indicative of many other conditions, including anticipated responses to cancer therapy. Therefore, assessment is targeted at patients whose clinical features and underlying malignant conditions suggest pending hypercalcemia conditions.

Measurement of serum levels of calcium and electrolytes and the result of an electrocardiogram contribute to the diagnosis of hypercalcemia. Because cancer patients in advanced stages of their disease often have nutritional deficiencies (with low albumin levels from malnutrition), calculating a corrected serum calcium level is important. Figure 12-1 shows the formula for calculating a correct serum calcium level. It also provides an example of a corrected serum calcium level.

Other laboratory values may be affected when calcium soars. In addition to a serum calcium level greater than 11 mg/dl, lab values may show decreased serum levels of potassium, sodium, and

FIGURE 12-1: CALCULATING A CORRECTED SERUM CALCIUM LEVEL

Calculate an additional 0.8 mg/dl of calcium for every 1.0 g/dl of albumin below normal (commonly 4.0 g/dl of albumin is used as normal or corrected total serum calcium [TSC]).

Ca (corrected mg/dl) =

Ca (measured mg/dl) + [0.8 X (4 – albumin concentration g/dl)]

1. **Determine albumin value**

	4.0	Normal albumin (low normal)
	− 2.0	Reported albumin value
	= 2.0	Amount of albumin below normal

2. **Correct for Ca++**   2.0 x 0.8 = 1.6 mg/dl Ca++

3. **Corrected Ca++**

	10.5 mg/dl	Measured TSC
	+1.6 mg/dl	Correction
	= 12.1 mg/dl	Corrected

phosphorus; increased levels of blood urea nitrogen; and increased creatinine. Also, the patient's condition may cause cardiac changes (Richerson, 2004).

In addition, antidiuretic hormone (ADH), normally responsible for urine concentration in the renal distal tubules, decreases in the presence of an elevated calcium level. This results in polyuria, accompanied by dehydration and a decrease in glomerular filtration rate. As a result, the kidneys are unable to excrete the calcium. Polyuria also causes the loss of magnesium and phosphorus (Shuey & Brant, 2004).

Signs and Symptoms

Hypercalcemia usually is not an initial indication of a malignant tumor, except in cases of multiple myeloma and some other rare conditions. Signs and symptoms of hypercalcemia can be general or vague. Table 12-1 lists common early signs and symptoms. The most common early signs of hypercalcemia are nausea and constipation. As hypercalcemia advances, the patient may experience muscle weakness, hyporeflexia, lethargy, and confusion. If left untreated, these symptoms can progress dramatically. The patient's mental status and level of consciousness are affected when hypercalcemia becomes critical. Then the patient's symptoms progress further. These symptoms can include severe arrhythmias, heart block, seizures, psychosis, coma, renal failure, and—ultimately—death.

TABLE 12-1: EARLY SIGNS AND SYMPTOMS OF HYPERCALCEMIA

- Fatigue (tired feeling)
- Excessive sleepiness
- Confusion
- Coma
- Extreme muscle weakness
- Loss of appetite
- Nausea and vomiting
- Stomach pain
- Constipation
- Changes in heartbeat (too slow or too fast)
- Frequent urination
- Excessive thirst
- Dry mucous membranes

Interventions

If hypercalcemia is mild, initial therapy includes hydration with intravenous (IV) normal saline solution and measures to increase urinary output. Patient activity is encouraged, particularly weight-bearing exercises. These exercises also maintain or increase the patient's level of mobility. Medications that promote high serum levels of calcium, such as estrogen therapy and thiazide diuretics, are avoided and a decrease in oral intake of calcium is encouraged (Gobel, 2005; Shuey & Brant, 2004).

Meantime, the patient's cancer continues to be treated. Killing of tumor cells results in gradual decreases in serum levels of calcium. For patients with pronounced hypercalcemia, aggressive therapy may be indicated. Specifically, a strategy for hypercalcemia treatment follows:

1. **Rapid IV hydration** (more than 250 ml/hr). (Do not start diuretics again until rehydration and electrolyte replacement are complete.)

2. **Administration of pharmacologic agents** that reduce calcium. Drugs prescribed for hypercalcemia include plicamycin (Mithramycin), calcitonin, etidronate disodium (Didronel), and prednisone; all interfere with bone resorption. Several types of bisphosphonates can inhibit bone resorption and decrease calcium absorption from the intestine, including pamidronate (Aredia) and zoledronic acid (Zometa).

Some patients require multiple treatments to correct the calcium imbalance. Long-term therapy, including dialysis, may be necessary for refractory or serious cases of hypercalcemia (Gobel, 2005; Shuey & Brant, 2004).

SUPERIOR VENA CAVA SYNDROME

SVCS is most commonly associated with lung cancers and mediastinal lymphomas. Certain nonmalignant conditions, including tuberculosis, aneurysm, and thrombus from central venous catheters, may also cause SVCS. Some patients have a rapid onset of SVCS with classic signs and symptoms. In others, the onset is more gradual with less dramatic signs and symptoms. If the superior vena cava compresses slowly over time, collateral circulation can develop that compensates for the ongoing compression (Hunter, 2005; Walton, 2005).

At Risk

Patients at risk are those diagnosed with lung cancers (75%) and mediastinal lymphomas, including Hodgkin's disease (10% to 15%) (Walton, 2005).

Pathophysiology

As a mechanical, structural problem, the pathophysiology of SVCS is straightforward. The superior vena cava is a low-pressure vessel surrounded by a variety of anatomic structures, including the trachea, sternum, mediastinum, vertebrae, and other large vessels. It is easily compressed by a mediastinal mass. Because of its critical role in venous return to the heart, compression of this vessel can impair blood return from the head, the upper extremities, and the upper part of the thorax, causing diminished cardiac output (see Figure 12-2).

Signs and Symptoms

The classic signs and symptoms of SVCS are obvious engorgement of the thoracic and neck veins, facial edema, shortness of breath, headache, and confusion or changes in level of consciousness. When these symptoms appear, patients report them as swelling of the arms, neck, hands, and face—especially when the patient rises after lying down. The swelling may decrease in a few hours. Patients also report tightness of clothes, rings, and jewelry; dizziness; protruding blood vessels; and bulging eyes. The veins may be pronounced when the patient is at rest. Approximately 60% of patients show symptoms on clinical examination (Walton, 2005).

FIGURE 12-2: SUPERIOR VENA CAVA SYNDROME

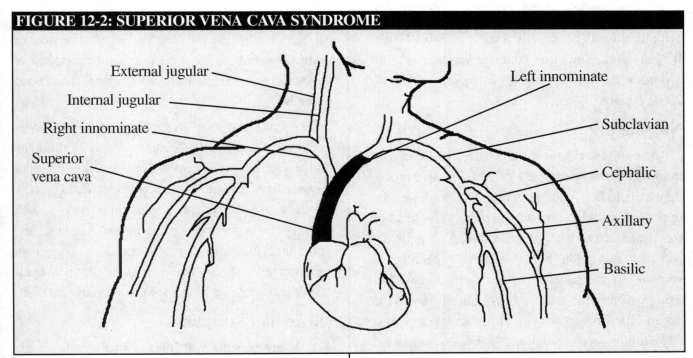

Diagnosis

A SVCS diagnosis is based on signs and symptoms and when those signs and symptoms first appear. If collateral circulation has developed, radiologic evaluation may be necessary. If SVCS is the initial indication of a malignant condition, a tissue biopsy is necessary to establish the diagnosis and plan appropriate interventions. When radiation therapy (RT) is the treatment of choice, additional computed tomography (CT), magnetic resonance imaging (MRI), or other radiologic studies may be ordered to best plan therapy.

For tumors that are highly responsive to chemotherapy, such as lymphoma, and small-cell lung cancer, chemotherapy may be the primary treatment rather than RT (Hunter, 2005; Walton, 2005).

Interventions

SVCS can be considered a life-threatening condition. In most cases, immediate RT is the primary effective treatment. Therapy should begin immediately when any of these conditions exists:

- the upper part of the airway is obstructed by edema

- cardiac output is severely compromised

- lack of venous return causes brain edema

- the patient has non-small-cell lung cancer or certain types of lymphoma.

With high doses of RT, rapid resolution and relief of signs and symptoms usually occur within 2 weeks. More conventional doses address symptoms less rapidly.

Combination chemotherapy is the treatment of choice when a histologic diagnosis confirms a tumor, such as small-cell lung cancer or lymphoma. Chemotherapy can be effective when the tumor is widely disseminated or when mediastinal radiation has been previously used. In some cases, the treatment plan includes chemotherapy plus RT. After therapy begins, persistent or progressive signs and symptoms may continue because of tumor necrosis rather than tumor progression.

Corticosteroids may decrease edema associated with cell death from treatment. If SVCS is associated with the use of a venous access device, the device needs to be removed. Then anticoagulant therapy should be started to dissolve the thrombus obstructing the superior vena cava (Hunter, 2005; Walton, 2005).

With treatment of the cause of the obstruction, symptoms of SVCS usually resolve in 7 to 10 days. If signs and symptoms continue or increase, the syndrome is not responding to therapy (Walton, 2005; Hunter, 2005).

Nursing Care

Nursing interventions for SVCS should support minimizing the syndrome's effects. Invasive procedures, including obtaining blood pressure in the upper extremities, should be avoided. The head of the patient's bed should be elevated to help the patient breathe. The nurse needs to explain interventions to the patient to decrease anxiety. After therapy begins, the nurse should carefully assess the patient for progression of signs and symptoms. Also, tumor necrosis may necessitate corticosteroid administration.

CARDIAC TAMPONADE

Cardiac tamponade starts with the extension of the tumor into adjacent tissue; usually, the tumor originates in a lung or the mediastinum or has spread as metastases from other sites.

At Risk

An estimated 20% of cancer patients have tumor involvement of the heart or pericardium at the time of death (Hunter, 2005).

Pathophysiology

In cardiac tamponade, the cavity between the two layers of the pericardium fills with malignant pericardial fluid, leading to an effusion. As intrapericardiac pressure increases, the heart constricts. Thus, its ability to pump effectively is impaired, affecting cardiac function.

Normally, the pericardial space holds about 50 ml of fluid between the layers of the pericardium. An increase in the volume of this fluid leads to increased intrapericardiac pressure. This pressure compresses the heart, compromising cardiac output, circulation,

and the ability of the heart muscle to pump effectively. Intrapericardiac pressure can also increase because of direct invasion of the tumor into cardiac tissue or because of changes in the heart or tissue inflammation after RT.

A combination of factors increases the severity of cardiac tamponade. A small volume of fluid can have a serious effect on cardiac function if tumor invasion or pericarditis is also present. If fluid accumulates gradually, the pericardium may stretch slowly and accommodate the increased volume and pressure. Compensatory tachycardia and peripheral vasoconstriction can occur in an effort to increase cardiac output and blood volume (Hunter, 2005).

Signs and Symptoms

Many patients with tumor involvement of the heart remain asymptomatic. When signs and symptoms of cardiac tamponade occur, they can include dyspnea or tachypnea, tachycardia, cough, hoarseness, and retrosternal pain in the chest that increases when the patient is supine. The patient may also have peripheral cyanosis, hiccups, and a weak or nonexistent apical pulse. If cardiac output is severely compromised, additional symptoms include reduced urinary output, edema, and decreased cerebral oxygenation resulting in changes in the patient's level of consciousness (Hunter, 2005).

Diagnosis

The diagnostic workup includes a chest radiograph or other imaging procedures. Usual findings are mediastinal widening, cardiac enlargement, and hilar adenopathy. Generally, an echocardiogram is the most accurate test for cardiac tamponade and shows two echoes if this condition is present. Other procedures include CT, electrocardiography, and pericardiocentesis or pericardial window; these procedures provide data for both the cytologic diagnosis and therapeutic management of cardiac tamponade.

Interventions

If fluid causes compromised cardiac output, the physician will order an emergency pericardiocentesis or pericardial window. If fluid reaccumulates, cardiac tamponade can reoccur within 24 to 48 hours. Medications (antibiotics or antineoplastics) are administered for sclerosis. To drain the fluid, the physician inserts a pericardial catheter. Then the sclerosing agent is administered. If needed, the process is repeated daily for several days.

Surgical approaches to cardiac tamponade may include either forming a pericardial window to allow fluid drainage or total pericardiectomy (removing the entire pericardial sac). Total pericardiectomy is usually reserved for cardiac tamponade caused by radiation-induced pericarditis. If tumor involvement of the heart is extensive, surgery as a treatment strategy is rare because morbidity and mortality from surgery is high.

If RT is contraindicated, the treatment option is to administer cytotoxic chemotherapy to reduce the size of the tumor. If this works, the response is quick. Administration of corticosteroids may reduce the inflammation associated with tamponade and pericardial sclerosing. If patients have extensive cardiac metastases, few treatment options are available (Hunter, 2005).

SPINAL CORD COMPRESSION

SCC is a serious complication of cancer. It is caused by pressure of a tumor on the spinal cord—the bundle of nerves running inside the backbone to the brain. Compression of the spinal cord is a true emergency and requires rapid, definitive therapy. Serious neurologic deficits from the compression—such as paraplegia—can be permanent (Hunter, 2005).

At Risk

Patients at risk are those with cancers of the lung, breast, and prostate and other cancers that may spread to the bone, such as multiple myeloma and lymphoma. Nonmalignant causes of SCC include herniated discs (Hunter, 2005).

Pathophysiology

SCC is usually a mechanical problem. As the tumor invades the spinal region from adjacent tissues or arises from and surrounds the spinal cord itself, increased pressure on the cord and nerve roots develops. Compression causes ischemia or hemorrhage and can lead to changes in motor, sensory, and autonomic function. Prolonged or severe compression can cause permanent paralysis (Hunter, 2005).

SCC can arise from primary tumor growth within the spinal column and its layers or from metastatic disease. When compression is caused by tumor cells within the cord, it is called *intramedullary*; tumors from the layers protecting the cord are *extramedullary-intradural*. Metastasis to the spine can be intramedullary (within the spine), leptomeningeal (within the cord's lining), or epidural (outside the cord's lining) (Flaherty, 2006).

Signs and Symptoms

Back pain is usually the first presenting symptom, and it may move to the side. The pain worsens when the patient lies down, coughs, sneezes, or moves and may not respond to pain medication. Numbness and tingling in the toes or fingers may also occur.

Later signs and symptoms of SCC include:

- leg weakness
- changes in gait
- changes in bowel or urinary habits, such as constipation or inability to empty the bladder
- bowel or bladder incontinence (Hunter, 2005)
- decreased sensation for deep pain and vibration and paralysis masked as atrophy.

Diagnosis

A complete physical assessment, including a thorough neurologic examination, helps define the location of SCC and the extent of neurologic impairment. Radiologic studies may include MRI, CT, myelography, radiography of the spine, and bone scan.

MRI is the procedure of choice for diagnosis of compression. In most cases, its specificity, sensitivity, and overall accuracy exceed those of other radiologic techniques (Wilkes, 2004). The primary disadvantage of MRI is that patients must lie still for an extended time during the procedure. If a patient has severe, deep back pain, lying still for a long period may be impossible (Wilkes, 2004). To successfully complete an MRI, the patient may require administration of conscious sedation or analgesic agents.

A combination of radiologic techniques may be indicated to determine the exact existence, location, or extent of the tumor. Once the extent and site or sites of the compression have been determined, a lumbar puncture may be ordered. This procedure allows a sampling of cerebrospinal fluid to evaluate malignant cells, leptomeningeal cells, infection, or other conditions affecting the central nervous system (Wilkes, 2004).

Interventions

Immediate consultation with a radiation oncologist and neurosurgeon is required to consider treatment options. Treatment usually does not affect the patient's prognosis, but it can significantly affect the patient's quality of life.

Corticosteroids administered before radiation treatments can relieve edema and pain. Then, on an emergency basis, RT begins if the tumor is radiosensitive, the spine is stable, and the spine has not been subjected to maximum radiation. Radiation is the primary and most common intervention for SCC; doses are 30 to 40 Gy over 2 to 4 weeks (Hunter, 2005; Wilkes, 2004). Early treatment can prevent

serious problems. Follow-up rehabilitation and physical therapy can minimize loss of function.

If additional radiation is not an option, surgery may be considered. If SCC is the initial indication of cancer, laminectomy is a primary option for treatment to relieve compression and simultaneously obtain tissue for pathologic diagnosis (Hunter, 2005; Wilkes, 2004).

Decompression of the area by laminectomy often gives prompt, temporary relief, but resection of the tumor is frequently impossible. Consequently, postoperative RT further relieves signs and symptoms and reduces tumor volume. If vertebral bodies have collapsed, surgery may be contraindicated because it may produce further spinal instability.

Chemotherapy added to RT or surgery can reduce the size of a tumor. If the tumor is responsive to chemotherapy—such as lymphoma or neuroblastoma—administering chemotherapy agents may be beneficial. If treatment is effective (RT, surgery, or chemotherapy), recovery of neurologic function is usually prompt.

Patients with severe neurologic deficits before therapy rarely show significant improvement after treatment. Initial strategies are RT or surgery. If neurologic impairment (including paralysis) is extensive, prospects for recovery generally are poor (Hunter, 2005; Wilkes, 2004).

Transverse myelitis (TM) is a neurologic syndrome caused by inflammation within the spinal cord, usually caused by infection, RT (total dose > 4500 cGy), or an autoimmune response. TM is uncommon but not rare. Symptoms include limb weakness, sensory disturbance, bowel and bladder dysfunction and disturbance, and back pain. TM symptoms can develop rapidly over several hours to several weeks. About one-half of patients with TM have their symptoms worsen within 24 hours of onset (Krishnan, Kaplin, Deshpande, Pardo, & Kerr, 2004).

TM, rather than SCC, may be the cause of symptoms. Diagnosis starts with MRI and can include further studies to identify infection. TM can be a central nervous system complication of non-Hodgkin's lymphoma (Krishnan et al., 2004).

Nursing Care

The nurse's role in the evaluation of SCC is critical. A nurse is usually the first health care provider to notice changes in neurologic function and to assess changes in a patient's neurologic status. Early on, patient complaints about pain can be subtle. Later symptoms of compression include weakness and changes in bowel and bladder habits. In an inpatient setting, the nurse is responsible for maintaining the stability of the spine and providing support to maintain or improve mobility.

After treatment of the compression, nurses should collaborate with physical therapists and other specialists in rehabilitation medicine to develop strategies to help patients regain their loss of function (Wilkes, 2004).

BRAIN METASTASIS

Brain metastasis is when cancer cells have spread to the brain from other primary cancer sites. Brain metastasis occurs in 20% to 40% of individuals diagnosed with cancer (Belford, 2006). Brain metastasis is an oncology emergency because early diagnosis and management can lead to the prompt initiation of therapy. Therapy started early gives patients a better opportunity for treatment response.

At Risk

Patients most at risk for brain metastasis include those diagnosed with lung cancer, breast cancer, melanoma, kidney cancer, or colon cancer. Lung cancer is the most common primary site of origin. In addition, almost 40% of patients with melanoma develop brain metastasis (Belford, 2006).

Pathophysiology

Brain metastasis occurs when cancer cells break away from the primary tumor and, through the bloodstream, take up residence in the brain (National Brain Tumor Foundation [NBTF], 2006). As tumor cells grow within the brain, they push against normal brain tissue, eventually destroying it.

Signs and Symptoms

Signs and symptoms of brain metastasis include headaches, seizures, speech impediments, weakness, poor vision, pain and numbness, decreased coordination and mobility, paralysis, nausea, and vomiting (NBTF, 2006). Eventually, brain metastasis causes the patient to feel more tired; the patient can also have problems sleeping, reading, and talking.

Diagnosis

In addition to physical examination, brain metastasis is diagnosed by MRI, CT, positron-emission tomography, and biopsy.

Symptoms of brain metastasis sometimes occur during treatment for primary cancer or after patients have completed treatment. These symptoms suggest cancer recurrence, so further systemic testing with imaging, laboratory work, and biopsy may be ordered to confirm tumor spread.

Interventions

Treatment options for brain metastasis are limited. If only one brain tumor is detected and it can be easily reached, surgery is commonly the treatment of choice. Whether surgery is an appropriate treatment decision is based on the tumor type, size, and location.

RT typically follows surgical treatment and is the best solo modality treatment when multiple tumors are present or the tumor is inaccessible via surgery. RT can also relieve symptoms (swelling, neurologic deficits). Types of RT for brain metastasis include whole brain radiation, a strategy that can treat large tumors as well as small, undetectable brain tumors. Side effects of whole brain radiation include nausea, vomiting, headaches, fever, memory loss, and problems with concentration (Machtay, 2006).

Stereotactic radiosurgery—also called *gamma knife* or *cyberknife treatment*—allows administration of a focused, precise, high dose of radiation to a tumor, usually in one session. The radiation beam is generated from many angles, targeting the tumor. The tumor needs to be small or few in number (e.g., less than three) for stereotactic radiosurgery to be the appropriate treatment strategy.

Few chemotherapies have been shown to be effective treatments for brain metastasis because chemotherapy has difficulty penetrating the blood-brain barrier. Examples of oral chemotherapy for brain metastasis include temozolomide (Temodar), procarbazine (Matulane), and lomustine (CeeNU).

IV chemotherapy for brain metastasis includes vincristine (Oncovin, Vincasar PFS), cisplatin (Platinol), carmustine (BiCNU), and carboplatin (Paraplatin). Methotrexate (Rheumatrex) may be administered orally, by injection, or intrathecally (injected directly into the spinal fluid) via an Ommaya reservoir (NBTF, 2006).

Strategies to treat the symptoms of brain metastasis can include administration of corticosteroids (to reduce swelling and brain inflammation, help with sleep, lessen pain, and improve cognition). Antiseizure medications and anticonvulsants may also be ordered to offset brain tumor–related seizures (NBTF, 2006)

DISSEMINATED INTRAVASCULAR COAGULATION

Coagulation involves a finely maintained balance between the formation and destruction of a blood clot. Alterations in this balance can cause disarray in the coagulation pathways. Several conditions can result from this imbalance, including DIC (Gobel, 2005).

At Risk

Although DIC is most often associated with acute promyelocytic leukemia (Gobel, 2005), its overall prevalence in cancer patients is approximately 10%. Any patient with cancer is at risk for DIC, particularly patients who have sepsis, trauma, or transfusion reactions (Gobel, 2005).

Pathophysiology

The pathophysiology underlying DIC appears to be an improbable reversal of the body's regulatory systems: bleeding occurring in response to a massive release of clotting factors. In reality, both formation of a thrombus and hemorrhage are occurring simultaneously. The coagulation pathways determine the release of intrinsic clotting factors (factors VIII, IX, XI, and XII) as well as extrinsic factor (factor VII) to produce prothrombin, thrombin, fibrinogen and, ultimately, platelet aggregation and clot formation.

The tumor or infection stimulates the coagulation pathways, which increase formation and deposition of fibrin clots. As quickly as coagulation factors appear, they are consumed. Thus, in DIC, coagulation is ineffective. At the same time, however, fibrinolysis is triggered, which breaks down the thrombi formed.

By-products of this process (fibrin degradation products) are not totally cleared from the system. Thus, while clotting factors accumulate, they are also being disseminated. They further inhibit platelet formation. As a result, minor localized bleeding can progress to severe hemorrhaging as DIC continues (Gobel, 2005).

Signs and Symptoms

In addition to frank bleeding, patients may have bruising, petechiae, hematuria, guaiac-positive stool or emesis, hemoptysis, or other evidence of poor coagulation or blood loss.

Diagnosis

Laboratory tests indicate blood loss or a dysfunction in coagulation. Platelet count, hemoglobin level, hematocrit, and fibrinogen level are decreased, whereas prothrombin time, activated partial thromboplastin time, thrombin time, and the level of fibrin-split products increase.

As DIC becomes more severe, patients may have signs and symptoms indicative of critical blood loss, including tachycardia, dyspnea, changes in level of consciousness, renal failure, and signs of shock (Gobel, 2005).

Interventions

The basic goal in treating DIC is to correct the underlying condition. Therefore, the patient receives chemotherapy for the cancer or antibiotics for sepsis. A secondary goal is to control signs and symptoms. Transfusions of red blood cells and fluid replace blood loss; transfusions of platelets, fresh frozen plasma, or cryoprecipitate restore missing or malfunctioning coagulation factors.

Nursing Care

The signs and symptoms of DIC may be subtle or may appear as common side effects associated with cancer therapy. Therefore, the nurse's judgment may be critical in evaluating physical indications and in reporting routine laboratory data.

Minor bleeding, anemia, and thrombocytopenia are prevalent among cancer patients. Key roles for the nurse related to DIC are recognition of patients at highest risk for DIC and administration of blood products and fluids to offset losses (Gobel, 2005).

SEPSIS

Septic shock is the body's response to an overwhelming infection.

At Risk

When a patient becomes granulocytopenic or neutropenic as a result of chemotherapy, the source of sepsis is usually the patient's own flora, such as *Escherichia coli, Pseudomonas,* or *Klebsiella* (Gobel, 2005).

Pathophysiology

Most cases of septic shock are caused by Gram-negative bacteria (40%) (Gobel, 2005). Other organisms contributing to sepsis include fungi (*Candida, Aspergillus*), anaerobes, viruses, and protozoa. Cancer patients are especially susceptible to sepsis because of aggressive treatments, which lead them to have immunocompromised conditions.

Signs and Symptoms

Early signs and symptoms of impending sepsis are irritability and confusion. Then, as septic shock develops, the patient experiences chills and fever; warm, flushed skin; increased heart rate (which can soon progress to bradycardia); decreased blood pressure; and decreased urine output. Table 12-2 lists the stages of sepsis and its clinical signs and symptoms.

Interventions

Blood and fluid cultures are drawn to determine the most accurate antibiotic regimen. While waiting for culture results, treatment begins with broad-spectrum antibiotics, fluid boluses of normal saline solution, and oxygen administration (Gobel, 2005). The strategy is to not change the antibiotic regimen for 72 hours, unless developing culture results discount initial antibiotic choices or the patient shows signs of shock. Empiric antifungal treatment (usually amphotericin B or other antifungals) starts when the patient is afebrile (5 to 7 days after initial administration of antibiotics begins) (Gobel, 2005).

TABLE 12-2: CLINICAL PRESENTATION OF SEPSIS

EARLY/COMPENSATORY	LATE/REFRACTORY
Signs and Symptoms	
Blood pressure < 90 mm Hg or > 40 mm Hg below baseline	Profound hypotension
High cardiac output	Low cardiac output
Low systemic vascular resistance	High systemic vascular resistance
Urine output < 0.5 ml/kg/hr	Anuria
Warm, flushed, dry skin	Cold, pale, clammy skin
Increased heart rate	Tachycardia, arrhythmias
Bounding pulses	Weak, thready pulse
Fever	Decreased core body temperature
Decreased level of consciousness	Decreased level of consciousness
Increased respiratory rate	Shortness of breath
Decreased respiratory depth	Decreased respiratory depth
Crackles	Crackles, wheezes
Diagnostic Tests	
Increased white blood cell (WBC) count	Increased or decreased WBC count
Hyperglycemia	Hypoglycemia, increased serum amylase and lipase
Metabolic acidosis, respiratory alkalosis	Metabolic acidosis, respiratory acidosis
Hypoxemia: $SvO_2 > 80\%$ (tissue extraction increased)	Refractory hypoxemia: $SvO_2 < 60\%$ (tissue extraction decreased)
Prolonged thrombin time	Decreased clotting factors
Decreased clotting factors	Increased hepatic transaminases
Increased fibrin split products	Increased bilirubin, blood urea nitrogen, creatinine

(Gobel, 2005; Wujcik, 2004)

SYNDROME OF INAPPROPRIATE ANTIDIURETIC HORMONE (SIADH)

At Risk

SCLC is the tumor type most commonly associated with SIADH (Gobel, 2005). SIADH can also be caused by treatment regimens that include vincristine and cyclophosphamide (Cytoxan) (Gobel, 2005).

Pathophysiology

SIADH occurs when a tumor releases ectopic ADH. It is classified as an endocrine paraneoplastic syndrome. High levels of ADH in plasma prompt the body to reabsorb water. (The fluid reabsorbed goes into the intracellular fluid and extracellular fluid compartments.) With the kidneys reabsorbing more water, the patient has a decreased urine output and expanding fluid volume.

Signs and Symptoms

The earliest signs and symptoms of SIADH are caused by a low sodium level and include weakness, muscle cramps, anorexia, nausea, diarrhea, headache, and confusion (Gobel, 2005). The patient may also gain weight. Fluid intake may exceed urine output. No peripheral edema may develop because excess fluid accumulates in the vascular system. Brain cells may swell and the patient may become lethargic; personality changes and seizures may develop and, without treatment, the patient can become comatose.

Diagnosis

The diagnostic criteria for SIADH are listed in Table 12-3.

Interventions

The patient with SIADH is placed on fluid restriction. The clinical treatment plan includes IV infusion of half-normal saline solution. This should correct the sodium imbalance and pull water out of swollen brain cells. Demeclocycline hydrochloride (Declomycin) is an agent used in treatment (Gobel, 2005).

Treatment of the underlying condition of SIADH includes chemotherapy for the malignancy or antibiotics for an infection (Gobel, 2005).

TUMOR LYSIS SYNDROME

TLS is characterized by hyperphosphatemia, hyperkalemia, hyperuricemia, and hypocalcemia. The patient is at high risk for renal failure and cardiac arrest (Cope, 2004; Gobel, 2005).

At Risk

At risk for TLS are patients diagnosed with lymphoblastic leukemia, Burkitt's lymphoma, and other high-grade aggressive lymphomas, which carry a high tumor burden. TLS also can occur during blast crisis in patients with acute myelogenous and chronic myelogenous leukemias.

TABLE 12-3: DIAGNOSTIC CRITERIA FOR SYNDROME OF INAPPROPRIATE ANTIDIURETIC HORMONE

Laboratory tests	
• Serum sodium	< 135 mEq/L (hyponatremia)
• Plasma osmolality	< 275 mOsm/kg (hypoosmolality)
• Urine osmolality	> 300 mOsm/L
• Specific gravity	> 1.015
• Urine sodium	> 30 mmol/L
• Blood urea nitrogen	< 8 mg/dl
• Creatinine	< 0.5 mg/dl
• Uric acid	< 2.4 mg/dl
Physical findings	
• Euvolia	
• Absence of edema	
Differential diagnosis	
• Exclude hypovolemia	
• Exclude hypervolemia	
Workup	
Normal thyroid, adrenal, cardiac, hepatic, and renal function	
No recent or current use of diuretics	

(Gobel, 2005)

Pathophysiology

TLS develops when rapidly growing, bulky tumors release intracellular electrolytes spontaneously during or after chemotherapy treatment. As cells die and lyse from chemotherapy treatment, large amounts of intracellular electrolytes and chemicals enter the bloodstream. Both rapid cell destruction and rapid cell reproduction are factors in TLS (Cope, 2004; Gobel, 2005).

Signs and Symptoms

Clinical manifestations of TLS include oliguria, weakness, bradycardia, nausea, vomiting, tetany, and ventricular failure.

Diagnosis

Diagnosis includes elevated uric acid and lactate dehydrogenase (LDH) levels, renal insufficiency or failure, and volume depletion. (Elevated uric acid levels occur because of a breakdown in nucleic acids.) Other factors in diagnosis are elevated levels of potassium and phosphate and decreased serum calcium level. (See Table 12-4.)

TABLE 12-4: LABORATORY AND CLINICAL FINDINGS OF TLS

- Hyperuricemia
- Hyperkalemia
- Hyperphosphatemia
- Hypocalcemia
- Increased LDH
- Decreased creatinine clearance
- Increased creatinine
- Increased blood urea nitrogen
- Decreased bicarbonate
- Decreased pH
- Decreased urine output
- Uric acid crystals on urinalysis

(Cope, 2004; Gobel, 2005)

Interventions

Treatment includes the administration of fluids (with sodium bicarbonate) to prevent uric acid from crystallizing and to maintain an alkaline urine pH. These fluids are administered rapidly. Dialysis may be necessary to prevent or control renal failure. Treatment also includes allopurinol. If hyperkalemia is suspected, withhold potassium (Cope, 2004; Gobel, 2005).

PLEURAL EFFUSION

Pleural effusion is the abnormal accumulation of fluid in the pleural cavity.

At Risk

Patients with lung, breast, GI, or ovarian tumors; lymphoma; or leukemia are at risk for pleural effusion.

Pathophysiology

A common complication of malignancy, pleural effusion is the result of metastases to the pleurae or mediastinal lymph nodes. Before a pleural effusion is diagnosed, a slowly developing pleural effusion can produce a large amount of fluid (Shuey & Payne, 2005).

Diagnosis

Pleural effusion is usually detected by physical examination findings, such as reduced breath sounds and dullness on percussion. A chest X-ray can confirm physical exam findings. To determine if malignancy is involved, a thoracentesis allows fluid withdrawal for cytology.

Signs and Symptoms

Clinical features of malignant pleural effusion include dyspnea on exertion or at rest; a dry, nonproductive cough; heaviness in the chest; weight loss; anxiety; a need to lie on the affected side; and diminished or absent breath sounds over the affected area. As much as 1 L of fluid can move through the pleural space in a 24-hour period (Shuey & Payne, 2005).

Interventions

Treatment targets the underlying tumor and may include chemotherapy to prevent fluid accumulation, RT (if the cause is lymphoma or certain types of lung cancer), pleurodesis (chemical sclerosing—with talc or chemotherapy—of the two pleural membranes), or pleurectomy (surgical removal of the parietal pleura with abrasion of the visceral pleura). An additional treatment strategy is to place a pleural catheter, which allows the patient to regularly drain fluid from the pleural space.

For palliative care, thoracentesis is the treatment of choice, providing temporary relief of symptoms. Unfortunately, with malignancy and its accompanying tumor cell spread, fluid can start accumulating again in as little as a day, with reaccumulation of all fluid within several days (Shuey & Payne, 2005).

Nursing Care

As the effusion decreases, nursing care should include assessment of the patient's respiratory status. If sclerosis is part of the treatment plan, the nurse manages the patient's chest tubes and provides patient teaching and comfort care (Shuey & Payne, 2005).

BONE METASTASIS

When a tumor spreads to the bone, it establishes secondary tumors in the bone called *bone metastases*. Spread of the primary tumor to the bone, through the bloodstream or lymphatic system, can damage bone and cause symptoms of bone pain.

At Risk

Patients at risk for bone metastasis include those with cancers of the breast, kidney, lung, prostate, or thyroid and those with multiple myeloma.

Pathophysiology

Bone metastasis compromises the structural support that bones provide. Bone lesions can be osteolytic (in which the tumor eats away at areas of the bone, making the bone fragile and weak) or osteoblastic (in which the tumor affects bone-forming cells, creating abnormal buildup of bone—called *osteosclerotic lesions*—that make bone weak and unstable). Metastasis of tumor cells affects how bone cells form, break down, and resorb. Sites of metastasis include the limbs, pelvis, rib cage, skull, and spine.

Diagnosis

Diagnosis is made by bone scan. Follow-up imaging can include CT, MRI, and chest X-ray.

Laboratory tests include calcium, magnesium, phosphorus, and sodium levels.

Signs and Symptoms

Clinical features of bone metastasis can include bone pain, broken bones, pathologic fractures, numbness or weakness in the legs, problems urinating or passing stool, numbness in the abdomen, loss of appetite (with nausea, thirst, and constipation), fatigue, and confusion.

Treatments

Bisphosphonates are agents that slow bone destruction, thereby reducing the risk of fractures, bone pain, and hypercalcemia. Examples of bisphosphonates are pamidronate (Aredia) and zoledronate (Zometa).

RT can ease pain, prevent fractures, and kill tumor cells at specific sites of spread. Typical RT comprises 10 treatments over a 2-week period (CancerSource, 2005). Radiopharmaceuticals used as palliative treatment for bone metastasis include strontium chloride and sarmarium 153.

Other treatments may include systemic chemotherapy (targeting the primary tumor cells), administration of nonsteroidal anti-inflammatory drugs, surgery to stabilize potential fracture areas, physical therapy, and nonpharmacologic treatments, such as relaxation and heat and cold therapy to control pain.

Nursing Care

With bone metastasis, nursing care includes vigilance in observation—noticing patient symptoms, monitoring laboratory values, alerting the physician to areas of possible metastasis, preventing falls, preventing fractures, and administering treatment (CancerSource, 2005).

SUMMARY

Patients diagnosed with malignancies may develop a condition that becomes an oncology emergency. Examples of oncology emergencies include hypercalcemia, SVCS, cardiac tamponade, SCC, brain metastasis, DIC, sepsis, SIADH, TLS, pleural effusion, and bone metastasis. Nurses caring for cancer patients should be aware of the early signs of these emergencies and know appropriate, timely interventions.

EXAM QUESTIONS

CHAPTER 12
Questions 47-51

Note: Choose the option that BEST answers each question.

47. Patients at risk for hypercalcemia are those with

    a. renal cell cancer.
    b. brain cancer.
    c. testicular cancer.
    d. skin cancer.

48. An early sign of superior vena cava syndrome (SVCS) is

    a. cramping in both legs.
    b. facial edema.
    c. rash.
    d. diarrhea.

49. A common initial symptom of spinal cord compression (SCC) is

    a. tightness in the collar.
    b. swollen fingers.
    c. back pain.
    d. persistent cough.

50. An early sign of sepsis is

    a. warm, flushed, dry skin.
    b. urine output greater than 40 ml/hr.
    c. slow respiratory rate.
    d. dystonia.

51. Interventions for tumor lysis syndrome (TLS) include

    a. physical therapy.
    b. IV fluids.
    c. defibrillation.
    d. fluid restriction.

REFERENCES

Belford, K. (2006). Central nervous system cancers. In C. Yarbro, M. Frogge, & M. Goodman (Eds.), *Cancer nursing: Principles and practice* (6th ed., pp. 1089–1136). Sudbury, MA: Jones & Bartlett.

CancerSource. (2005). *Understanding bone metastasis—When cancer spreads to the bone.* Retrieved April 17, 2007, from http://www.cancersource.com/Search/34,25952-1

Cope, D. (2004). Tumor lysis syndrome. *Clinical Journal of Oncology Nursing, 8*(4), 415–416.

Flaherty, A. (2006). Spinal cord compression. In C. Yarbro, M. Frogge, & M. Goodman (Eds.), *Cancer nursing: Principles and practice* (6th ed., pp. 910–924). Sudbury, MA: Jones & Bartlett.

Gobel, B. (2005). Metabolic emergencies. In J. K. Itano & K. N. Taoka (Eds.), *Core curriculum for oncology nursing* (4th ed., pp. 383–421). St. Louis: Elsevier.

Hunter, D. (2005). Structural emergencies. In J. K. Itano & K. N. Taoka (Eds.), *Core curriculum for oncology nursing* (4th ed., pp. 422–439). St. Louis: Elsevier.

Krishnan, C., Kaplin, A.I., Deshpande, D., Pardo, C.A., & Kerr, D.A. (2004). Transverse myelitis: Pathogenesis, diagnosis and treatment. *Frontiers in Bioscience, 9,* 1483-1499. Available from http://www.myelitis.org/newsletters/v6n1/Frontiers%20in%20Bioscience%20review%20article.pdf

Machtay, M. (2006). *Treatment for brain metastasis.* Retrieved October 31, 2006, from http://www.oncolink.com/custom_tags/print_ARTICLE.cfm?Page=2&id=1815&Section=Ask_The _Experts

National Brain Tumor Foundation. (2004). *The essential guide to brain tumors.* Retrieved April 17, 2007, from http://www.braintumor.org/patient _info/publications/brochures/documents/guide_wpics.pdf

Richerson, M. (2004). Electrolyte imbalances. In C. Yarbro, M. Frogge, & M. Goodman (Eds.), *Cancer symptom management* (3rd ed., pp. 440–460). Sudbury, MA: Jones & Bartlett.

Shuey, K. (2004). Hypercalcemia of malignancy: Part I. *Clinical Journal of Oncology Nursing, 8*(2), 209–211.

Shuey, K., & Brant, J. (2004). Hypercalcemia of malignancy: Part II. *Clinical Journal of Oncology Nursing, 8*(3), 321–323.

Shuey, K., & Payne, Y. (2005). Malignant pleural effusion. *Clinical Journal of Oncology Nursing, 9*(5), 529–532.

Walton, A. (2005). Superior vena cava syndrome: An education sheet for patients. *Clinical Journal of Oncology Nursing, 9*(4), 479–480.

Wilkes, E. (2004). Spinal cord compression. In C. Yarbro, M. Frogge, & M. Goodman (Eds.), *Cancer symptom management* (3rd ed., pp. 359–373). Sudbury, MA: Jones & Bartlett.

Wujcik, D. (2004). Infection. In C. Yarbro, M. Frogge, & M. Goodman (Eds.), *Cancer symptom management* (3rd ed., pp. 252–275). Sudbury, MA: Jones & Bartlett.

CHAPTER 13

LUNG CANCER

CHAPTER OBJECTIVE

After completing this chapter, the reader will be able to describe issues relevant to the care and treatment of the patient with lung cancer.

LEARNING OBJECTIVES

After studying this chapter, the reader will be able to

1. describe the incidence of and death rates for lung cancer in the United States.

2. identify two risk factors for lung cancer.

3. identify two symptoms of late-stage lung cancer.

4. name two chemotherapies that are used in treating lung cancer.

INTRODUCTION

Lung cancer remains one of the most difficult cancers to treat, with major treatment break-throughs elusive. Lung cancer remains a mostly silent killer, because patients often do not experience early symptoms and can present at diagnosis at an advanced stage. Yet promising strategies to improve lung cancer diagnosis and treatment offer hope; they include multimodality approaches—especially adding novel and targeted therapies to chemotherapy. This chapter reviews the epidemiology of lung cancer, well-known risk factors, screening strategies, and the most common treatments.

EPIDEMIOLOGICAL TRENDS

Lung cancer is the leading cause of cancer death among men and women in the United States. (American Cancer Society [ACS], 2006). In 2006, about 174,470 people were diagnosed with lung cancer and about 162,460 people died of the disease—more deaths than the mortality estimates for colorectal, breast, and prostate cancers combined (ACS, 2006). Lung cancer is the leading cause of death for women and men. In men, it accounts for 14% of new cases and 32% of cancer deaths. In women it accounts for 12% of new cases and 25% of cancer deaths (Flannery, 2005).

Although many factors have been associated with this major national and worldwide health problem, cigarette smoking has been estimated to cause 90% of all lung cancer deaths. (Flannery, 2005). Risk is related to:

- amount smoked (pack years = # of cigarette packs smoked/day x # years person smoked)

- age of smoking onset

- product smoked (tar and nicotine content, filters)

- depth of inhalation

- gender.

Symptoms at presentation include:

- cough

- dyspnea
- hemoptysis
- recurrent infections
- chest pain.

Cough and dyspnea are the most common presenting symptoms (lungcancer.org, 2005), accompanied by fatigue. Hemoptysis is also reported, especially in middle-age or older persons. Chest and shoulder pain may also occur and may be indicative of the tumor location, called *pancoast tumor* (lungcancer.org, 2005). Symptoms secondary to distant metastases include pain and weight loss. Figure 13-1 shows the anatomy of the lungs.

Compared with rates for nonsmokers, lung cancer rates are 22 times higher for male smokers and 12 times higher for female smokers (Flannery, 2005). Lung cancer continues to cause more than 2.5 times more deaths in men than prostate cancer, the second leading cancer killer among men in the United States (ACS, 2006; Jemal, 2006). In addition to being a killer of men, lung cancer now kills more women than any other cancer in the United States. The highest incidence of lung cancer for both sexes is in the elderly (ACS, 2006).

Lung cancer incidence and mortality are increasing in non-Caucasian groups. In Caucasian men, the rates have declined or stabilized (Flannery, 2005). As of 2006, incidence rates for lung cancer declined significantly in men and have somewhat stabilized in women (ACS, 2006; Houlihan, Inzeo, Joyce, & Tyson, 2004; lungcancer.org, 2005). (See Chapter 1, Figure 1-1.)

PREVENTION, SCREENING, AND EARLY DETECTION

Prevention of lung cancer requires successful strategies to help patients not start smoking or to stop smoking if they are smokers. If smoking were totally eliminated, 85% of lung cancers would disappear (ACS, 2006). Chapter 3 (Table 3-3) provides some suggested strategies to help individ-

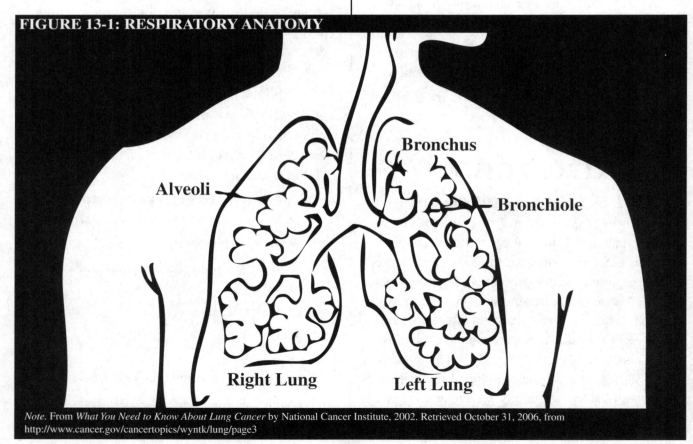

FIGURE 13-1: RESPIRATORY ANATOMY

Bronchus

Alveoli

Bronchiole

Right Lung

Left Lung

Note. From *What You Need to Know About Lung Cancer* by National Cancer Institute, 2002. Retrieved October 31, 2006, from http://www.cancer.gov/cancertopics/wyntk/lung/page3

uals quit smoking. Additional efforts to prevent smoking continue to focus on antismoking education, legislation, and taxation of cigarettes.

High-intensity smokers who take pharmacological doses of beta-carotene have an increased lung cancer incidence and mortality that is associated with taking the supplement (National Cancer Institute [NCI], 2006). Taking vitamin E supplements does not affect the risk of lung cancer (NCI, 2006). In time, a genetic link may be established for those diagnosed with lung cancer who have never smoked.

Other lung cancer prevention strategies include the avoidance of sources of asbestos, radon, and selected occupational agents. As a secondary prevention strategy, chemoprevention or chemo-prophylaxis is being studied; the findings so far have been inconclusive (NCI, 2006). Chemo-prevention agents, such as retinoids, carotenoids (synthetic forms of vitamin A), and selenium, target the epithelial tissue exposed to carcinogens; the agents seek to prevent or reverse the promotion phase of carcinogenesis.

Standard screening tests (chest X-rays, sputum cytology at regular intervals) have not proven to be effective for early detection of lung cancer. Spiral computed tomography (CT) and positron-emission tomography have been shown to detect lung cancer at an earlier stage.

In 2006, the results of a large collaborative study (for the period 1994–2005) of asymptomatic persons at risk for lung cancer were published. Those studied received low-dose spiral screening CTs at baseline and at 7 and 19 months from baseline. A cohort of screening CTs for these individuals were able to show early-stage lung cancer; those diagnosed went on to receive prompt treatment (surgical resection). Survival rates (92%) for the treated patients indicated that this approach to screening can detect lung cancer early enough so that it is curable (International Early Lung Cancer Action Program Investigators, 2006). Based on these promising data, efforts will continue to make mass CT screenings for at-risk individuals cost-effective.

STAGING SCHEMA, PATTERNS OF METASTASIS

Lung cancer histological staging includes two main tumor classes:

1. Non-small-cell lung cancer (NSCLC). NSCLC has three types:
    –   adenocarcinoma
    –   squamous cell carcinoma
    –   large-cell carcinomas.

    NSCLC accounts for 80% of bronchogenic cancers (NCI, 2006).

2. Small-cell lung cancer (SCLC). SCLC accounts for about 20% of bronchogenic cancers (NCI, 2006). SCLC is also referred to as *oat-cell cancer.*

Non-Small-Cell Lung Cancer

The American Joint Committee on Cancer staging schema uses eight stages for NSCLC. Each stage is distinct in its characteristics and what it determines as a statistically based response to treatment and 5-year survival outcomes (see Table 13-1).

The pattern of metastasis for lung cancer spread is to:

*   lymph nodes
*   brain
*   bones
*   liver
*   other lobes of lungs and pleurae
*   adrenal glands.

Factors that correlate with adverse prognosis include:

*   presence of pulmonary symptoms
*   large tumor size (greater than 3 cm)
*   nonsquamous histology

TABLE 13-1: STAGING OF LUNG CANCER

Lung cancer is the most common cause of cancer-related death in men and women; approximately 174,470 new cases were diagnosed in 2006. This disease is one of the most difficult cancers to treat; 5-year survival rates are approximately 15% (ACS, 2006). Bronchoscopy is an important procedure for accurate staging prior to therapy. Surgery and radiation therapy are the primary modalities of treatment for localized or regional disease. The primary tumor may be squamous cell carcinoma or adenocarcinoma. Metastatic spread occurs to intrathoracic lymph nodes, followed by cervical lymph nodes, liver, brain, bones, adrenal glands, kidneys, and the contralateral lung.

Primary Tumor (T)

TX   Primary tumor cannot be assessed

T0   No evidence of primary tumor

Tis   Carcinoma in situ

T1   Tumor $\leq$ 3 cm without invasion more proximal than the lobar bronchus

T2   Tumor > 3 cm in size; involves main bronchus $\geq$ 2 cm distal to the carina; invades visceral pleura

T3   Direct invasion of chest wall, diaphragm, pericardium; involves main bronchus; < 2 cm distal to the carina

T4   Tumor invades mediastinum, heart, great vessels, trachea, esophagus, vertebral body, carina; or separate tumor nodules in the same lobe; or tumor with a malignant pleural effusion

Regional Lymph Nodes (N)

NX   Regional lymph nodes cannot be assessed

N0   No regional lymph node metastasis

N1   Metastasis in ipsilateral peribronchial and/or ipsilateral hilar lymph nodes

N2   Metastasis in ipsilateral mediastinal and/or subcarinal lymph nodes

N3   Metastasis in contralateral mediastinal, contralateral hilar, ipsilateral or contralateral scalene, or supra-clavicular lymph node(s)

Distant Metastasis (M)

MX   Distant metastasis cannot be assessed

M0   No distant metastasis

M1   Distant metastasis

Stage Grouping

Stage 0	Tis	N0	M0
Stage IA	T1	N0	M0
Stage lB	T2	N0	M0
Stage IIA	T1	N1	M0
Stage IIB	T2	N1	M0
	T3	N0	M0
Stage IIIA	T1	N2	M0
	T2	N2	M0
	T3	N1, N2	M0
Stage IIIB	Any T	N3	M0
	T4	Any N	M0
Stage IV	Any T	Any N	M1

Note. Used with the permission of the American Join Committee on Cancer (AJCC), Chicago, Illinois. The original source for this material is the *AJCC Cancer Staging Manual,* Sixth Edition (2002), published by Springer-New York, www.springeronline.com.

- metastases to multiple lymph nodes within a TNM-defined nodal station

- vascular invasion

- increased numbers of tumor blood vessels in the tumor specimen (NCI, 2006).

Treatments

Surgery

Standard treatment for stage I and II NSCLC is surgical resection with the goal of cure. Thoracotomy is used for pulmonary resection. The type and location of the incision depends on the stage of disease. Lobectomy and pneumonectomy have been the principal types of thoracotomy for decades.

Lobectomy (the removal of a lobe of the lung) is associated with lower morbidity and mortality rates than pneumonectomy (the removal of one lung). For small tumors, lobectomy is the preferred treatment. If the tumor is confined to a single lobe, the tumor is removed with a lobectomy.

Pneumonectomy is now performed only if a tumor cannot be completely excised by lobectomy. Pneumonectomy complications can include perfusion and ventilation problems, such as circulatory overload and pulmonary hypertension (Flannery, 2005). Other more-involved surgeries might be considered when the tumor has spread to adjacent areas of the bronchial tree.

The 5-year survival rates following surgical resection exceed 50% for stage I and 35% for stage II tumors (Flannery, 2005; NCI, 2006).

For stage IIIA, IIIB, and IV NSCLC, surgery can be ineffective so it is not the treatment of choice.

Radiation Therapy

For stage I and stage II NSCLC, radiation therapy (RT), utilizing either external beam or brachytherapy, is a viable option for those who cannot tolerate or refuse surgical resection. RT is generally delivered in fractions 5 days a week over 5 to 6 or more weeks. This therapy is often the best chance to cure the disease if the patient is not a surgical candidate.

The standard of care for selected stage IIIA patients after surgery and those with unresectable stage III NSCLC is RT. The combined-modality treatment (chemotherapy and RT) can lower recurrence rates and appears to confer a modest survival advantage over chemotherapy alone.

As a palliative measure, RT can be effective, especially for the symptoms of metastatic lung cancer (Flannery, 2005).

Chemotherapy

Chemotherapy is a treatment option for selected stage III and stage IV NSCLC, usually offered after RT. The standard of treatment includes cisplatin (Platinol)–based chemotherapy protocols. Other agents used in the treatment of NSCLC include paclitaxel (Taxol), docetaxel (Taxotere), etoposide (VePesid), gemcitabine (Gemzar), vinorelbine (Navelbine), and irinotecan (Camptosar). Patients with distant metastases (stage IV) can be treated with either chemotherapy alone or supportive care.

In 2006, the U.S. Food and Drug Administration (FDA) approved bevacizumab (Avastin)—added to cisplatin and paclitaxel—as a first-line treatment for NSCLC (Genentech, 2006). This combination regimen is indicated for unresectable, locally advanced, recurrent or metastatic NSCLC.

Studies have suggested that patients presenting with early-stage lung cancer have a survival advantage when treated with surgery and adjuvant platinum-based chemotherapy (Maltzman, 2004).

Targeted therapies added to treatment protocols include gefitinib (Iressa) and erlotinib (Tarceva). Gefitinib inhibits an enzyme (tyrosine kinase) present in lung cancer cells and has been used as a single agent for the treatment NSCLC that has progressed after or failed to respond to two other types of chemotherapy. In 2005, the FDA issued new labeling requirements for gefitinib that limits the indication to cancer patients who, in the opinion of their treating physician, are currently benefiting or have previously benefited from gefitinib treatment (FDA, 2005).

Erlotinib is indicated for patients with locally advanced or metastatic NSCLC after failure of at least one prior chemotherapy regimen. It blocks tumor cell growth in NSCLC by targeting the protein HER1/epidermal growth factor receptor (EGFR), a protein that is present on the surface of some cancer cells and normal cells (Genentech, 2006).

Small-Cell Lung Cancer

SCLC is the most aggressive lung cancer. It is responsive to chemotherapy and RT, but the recurrence rate is high even in its early stage. Cell types of SCLC include oat cell, intermediate, and combined.

For SCLC, many clinicians use a simple two-stage system when diagnosing patients—limited-stage disease (tumor in one hemithorax and regional lymph nodes with or without pleural effusion) and extensive-stage disease (tumor has spread beyond areas of limited stage disease).

Untreated SCLC has a prognosis of approximately 12 weeks (NCI, 2006).

Treatments

For some selected, limited SCLC patients with small masses and no lymph node involvement or metastasis, surgery may be the treatment of choice, followed by chemotherapy. For limited stage disease—when radiation is added to the treatment protocol—the usual dosage of chest RT is 45 to 50 Gy over 3 to 4 weeks. Protocols can include up to 60 Gy over 6 weeks.

SCLC is sensitive to chemotherapy as a treatment option. Chemotherapy, with or without RT, has been the mainstay of treatment for many years. Induction therapy includes etoposide and cisplatin-based protocols (mainly carboplatin).

Other agents used in treatment include cyclophosphamide (Cytoxan), doxorubicin (Adriamycin), mitomycin (Mutamycin), vincristine (Oncovin), cisplatin, paclitaxel, gemcitabine, and topotecan (Hycamtin) (Flannery, 2005; NCI, 2006).

FUTURE STRATEGIES FOR TREATMENT

Because effective treatment for lung cancer remains elusive, patients should be encouraged to enroll in clinical trials (NCI, 2006). Areas of study include angiogenesis inhibitors, biological therapies (e.g., monoclonal antibodies, vaccines), inhaled chemotherapy, cryotherapy, gene therapy, molecularly targeted therapies (e.g., EGFR inhibitors and mutations research), photodynamic therapy, radiofrequency ablation, and radiation techniques (e.g., stereotactic). Studies are also looking at reliable tumor markers to identify disease-causing proteins, diagnose lung tumors early, and measure treatment effectiveness (lungcancer.org, 2005). For example, one approach to lung cancer therapy involves the mechanism of estrogen. Since 1930, the rate of lung cancer deaths in women has increased 600%, so some experts believe that women are more susceptible to lung cancer than men because of estrogen and its effects. The newest and most effective treatments for lung cancer may need to be able to block the effects of estrogen on lung cancer (Hogle & McLemore, 2005).

SUMMARY

With the prevalance of smoking increasing among adolescents, the incidence of lung cancer is not abating. Moreover, long-term effective treatments for lung cancer are still not available. Considerable attention from the research community suggests that those diagnosed with lung cancer may eventually have promising treatment options. Until then, lung cancer diagnosed at an advanced stage remains a very difficult cancer diagnosis with limited treatment options.

EXAM QUESTIONS

CHAPTER 13
Questions 52-55

Note: Choose the option that BEST answers each question.

52. Lung cancer is the leading cause of death among

    a. only women.
    b. only men.
    c. women and men.
    d. youth under age 16.

53. Smoking as a risk factor for lung cancer also depends on

    a. exposure to sunlight.
    b. age when a person started smoking.
    c. level of physical activity.
    d. eating a diet high in vitamin C.

54. Symptoms of metastatic lung cancer include pain and

    a. weight loss.
    b. constipation.
    c. dizziness.
    d. dysphagia.

55. A chemotherapy used in treating lung cancer is

    a. trastuzumab.
    b. cisplatin.
    c. dexamethasone.
    d. morphine.

REFERENCES

American Cancer Society. (2006). *Cancer facts & figures 2006.* Atlanta: Author.

American Joint Committee on Cancer. (2002). *AJCC cancer staging manual* (6th ed.). New York: Springer-Verlag.

Flannery, M. (2005). Nursing care of the client with lung cancer. In J. K. Itano & K. N. Taoka (Eds.), *Core curriculum for oncology nursing* (4th ed., pp. 512–523). St. Louis: Elsevier.

Genentech. (2006). *Products.* Retrieved April 17, 2007, from http://www.gene.com/gene/products/index.jsp

Hogle, W., & McLemore, M. (2005). Treatments that block estrogen may increase survival from lung cancer. *Clinical Journal of Oncology Nursing 9*(4), 401.

Houlihan, N., Inzeo, D., Joyce, M., & Tyson, L. (2004). Symptom management of lung cancer. *Clinical Journal of Oncology Nursing, 8*(6), 645–652.

International Early Lung Cancer Action Program Investigators. Henschke, C., Yankelevitz, D., Libby, D., Pasmantier, M., Smith, J., & Miettinen, O. (2006). Survival of patients with stage I lung cancer detected on CT screening. *New England Journal of Medicine, 355*(17), 1763–1771.

Jemal, A., Siegel, R., Ward, E., Murray, T., Xu, J., Smigal, C., et al. (2006). Cancer statistics, 2006. *CA: Cancer Journal for Clinicians, 56(2),* 106–130.

Lungcancer.org. (2005). *Lung cancer 101.* Available from http://www.lungcanceronline.org/patients/fs_patient_caregivers.htm

Maltzman, J. (2004). *New paradigm in early stage lung cancer.* Available from http://www.oncolink.upenn.edu

National Cancer Institute. (2002). *What you need to know about lung cancer.* Retrieved October 31, 2006, from http://cancer.gov/cancertopics/wyntk/lung

National Cancer Institute. (2006). *Lung Cancer.* Retrieved October 31, 2006, from http://cancer.gov/cancertopics/types/lung

U.S. Food and Drug Administration. (2005). *Gefitinib (marketed as Iressa) information.* Retrieved October 31, 2006, from http://www.fda.gov/CDER/DRUG/infopage/gefitinib/default.htm

CHAPTER 14

BREAST CANCER

CHAPTER OBJECTIVE

After completing this chapter, the reader will be able to describe the screening strategies and treatments for breast cancer.

LEARNING OBJECTIVES

After studying this chapter, the reader will be able to

1. identify two risk factors for breast cancer.

2. recognize a staging workup for breast cancer.

3. name two chemotherapies that are used in treating breast cancer.

4. name a hormonal therapy for breast cancer.

INTRODUCTION

Breast cancer incidence and death rates continue to be high, although early screening via mammography, breast self-exams (BSEs), and clinical breast exams (CBEs) have allowed earlier and more effective treatments. This chapter reviews the epidemiology of breast cancer, its risk factors, prevention and detection strategies, staging, and treatment strategies. It also reviews hereditary risk factors that put some women at higher risk for breast cancer.

EPIDEMIOLOGICAL TRENDS

Breast cancer is the most frequently diagnosed cancer in women. It is second to lung cancer as the leading cause of all cancer deaths in women and is the leading cause of death for women 40 to 44 years of age (American Cancer Society [ACS]), 2006).

One in eight women will develop breast cancer over a lifetime. In the 1980s, the incidence of breast cancer increased rapidly due to increased use of mammography. The incidence is still increasing, although its rate has somewhat slowed. The increase in incidence is notable in the older than 50 age-group. More than 75% of all breast cancer occurs in women who are 50 years of age or older (ACS, 2006).

In 2006, an estimated 212,920 new cases of invasive disease were diagnosed and 41,430 people died of breast cancer. Rates of women who died of breast cancer have declined 2.3% from 1990 to 2002 (ACS, 2006). Breast cancer also occurs in men (less than 1% of cases). In 2006, an estimated 1,720 new cases were diagnosed in men.

In 2006, new cases of early stage in situ breast cancer totaled 61,980. Of these early stage cases, approximately 85% were ductal carcinoma in situ (DCIS). This increase in new DCIS cases is thought to be due to wider use of screening mammography (ACS, 2006; Jemal et al.,2006).

TYPES OF BREAST TUMORS

Cancer cells in breast tissue can be found in the lobes or smaller lobules (lobular cancer) and in the ducts (ductal cancer).

Carcinoma in situ is a premalignant lesion. With in situ forms of cancer, tumor cells have not yet invaded into the ducts or lobes. Thus, they are contained. However, the diagnosis of DCIS or lobular carcinoma in situ (LCIS) can be high-risk markers for developing breast cancer. Figure 14-1 is a schematic of DCIS.

FIGURE 14-1: DUCTAL CARCINOMA IN SITU

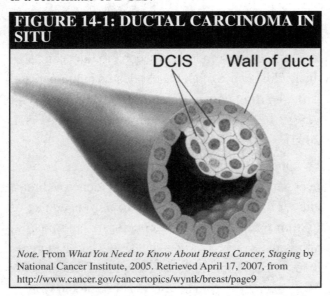

Note. From *What You Need to Know About Breast Cancer, Staging* by National Cancer Institute, 2005. Retrieved April 17, 2007, from http://www.cancer.gov/cancertopics/wyntk/breast/page9

Invasive breast cancer is usually adenocarcinoma. Figure 14-2 is a schematic of invasive breast cancer.

The most common type of breast cancer is ductal carcinoma. It begins in the lining of the ducts. Infiltrating ductal carcinoma occurs in two-thirds of women presenting with breast cancer. It is aggressive in the speed of its spread and ability to go to distant sites.

Inflammatory breast cancer is rare and involves the lymphatics and skin. Its spread is very aggressive and requires equally aggressive treatment.

FIGURE 14-2: INVASIVE BREAST CANCER

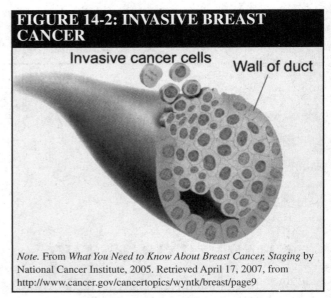

Note. From *What You Need to Know About Breast Cancer, Staging* by National Cancer Institute, 2005. Retrieved April 17, 2007, from http://www.cancer.gov/cancertopics/wyntk/breast/page9

RISK FACTORS

Defining risk factors for breast cancer continues to be problematic. Women who get breast cancer do not necessarily have the following risk factors, but studies have suggested the following factors put women at higher risk (National Cancer Institute [NCI, 2006]). Therefore, a combination of factors appears to increase a woman's risk of breast cancer.

Age

Breast cancer risk increases with age. Breast cancer is uncommon among women younger than 35 years, and risk increases among those older than 60 years (NCI, 2006). Approximately 77% of women with breast cancer are older than age 50. (ACS, 2006).

Race

Incidence rates are higher for Caucasian women than for women from other ethnic groups. However, these statistics may be skewed by study methodologies, which look at Caucasian women more often than other groups. Even taking into account economic factors (better access to care), Caucasian women were not always diagnosed early (ACS, 2006).

Sex

Men can develop breast cancer, but this disease is about 100 times more common among women than men.

Personal History

Risk increases for women who have been diagnosed with breast cancer before. Previous history of breast cancer increases a woman's risk three- to four-fold (NCI, 2006).

Family History

Risk increases if a woman's mother, sister, or daughter had breast cancer, especially when young (first-degree relative doubles the risk) (ACS, 2006). See "Genetic Alterations" section below.

Breast Changes

Certain breast changes, such as atypical hyperplasia LCIS, increase the risk. On a mammogram, these changes show as a high proportion of dense lobular and ductal tissue.

Genetic Alterations

So far, the syndromes most commonly associated with an autosomal dominant inheritance of breast cancer risk are hereditary breast and ovarian cancer due to BRCA1 or BRCA2 gene mutations, Li-Fraumeni syndrome due to p53 mutations, and Cowden syndrome due to PTEN mutations. Germline mutations in PTEN, a protein tyrosine phosphatase with homology to tensin, located on chromosome 10q23, are responsible for this syndrome (NCI, 2006, 2007).

BRCA1

In 1990, a susceptibility gene for breast cancer was mapped by genetic linkage. BRCA1 appears to be responsible for the disease in 45% of families with multiple cases of breast cancer only and up to 90% of families that have histories of both breast and ovarian cancer. Approximately 1 in 800 individuals in the general population may carry a pathogenic mutation in BRCA1. This susceptibility is more prevalent in Ashkenazi Jews (Bernice, 2005; NCI, 2006, 2007).

BRCA2

A second breast cancer susceptibility gene, BRCA2, was localized in families with multiple cases of breast cancer that were not linked to BRCA1. Mutations in BRCA2 are thought to account for approximately 35% of multiple case breast cancer families, and are also associated with male breast cancer, ovarian cancer, prostate cancer, and pancreatic cancer (Bernice, 2005; NCI, 2006, 2007).

Studies have shown that the likelihood of finding a BRCA1 or BRCA2 mutation is more than 50% if the patient has had bilateral breast cancer, both breast and ovarian cancer diagnoses, a diagnosis of breast cancer before age 40, or relatives with both breast and ovarian cancers (NCI, 2006).

These genetic mutations produce different clinical phenotypes of characteristic malignancies and, in some instances, associated nonmalignant abnormalities. Several other genetic syndromes that may include breast cancer are being studied.

Genetic testing and counseling can help women look at their family history. Then data and trends from the history can contribute to a profile, indicating whether a woman has an increased susceptibility to breast cancer. The focus of counseling is usually on women with mothers or sisters with breast cancer. Additional focus is on those with second-degree relatives with breast cancer (NCI, 2007).

Estrogen

Long-term exposure to estrogen increases the risk of breast cancer. This includes women who began menstruation before age 12, experienced menopause after age 55, never had children, or took hormone replacement therapy for long periods.

Late Childbearing

Risk increases if the first born was born after the mother turned 30.

Radiation Therapy

Radiation therapy (RT) exposure (e.g., for Hodgkin's disease) before age 30 increases the risk.

Weight Gain and Other Lifestyle Factors

Especially after menopause, risk increases for those who consume high-fat diets, have sedentary lifestyles, or smoke. Studies also suggest that the more alcohol a woman drinks, the greater her risk of breast cancer (NCI, 2005d).

Unproven Risks

No evidence, to date, supports these factors as risks for breast cancer (NCI, 2006):

- antiperspirants
- underwire bras
- induced abortion
- breast implants
- night work.

As a review, Table 14-1 highlights breast cancer risk factors.

PROTECTIVE MEASURES

To mitigate risk factors, researchers are looking at protective agents as well as behaviors to prevent breast cancer. Among areas of focus are exercise, diet, and chemoprotective agents. To date, no one strategy or combination of strategies has emerged to prevent breast cancer. These factors suggest a protective effect again breast cancer, but few hard data are available.

Prophylactic Mastectomy

Some women with an inherited risk of developing invasive breast cancer choose to have prophylactic mastectomies. The advantage of this strategy is not clear. Few prospective data exist regarding the benefit of prophylactic mastectomy among these women.

TABLE 14-1: SELECTED BREAST CANCER RISK FACTORS

(Note: 70% of women diagnosed with breast cancer have no known risk factors.)

- Gender (women are 100 times more likely to develop breast cancer than men)
- Early menarche (before age 12)
- Nulliparity or parity after age 30
- Late menopause (after age 55)
- Familial (20%) and hereditary breast cancer (9%) account for a very small proportion of diagnosed cases
    - Inheritance of the BRCA1 susceptibility gene is associated with a strong likelihood that the effect of the mutation leads to disease (90% for families with multiple breast and ovarian cancers and 70% for those with breast cancers diagnosed before age 45).
    - BRCA2 has been identified on the long arm of chromosome 13 (13q12-13). This mutation appears to be associated with male breast cancer and early-onset female breast cancer.
- Obesity slightly increases overall risk, especially for postmenopausal women.
- Alcohol risk related to breast cancer is greatest for women who drink more than two drinks per day.
- Radiation
    - Survivors of atomic bombs exhibit an increased prevalence of breast cancer as well as other cancers.
    - Breast cancer risk has been associated with RT. The risk increases with dosage, especially if a woman is exposed in the period of young adulthood.

(Bernice, 2005; NCI, 2005a, 2006)

Hormonal Therapy as Chemoprevention

Tamoxifen (Nolvadex) is an antiestrogen hormone that helps prevent breast cancer. It blocks the action of estrogen in breast tissue, thereby preventing estrogen from stimulating the proliferation of breast cancer cells (Johansen, 2005; Mahon, 2004).

Studies have confirmed the benefit of adjuvant tamoxifen in estrogen receptor (ER)–positive premenopausal women. (See "Hormonal Treatment" later in chapter.) A study published in 2003 reported that women at high risk for breast cancer who took tamoxifen were 28% less likely to be diagnosed with benign breast conditions (NCI, 2006). In another study from the Breast Cancer Prevention Trial, women who took tamoxifen for 5 years had a 49% reduction in new cases of breast cancer (Bernice, 2005; Harwood, 2004; NCI, 2006).

Results from the National Surgical Adjuvant Breast and Bowel Project B-14 study, which compared 5 years of adjuvant tamoxifen to 10 years of adjuvant tamoxifen for women with early-stage breast cancer, indicate no advantage for continuation of tamoxifen beyond 5 years in women with node-negative, ER-positive breast cancer (NCI, 2006). The optimal duration of tamoxifen treatment for node-positive women is still controversial and is being studied in ongoing clinical trials (NCI, 2006).

Tamoxifen may cause weight gain, hot flashes, vaginal discharge or irritation, nausea, and irregular periods. Women who are still menstruating and have irregular periods may become pregnant more easily when taking tamoxifen (NCI, 2005b). Blood clots and development of cataracts are rare but significant side effects. And some studies show that tamoxifen can slightly increase the risk of developing endometrial cancer. (Risk is two to seven times greater in women taking tamoxifen than in those who are not.)

Tamoxifen is also a treatment for metastatic breast cancer.

SIGNS AND SYMPTOMS

Breast cancer tumor cells are usually an abnormality detected with mammography before a mass is felt by the woman or health care professional (ACS, 2006). With larger tumors, a mass can be detected as a lump, swelling, distortion, tenderness, skin irritation, dimpling, nipple pain, scaliness, ulceration, retraction, or spontaneous discharge (ACS, 2006).

SCREENING AND DETECTION STRATEGIES

Breast Self-Examination

BSE has long been a means for patients to have control and an early awareness of breast changes. Despite BSE being an accepted and effective strategy for early breast cancer detection, studies report that BSE is not universally practiced (NCI, 2005a). Evidence is limited about whether BSE is actually practiced by many women at risk for breast cancer. In addition, it is unknown if women who practice BSE universally practice with good technique (Weiss, 2007). Thus, BSE as a widely accepted method of prevention is in question.

Clinical Breast Examination

CBE is a manual breast exam performed by a trained clinician. Although recommended at regular intervals for women at risk for breast cancer, few studies show that CBE is effective in reducing incidence and mortality (NCI, 2006). CBE is recommended, especially for women who carry the BRCA1 or BRAC2 high-risk mutation.

Mammography

A mammogram is a low-dose X-ray of the breast. Screening mammography is widely used to look for breast disease in women who are asymptomatic. Mammograms can show masses, cysts, or small deposits of calcium in the breast. Although most calcium deposits are benign, microcalcifications may be an early sign of cancer.

Although breast X-rays have been performed for more than 70 years, modern mammography has only existed since 1969. That was the first year X-ray units specifically for breast imaging were available. Modern mammography equipment designed for breast X-rays uses very low levels of radiation, usually a dose of about 1 mGy to 2 mGy (100 to 200 mrad) per view, or 2 mGy to 4 mGy (200 to 400 mrad) per two-view exam. Mammography has never been shown to be harmful to women or to increase the risk of breast cancer.

To put the X-ray dose for mammography into perspective, if a woman has yearly mammograms beginning at age 40—continuing until she is 90—she will receive 20 to 40 rads of radiation. If treated with RT for breast cancer, she will receive several thousand rads. Another way to clarify the risk: One mammogram exposes a woman to about the same amount of radiation as flying from New York to California on a commercial jet (NCI, 2005a, 2006).

Improved mammography technology allows digital recording of the radiographic image so that it can be stored in a computer, magnified in size, and made available for comparison over time with the patient's most recent digital mammography images.

Mammography Screening

In the general population, strong evidence suggests that regular mammography screening of women ages 50 to 59 years leads to a 25% to 30% reduction in breast cancer mortality (NCI, 2006). Table 14-2 lists the latest mammography and CBE recommendations from the ACS and NCI.

For women who begin mammographic screening at ages 40 to 49 years, a 17% reduction in breast cancer mortality is seen, based on 15 years of data after the start of screening. The reduction rate is lower for women ages 30 to 49 with a first-degree relative with breast cancer (due to the

---

TABLE 14-2: RECOMMENDED SCREENING GUIDELINES

- Women should undergo yearly mammograms starting at age 40 and continuing for as long as they are in good health.

- CBE should be part of a periodic health exam, about every 3 years for women in their twenties and thirties and every year for women age 40 and older.

- BSE is an option for women starting in their twenties. Women should promptly report any breast change to their health care provider.

- Women at increased risk (e.g., family history, genetic tendency, past breast cancer) should talk with their doctors about the benefits and limitations of starting mammography screening earlier, having additional tests (e.g., breast ultrasound or magnetic resonance imaging), or having more-frequent exams.

(ACS, 2006; NCI, 2006)

---

lower sensitivity rate of mammography for younger women) (NCI, 2005a).

Studies have concurred that the positive predictive value of mammography increases with age and is highest among older women and among women with a family history of breast cancer. Other studies show that CBE or CBE with mammography have been more effective than mammography alone in detecting breast cancers over time (NCI, 2005a).

For the best mammography results, women should have their films taken at a consistent location so they can be compared. The experience of the radiologist reviewing films is also important.

False-Positives

Approximately 10% of women require additional mammograms due to false-positives. Yet only 8% to 10% of those women will need a biopsy, and 80% of those biopsies will not show cancer (NCI, 2006).

Mammography sensitivity ranges between 70% and 90%, depending on the woman's age and the density of her breasts, which is affected by her genetic predisposition, hormone status, and diet. In studies based on an average sensitivity of 80%, mammograms miss approximately 20% of breast tumors during screening (false-negatives) (NCI, 2005a, 2006).

A retrospective analysis of 61,273 screening mammograms showed that 3.3% of studies had false-positives due to superimposition of normal breast structures. About half of these false-positives could be eliminated with two-view studies and 29% by additional diagnostic imaging (NCI, 2006).

Under the Mammography Quality Standards Act enacted by Congress in 1992, all facilities that perform mammography must be certified by the U.S. Food and Drug Administration. This mandate has resulted in improved mammography technique, lower radiation dose, and better training of personnel.

STAGING SCHEMA, PATTERNS OF METASTASIS

Breast cancer is considered to be a heterogenous, highly variable disease. Even among women with the same histological type, clinical stage, and treatment, some will be cured while others will develop metastatic disease within 6 months of therapy.

Aberrant cell clones have diverse growth rates. Moreover, their metastatic potential may, in part, account for differences seen in patients' clinical statuses.

When breast cancer metastasizes, it spreads widely and to almost all organs of the body. It primarily travels to the bone, lungs, lymph nodes, liver, and brain. The first sites of metastases are usually local or regional, involving the chest wall or axillary supraclavicular lymph nodes or bone.

Women with ER negative (ER–) disease are more likely to have recurrences in visceral organs. Women with ER positive (ER+) disease more often have recurrences in skin and bone (Bernice, 2005; NCI, 2006).

Table 14-3 reviews the common staging schema for breast cancer.

Staging

Tumor Size

There is a clear relationship between increasing tumor size and increased risk of recurrence. Prior to the more widespread use of mammography, less than 8% of women with node-negative breast cancer had tumors that were less than 1 cm in diameter, with a relative overall 5-year survival of nearly 99%. Patients with tumors measuring 1 to 3 cm have a relative 5-year survival of approximately 91%, whereas those with tumors measuring more than 3 cm have a 5-year survival of 85% (NCI, 2005b). However, recurrence rates for patients with tumors greater than 3 cm are more than 50% (NCI, 2005b).

Axillary Node Involvement

The involvement of the axillary nodes has long been recognized as a key feature in determining prognosis in breast cancer. Therefore, staging of breast cancer includes the status of the axillary lymph nodes (size, number, location, and method of detection of regional metastases), size of the tumor, metastatic spread, and hormone receptor levels (Singletary & Connolly, 2006).

Clinical assessment of the axillary nodes carries a 30% false-positive and false-negative rate. Pathological staging of the lymph nodes is mandatory. Seventy percent of patients with negative nodes survive 10 years. Prognosis worsens as the number of positive lymph nodes increases. Recurrence of disease is seen in approximately 75% of women with many positive nodes (NCI, 2006).

Sentinel node biopsy allows harvesting of a few lymph nodes so that staging information can be determined (University of Texas M.D. Anderson Cancer Center, 2003). This technique targets selected lymph nodes during biopsy. The procedure

TABLE 14-3: STAGING OF BREAST CANCER (1 OF 2)

Breast cancer is the most common malignancy in women. It is estimated that 212,920 new cases occurred during 2006 in the United States, with approximately 41,430 deaths attributed to the disease (ACS, 2006).

Many new adjuvant treatment protocols have been designed for patients with this disease. The size of the primary tumor and the presence or absence of regional lymph node involvement remain the most predictive factors of survival.

Pathologic staging no longer requires a modified radical mastectomy. Removal of the primary cancer with no gross tumor at the margins is now adequate. Dissection of at least the lowest level of axillary lymph nodes is required. Six or more lymph nodes are usually included for microscopic examination. Metastasis to ipsilateral supraclavicular lymph nodes is now considered M1 disease.

Primary Tumor (T)

TX	Primary tumor cannot be assessed
Tis	Noninvasive carcinoma (DCIS, LCIS) or Paget's disease of the nipple with no underlying tumor
T1	2 cm in maximal diameter
T1mic	Microinvasion ≤ 0.1 cm
T1a	0.1–0.5 cm
T1b	0.5–1.0 cm
T1c	1.0–2.0 cm
T2	2–5 cm in maximal diameter
T3	> 5 cm in maximal diameter
T4	Tumor of any size with direct extension to (a) chest wall or (b) skin, only as described below
T4a	Extension to chest wall, not including pectoralis muscle
T4b	Edema (including peau d'orange), or ulceration of the skin of the breast, or satellite skin nodules confined to the same breast
T4c	Both T4a and T4b
T4d	Inflammatory carcinoma

Regional Lymph Nodes (N)

NX	Unable to evaluate regional lymph nodes
N0	No involvement of regional lymph nodes
N1	Metastatic involvement of ipsilateral axillary lymph nodes (movable)
N2	Metastatic involvement of ipsilateral lymph nodes (fixed)
N3	Metastatic involvement of ipsilateral internal mammary lymph nodes

Distant Metastasis (M)

MX	Unable to evaluate distant metastasis
M0	No distant metastasis
M1	Distant metastasis present

Stage Grouping

Stage 0	Tis	N0	M0
Stage I	T1	N0	M0
Stage IIA	T0	N1	M0
	T1	N1	M0
	T2	N0	M0
Stage IIB	T2	N1	M0
	T3	N0	M0

TABLE 14-3: STAGING OF BREAST CANCER (2 OF 2)			
Stage IIIA	T0	N2	M0
	T1	N2	M0
	T2	N2	M0
	T3	N1, N2	M0
Stage IIIB	T4	Any N	M0
	Any T	N3	M0
Stage IIIC	Any T	N3	M0
Stage IV	Any T	Any N	M1

Note. Used with the permission of the American Joint Committee on Cancer (AJCC), Chicago, Illinois. The original source for this material is the *AJCC Cancer Staging Manual,* Sixth Edition (2002) published by Springer-New York, www.springeronline.com.

can spare extensive resection of the lymph nodes. Figure 14-3 identifies the drainage system of the axillary lymph nodes; Figure 14-4 shows a schematic of sentinel node mapping.

FIGURE 14-3: DRAINAGE

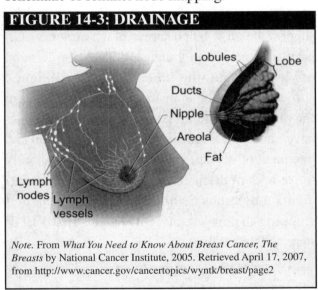

Note. From *What You Need to Know About Breast Cancer, The Breasts* by National Cancer Institute, 2005. Retrieved April 17, 2007, from http://www.cancer.gov/cancertopics/wyntk/breast/page2

Metastasis

Evaluation of metastatic spread of disease is the third main component of staging. Typically, a workup for metastatic spread includes chest, abdominal, and pelvic computed tomography (CT) scans; a bone scan, or a positron-emitted tomography scan. Major sites of breast cancer metastasis include the bone, lungs, liver, and brain. Bone is the most frequent site of distant metastasis (Bernice, 2005).

FIGURE 14-4: LYMPH NODE SENTINEL MAPPING

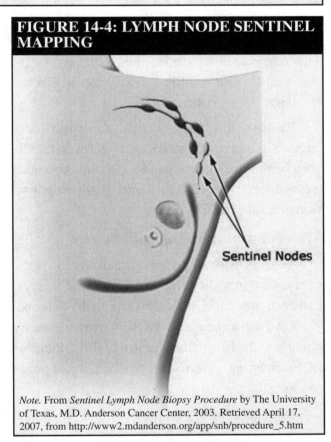

Note. From *Sentinel Lymph Node Biopsy Procedure* by The University of Texas, M.D. Anderson Cancer Center, 2003. Retrieved April 17, 2007, from http://www2.mdanderson.org/app/snb/procedure_5.htm

PATHOLOGIC PROGNOSTIC FACTORS

Hormone Receptor Status

Hormone receptor status is a pathologic prognostic factor. This information indicates whether breast cancer may respond to hormonal treatment as part of the treatment plan. Normal breast epithelium has hormone receptors and responds specifically to the stimulatory effects of estrogen and progesterone. A majority of breast cancers retain ERs. For these tumors, estrogen retains proliferative control over the malignant cells. The major benefit to knowing a woman's hormone receptor status concerns its value in predicting which patients will respond to hormone manipulation therapy.

A tumor cell with ERs on its surface is known as ER+. When the cell has progesterone receptors (PRs) on its surface, it is PR positive (PR+) (Mahon, 2004).

Tumors that are well differentiated or are of a lower grade tend to be ER+ and PR+. Tumors that are positive for both receptors (ER and PR) have a better than 75% response rate to endocrine therapy. This rate is compared to tumors that are positive only for ER (ER+ and PR–), which have a response rate under 35% (Mahon, 2004).

Tumors that lack receptor activity do not respond to hormonal therapy and tend to be tumors with higher histologic grades. Postmenopausal women tend to be ER+, whereas premenopausal women tend to be ER–.

Molecular and Biological Factors

Another pathologic prognostic factor is the expression of molecular and biological factors. Estrogen may exert inhibitory action on epidermal growth factor receptor (EGFR) production by binding to the ER. In the absence of this inhibition, EGFR may actually increase proliferation of breast cancer cells.

Overexpression or amplification of the human epidermal growth factor receptor-2 protein (HER2/neu) oncogene occurs in about 20% to 30% of human breast cancers and correlates positively with a poor prognosis in node-positive disease (Bernice, 2005; NCI, 2006). Overexpression of HER2/neu occurs more frequently in advanced tumors that are poorly differentiated. The more that is learned about the HER2/neu gene and other gene processes, the better targeting of patients for effective novel treatments will be. For example, in women with metastatic breast cancer and high

levels of HER2/neu, there is a correlation between poor response to some endocrine therapy and a favorable response to chemotherapy, especially cisplatin (Platinol), doxorubcin (Adriamycin), and paclitaxel (Taxol).

Overexpression of vascular endothelial growth factor (VEGF) is thought to be involved in tumor genesis and metastasis in primary breast cancer. Increased expression of VEGF is associated with decreased overall survival in women with node-negative breast cancer (NCI, 2005b, 2006). Primary tumors and metastases do not grow beyond 2 mm in diameter without an enhanced vascular supply.

In tumor cells, chemical signals called *cytokines* are thought to stimulate resting vascular endothelial cells into a rapid growth phase. Cytokines also support the growth and spread of the tumor. VEGF is an angiogenic factor that stimulates proliferation of vascular endothelial cells. Tumor-induced neovascularization appears to be a critical step in the oncogenic and metastatic cascades and may have important implications for the evaluation and treatment of women with breast cancer (especially those with node-negative disease). Future treatments may focus on understanding VEGF and stopping the proliferative processes that VEGF starts (NCI, 2005b).

Under normal circumstances, p53 is a tumor suppressor gene that contributes to a cell cycle regulation process that programs cell death. When this tumor suppressor gene is absent, aggressive tumor growth may increase. The p53 gene mutation appears to be an independent prognostic marker of early relapse (NCI, 2005b).

TREATMENT STRATEGIES

Surgery

The following are surgical treatment options for breast cancer.

Lumpectomy/Partial Mastectomy

The objectives of a lumpectomy or partial mastectomy are to remove the lump or area identified and then evaluate the tissue. The potential for breast conservation should be considered during planning of the biopsy procedure (Bernice, 2005). (See Figure 14-5.)

FIGURE 14-5: LUMPECTOMY

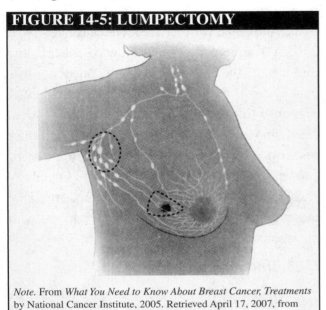

Note. From *What You Need to Know About Breast Cancer, Treatments* by National Cancer Institute, 2005. Retrieved April 17, 2007, from http://www.cancer.gov/cancertopics/wyntk/breast/page10

Radical Mastectomy

Mastectomy is surgical removal of the breast along with lymph nodes and some of the chest wall. Figure 14-6 shows the incisions for a radical mastectomy.

Modified Radical Mastectomy

A modified radical mastectomy involves removal the breast but spares some of the lymph nodes and chest wall. (See Figure 14-7.)

Radiation Therapy

RT usually is an adjuvant option of treatment after lumpectomy or mastectomy. Typical treatment protocols consist of 5000 to 6000 cGy over 5 to 6 weeks in daily doses. Palliative RT can relieve the symptoms of bone or brain metastasis (Bernice, 2005).

FIGURE 14-6: RADICAL MASTECTOMY

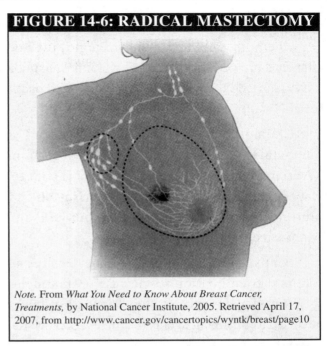

Note. From *What You Need to Know About Breast Cancer, Treatments,* by National Cancer Institute, 2005. Retrieved April 17, 2007, from http://www.cancer.gov/cancertopics/wyntk/breast/page10

FIGURE 14-7: MODIFIED RADICAL MASTECTOMY

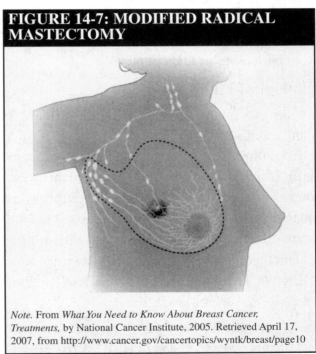

Note. From *What You Need to Know About Breast Cancer, Treatments,* by National Cancer Institute, 2005. Retrieved April 17, 2007, from http://www.cancer.gov/cancertopics/wyntk/breast/page10

Hormonal Treatment

Among hormonal treatment strategies are tamoxifen (Nolvadex), an antiestrogen; raloxifene (Evista), a selective estrogen receptor modulator; and aromatase inhibitors such as anastozole (Arimidex) and letrozole (Femara). A gonadotropin used in adjuvant breast cancer treatment is goserelin (Zoladex) (ACS, 2005; Mahon, 2004; NCI, 2006).

Chemotherapy

Chemotherapy treatment strategies include standard protocols that include cyclophosphamide (Cytoxan), doxorubicin (Adriamycin), and paclitaxel (Taxol).

Chemotherapy protocols for advanced or metastatic disease include doxorubicin (Adriamycin), paclitaxel, docetaxel (Taxotere), capecitabine (Xeloda), vinorelbine (Navelbine), mitomycin (Mutamycin), 5-fluorouracil, and vinblastine (Velban).

For patients with decreased bone density and skeletal complications of disease or treatment, bisphosphonates such as alendronate (Fosamax) are used as treatment agents (Bernice, 2005; Marrs, 2005). Aromatase inhibitors increase the patient's risk new or continuing osteoporosis. Therefore, bisphosphonates are typically ordered in tandem with hormonal therapy.

Biological Therapy

Approximately 25% of patients with breast cancer have tumors that overexpress HER2/neu (NCI, 2006). Trastuzumab (Herceptin) is an anti-HER2/neu antibody, approved as adjuvant treatment for patients with HER2-overexpressing cancers. Results from study data released in 2006 show that trastuzumab regimens—with or after chemotherapy— for patients with overexpressed HER2/neu lead to a significant improvement in disease-free survival (NCI, 2006).

Patients with metastatic breast cancer with substantial overexpression of HER2/neu are candidates for treatment with a combination of trastuzumab and paclitaxel or for clinical studies of trastuzumab combined with taxanes and other chemotherapeutic agents.

Another targeted therapy, bevacizumab (Avastin), in combination with standard chemotherapy (paclitaxel), increases the period before cancer progression in metastatic breast cancer patients compared with patients who receive the same chemotherapy without bevacizumab.

TUMOR MARKERS

A tumor marker (also called a *serum marker* or *biomarker*) is a substance found in higher-than-normal amounts in the blood, urine, or body tissues of people with certain kinds of cancer (NCI, 2005c). Tumor markers are produced either by the tumor or by the body as a result of cancer or other conditions. They are an additional measurement of response to treatment, joining with the clinical exam, imaging studies, and biopsies. In time, tumor markers will be able to detect and diagnose all cancers (American Society of Clinical Oncology [ASCO], 2002). The ASCO recommends tracking these tumor markers when caring for patients with breast cancer:

HER2/neu (c-erbB-2)

This marker is found in some breast cancer cells and may help indicate how a woman will respond to different types of treatment. ASCO recommends the use of HER2/neu for the diagnosis and prognosis of breast cancer.

Every patient with breast cancer should receive a test for HER2/neu either at time of diagnosis or recurrence. HER2/neu levels can identify women who are likely to benefit from trastuzumab treatment or anthracycline-based treatments (e.g., adriamycin, doxorubicin, epirubicin [Ellence]). HER2/neu levels should not be used to predict the risk of breast cancer recurrence.

Steroid Hormone Receptors

In both premenopausal and postmenopausal women, levels of ERs and PRs can predict women who are likely to benefit from hormone treatment. ER and PR status should be used with other data (e.g., size of the tumor and presence of cancer cells in lymph nodes) to evaluate whether hormone treatment may be appropriate.

CA 27.29

Levels of CA 27.29 can increase as a tumor grows and, therefore, can indicate a response to or failure of treatment. Very high levels of CA 27.29 may indicate advanced disease or metastatic cancer. Unfortunately, false-positives can occur.

CA 15-3

In breast cancer, CA 15-3 is a protein that can be used to monitor a patient's response to treatment. The level can rise with tumor growth and fall with treatment. Used with other tests (such as ER and PR, HER2/neu, BRCA1, BRCA2), CA 15-3 can further help determine the extent of cancer and its spread—for example, to liver and bones. CA 15-3 is not a screening tool for breast cancer.

SUMMARY

Breast cancer is the most frequently diagnosed cancer in women. Because of screening via mammography and regular CBEs, many breast cancers are found early enough for treatments to be effective. Surgery, RT, and chemotherapy remain the mainstays of treatment for breast cancer. In addition, hormonal and targeted therapies have been shown to be effective in some women, allowing those women (especially those with hormone-fed cancers) to live longer. In addition to clinical exams, imaging studies, and standard laboratory blood work, tumor markers have now become a regular component of breast cancer treatment monitoring.

CASE STUDY: BREAST CANCER

LT is a 68-year-old Chinese-American woman who presents to her primary care physician (PCP) after feeling a lump in her right breast when taking a shower. The lump, which is in the upper outer quadrant, is the size of a plum. LT's last mammogram was 4 years ago. The PCP palpates a 4-cm mass, measured by hand calibration, with irregular borders. The PCP orders an ultrasound-guided core needle biopsy and chest X-ray.

On ultrasound, the mass is noted to be 3.8 cm. Pathology evaluation reports that the mass is invasive ductal carcinoma. Further evaluation of the tumor cells indicates that the cells are ER+ and PR+ and HER2 negative. LT is referred to a surgical oncologist and radiation oncologist.

Further workup includes a bone scan and CT of the chest, abdomen, and pelvis. All tests were negative for cancer spread.

After discussion of treatment options with her surgical oncologist and radiation oncologist, LT opted to have a lumpectomy, followed by adjuvant RT. The lumpectomy procedure was unremarkable. (The excised nodule was 3.8 cm x 2 cm with clean margins.) Based on sentinel node mapping, LT was found to have no positive nodes. LT's breast cancer was staged at T2 N0 M0. She went home about 4 hours after the procedure.

Postoperatively, LT experienced some pain that resolved within a few days with oral hydrocodone twice a day. She also had some nausea because of anesthesia, which also resolved within 2 days of the procedure. She was instructed to reduce physical activity involving her right side for 7 to 10 days.

Adjuvant RT to her right breast began 4 weeks after surgery. A total of 6200 cGy was given (25 fractions) over 6 weeks (five times per week). LT complained of skin irritation from the RT, which started 2 weeks after her therapy began. She was counseled to manage her mild erythema by washing with gentle soap and water, avoiding heat, and using unscented creams on her breast. The erythema resolved about 2 weeks after her treatments ended.

Approximately 2 weeks after her RT sessions ended, LT returned to consult with her medical oncologist. The medical oncologist prescribed adjuvant hormonal treatment—anastrozole (Arimidex), daily. This hormonal treatment was to continue indefinitely, although studies of anastrozole show benefit for 5 years. On anastrozole, LT experienced joint pain. Because of her fixed income, she is reluctant to spend money on her hormonal therapy because the prescription has a large co-pay.

At 3 months after completion of RT, LT had a mammogram. The results were negative for any new masses.

Since her lumpectomy, LT noted some swelling in her right arm, especially upon waking. She was referred to a lymphedema specialist, who treated the swelling with massage two times perweek for 4 weeks. She was encouraged to use an arm compression sleeve to control the lymphedema.

Additional Information

LT started menopause at age 50. (She believes she started menstruation at age 13.) She is gravida 2, para 2. Her first child was born when she was 27 years old. She has never taken oral contraceptives.

She has an uncle who died of pancreatic cancer and has no history of breast cancer in her family.

Throughout her treatment, LT used Chinese herbs to "kill off the tumor." (Her children helped her purchase them on the Internet.)

LT, a grandmother of two, attended three support group sessions geared toward breast cancer patients. When she was first diagnosed, she cried easily around her family. She also had trouble sleeping and said she could not concentrate.

LT is pleased with her recovery but states she initially had second thoughts about whether she should have had her breast removed as treatment. Eventually, she believed she was able to regain control of her breast health by doing a monthly BSEs, getting her yearly mammogram, and receiving yearly check-ups.

LT, a widow, has resumed helping with child-care for her two grandchildren while her daughter

works. She finds that her stamina has increased over the last year.

Four years after her initial treatment and diagnosis, she takes pride in considering herself a breast cancer survivor. She plans to participate in a 3-day walk for breast cancer.

Questions

1. When is radiation treatment considered as a treatment for breast cancer?

2. Why is LT a candidate for adjuvant hormonal therapy?

3. From LT's history, which factors increase her risk of developing breast cancer?

4. What benefit or harm is known about taking Chinese herbs and breast cancer?

5. In addition to attending a support group and occasional use of sleeping medication, what additional strategies could help LT better cope with her diagnosis, treatment period, and recovery?

Answers

1. Surgery combined with RT is the standard treatment protocol for early-stage, localized breast cancer. Statistics show that surgery and RT reduce the likelihood of tumor recurrence in the breast. Adjuvant chemotherapy and hormonal therapy further increase survival rates for breast cancer patients. LT's tumor was greater than 2 cm; therefore, her breast cancer, staged at stage II, would be treated with surgery and RT. (Chemotherapy and hormonal therapy may also be recommended, based on the tumor pathology and lymph node spread.)

2. Because LT's ERs and PRs were positive, hormone therapy is a treatment option. Estrogen can control the proliferation of malignant cells. Therefore, manipulating the stimulatory effects of estrogen can reduce or limit malignancy growth. When patients are ER+ or PR+, they have a better than 75% response rate to hormonal therapy. If the patient is only ER+

then the response rate decreases to 35%. Examples of therapeutic hormones for breast cancer include tamoxifen (antiestrogen therapy) and anastrozole, letrozole, and exemestane (an aromatase inhibitor).

3. From what is known about LT's history, her risk factors for breast cancer includes age and sex. Other risk factors for breast cancer include race (Caucasians have a higher incidence rate), personal previous history of breast cancer, family history of breast cancer, breast changes, genetic alteration syndromes, estrogen exposure, weight gain and late childbearing.

4. No studies have shown definitive benefit or harm from taking Chinese herbs for breast cancer. The exact compounding of a particular Chinese herb remedy (content, dose, quality of ingredients) is unknown. Moreover, studies have shown that certain herbs should be avoided during chemotherapy treatment. For example, glucosamine should be avoided during some chemotherapy treatments (e.g., etoposide and doxorubicin) because glucosamine can induce resistance to the effects of those chemotherapies.

5. Other strategies to help LT cope with her cancer and recovery may include one-on-one counseling sessions (to reduce anxiety and depression and support emotional needs), encouraging recreational, and providing information and interventions (e.g., on side effect anticipation and management) to address LT's concerns.

EXAM QUESTIONS

CHAPTER 14
Questions 56-59

Note: Choose the option that BEST answers each question.

56. One risk factor for breast cancer is

    a. personal history of breast cancer.

    b. antiperspirant use.

    c. breast implants.

    d. breast-feeding.

57. A component of staging for breast cancer is

    a. weight at time of diagnosis.

    b. lymph node dissection.

    c. smoking history.

    d. complete blood count.

58. An agent used in treating breast cancer is

    a. brachytherapy.

    b. cytarabine.

    c. ciprofloxacin.

    d. trastuzumab.

59. A hormonal therapy used to treat breast cancer is

    a. sargramostim.

    b. rabeprazole.

    c. letrozole.

    d. leutinizing hormone.

REFERENCES

American Cancer Society. (2005). Hormonal therapy for breast cancer: Estrogen and estrogen receptors. *CA: Cancer Journal for Clinicians, 55,* 195-198.

American Cancer Society. (2006). *Cancer facts & figures 2006.* Atlanta: Author.

American Joint Committee on Cancer. (2002). *AJCC cancer staging manual* (6th ed.). New York: Springer-Verlag.

American Society of Clinical Oncology. (2002). *A patient guide: Understanding tumor markers for breast and colorectal cancers.* Retrieved April 17, 2007, from http://www.plwc.org/plwc/external_files/tmarker_fin.pdf

Bernice, M. (2005). Nursing care of the client with breast cancer. In J.K. Itano & K.N. Taoka (Eds.), *Core curriculum for oncology nursing* (4th ed., pp. 492-511). St. Louis: Elsevier.

Harwood, K. (2004). Advances in endocrine therapy for breast cancer: Considering efficacy, safety, and quality of life. *Clinical Journal of Oncology Nursing, 8*(4), 629-637.

Jemal, A., Siegel, R, Ward, E., Murray, T., Xu, J, Smigal, C., et al. (2006). Cancer statistics, 2006. *CA: Cancer Journal for Clinicians, 56(2),* 106-130.

Johansen, A. (2005). Breast cancer chemoprevention: A review of selective estrogen receptor modulators. *Clinical Journal of Oncology Nursing, 9*(3), 317-320.

Mahon, S. (2004). Chemoprevention of breast cancer. *Clinical Journal of Oncology Nursing, 8*(4), 421-423.

Marrs, J. (2005). Osteoporosis in the oncology setting. *Clinical Journal of Oncology Nursing, 9*(2), 261-263.

National Cancer Institute. (2005a). *Cancer trends progress report—2005 update.* Available from http://progressreport.cancer.gov

National Cancer Institute. (2005b). *Cancer trends progress report—2005 update. Breast cancer treatment.* Retrieved April 17, 2007, from http://progressreport.cancer.gov/doc_detail.asp?pid=1&did=2005&chid=24&coid=223&mid=

National Cancer Institute. (2005c). *Tumor markers: Questions and answers.* Retrieved April 17, 2007, from http://cancer.gov/cancertopics/fact sheet /detection/tumor-markers

National Cancer Institute. (2005d). *What you need to know about breast cancer.* Retrieved April 17, 2007, from http://www.cancer.gov/cancer topics/wyntk/breast/

National Cancer Institute. (2006). *Breast cancer.* Retrieved April 17, 2007, from http://cancer .gov/cancertopics/types/breast

National Cancer Institute. (2007). *Genetics of breast and ovarian cancer.* Retrieved May 31, 2007, from http://cancer.gov/cancertopics/pdq/genetics/breast-and-ovarian/Health Professional/page2#Section_97

Singletary, S., & Connolly, J. (2006). Breast cancer staging: Working with the sixth edition of the *AJCC Cancer Staging Manual. CA: Cancer Journal for Clinicians, 56*(1), 37-47.

University of Texas M.D. Anderson Cancer Center. (2003). *Sentinel lymph node biopsy.* Retrieved April 17, 2007, from http://www2.mdanderson .org/app/snb/procedure_5.htm

Weiss, M. (2007). *Ductal carcinoma in situ (DCIS).* Retrieved April 17, 2007, from http://www.breast cancer.org/ dcis_ductal_carcinoma_in_situ.html

CHAPTER 15

COLORECTAL CANCER

CHAPTER OBJECTIVE

After completing this chapter, the reader will be able to describe risk factors, screening methods, symptoms, and management of colorectal cancer.

LEARNING OBJECTIVES

After studying this chapter, the reader will be able to

1. recognize the incidence of and death rates for colorectal cancer in the United States.

2. identify two risk factors for colorectal cancer.

3. identify two symptoms of colorectal cancer.

4. name two chemotherapies that are used in treating colorectal cancer.

INTRODUCTION

Colorectal cancer remains one of the leading causes of cancer death in men and women. It is a frequent cause of cancer for at-risk populations. Yet promising treatments are improving survival statistics for those with early-stage colorectal cancer. This chapter highlights the risk factors for colorectal cancer, methods of colorectal screening and detection, and current treatments.

EPIDEMIOLOGICAL TRENDS

Colorectal cancer is the second leading cause of cancer death in men and women. In 2006, more than 106,680 new cases of colorectal cancer and 56,000 deaths were reported (National Cancer Institute [NCI], 2007). In 2005, 10% of all new cancer cases in men were colorectal cancer; for women, 11% of new cancer cases were colorectal cancer (Viale, Fung, & Zitella, 2005).

Colorectal cancer is the third most frequent cancer occurring in both sexes (American Cancer Society [ACS], 2006). One out of eighteen people in this country will develop colorectal cancer at some point in their lifetime (Maltzman, 2004a). Colon cancer is 2.5 times more common than rectal cancer (ACS, 2006). Approximately 7% of colorectal cancers occur in people younger than age 40.

Among African Americans, the incidence of colon cancer has increased by 30% since 1973 and is now higher than in Caucasians (ACS, 2006). African Americans are 30% more likely to die of the disease than other ethnic groups (Maltzman, 2004a).

The 5-year survival rate for colorectal cancer has increased to greater than 90% in the early localized stage. However, only 39% of colorectal cancers are diagnosed at an early stage (ACS, 2006). After spread to adjacent organs, the 5-year survival rate drops to 68%. When metastasis is distant, survival at 5 years is only 10% (ACS, 2006).

Incidence rates for colorectal cancer have been slightly decreasing, attributable to increased screening and polyp removal that prevents tumor progression (ACS, 2006). Unfortunately, more than 50% of new patients present with stage III or metastatic disease, and half of all people with colorectal cancer are diagnosed with recurrent or metastatic disease (Viale et al., 2005). Therefore, screening and early diagnosis are crucial in helping to reduce mortality.

New therapies for advanced colorectal cancer (reviewed later in this chapter) have almost doubled the life expectancy for patients. In a disease that has had very few changes in disease reduction and overall survival, new chemotherapy and biotherapy agents have led the way in providing effective treatment options for those diagnosed with colorectal cancer (Viale et al., 2005).

RISK FACTORS

The incidence of colorectal cancer is high in industrialized regions, such as North America, northwestern Europe, and Australia. Incidence is low in less-developed regions, such as Asia, Africa, and South America. Therefore, diet is a major focus of exploration to establish colorectal cancer risk factors.

Epidemiologic, experimental (animal), and clinical investigations suggest that diets high in total fat, protein, calories, alcohol, and meat (both red and white) and low in calcium and folate are associated with an increased incidence of colorectal cancer (NCI, 2007; Strohl, 2005). However, studies to date have shown that cereal fiber supplementation and diets low in fat and high in fiber, fruits, and vegetables do not reduce the rate of adenoma recurrence over a 3-year to 4-year period (NCI, 2007).

Cigarette smoking is another risk factor for colorectal cancer (NCI, 2007).

Patients are considered to be at high risk for colon cancer if they have a prior experience of colon cancer; a precursor lesion, such as a polyp; a history of chronic inflammatory bowel disease, such as Crohn's disease or ulcerative colitis; a strong family history of the disease; or the presence of certain gene markers.

More common conditions with an increased risk include a personal history of colorectal cancer or adenoma; first-degree family history of colorectal cancer or adenoma; and a personal history of ovarian, endometrial, or breast cancer. Yet these high-risk groups account for only 23% of all colorectal cancers (NCI, 2007).

Hereditary Risk Factors

Hereditary colon cancer syndrome is a set of signs that identify a genetic condition that predisposes people to colon cancer. There are three main categories of heredity colon cancer syndromes. They account for 10% to 15% of colorectal cancers (NCI, 2007). In familial adenomatous polyposis (FAP), patients grow hundreds of polyps, any of which may turn into cancer at any time. The growth of these polyps starts at an early age. Because of the early age of onset and the many polyps that develop, nearly all patients with FAP develop cancer at some point in their lives.

Those with attenuated familial adenomatous polyposis (AFAP) have fewer than 100 adenomatous polyps in their colon and rectum. AFAP tends to be diagnosed in patients later than FAP, approximately 10 to 15 years later. It has been recommended that AFAP patients have colonoscopies rather than sigmoidoscopies because adenomatous polyps are predominantly right-sided and beyond the reach of a sigmoidoscope (Lee, 2005).

In contrast, patients who are diagnosed with hereditary nonpolyposis colon cancer (HNPCC)—also called Lynch syndrome I and II—may develop fewer polyps. However, the polyps that do grow are very aggressive, with up to 80% of patients developing colon cancer. HNPCC-affected individuals are typically older than FAP patients at the time that they are diagnosed with colon cancer, but younger than those without a genetic predisposition (i.e., those who develop colon cancer sporadically) (Maltzman, 2004a).

Other cancers associated with HNPCC are endometrial, stomach, gallbladder, brain, and breast cancers.

Limiting screening or early cancer detection to only these high-risk groups discussed above would miss the majority of colorectal cancers (NCI, 2005a). Studies continue to look at those with a genetic susceptibility to colon cancer so that this population can be targeted for various prevention strategies. In the long-term, this research may lead to a better understanding of the biology of colorectal cancer and may result in new therapeutic and preventive techniques.

PREVENTION, SCREENING, AND DETECTION

Recommendations for primary prevention of colorectal cancer include dietary changes—decreasing saturated fat intake, increasing protein intake, and increasing the amount of fruits and vegetables in the diet (Strohl, 2005). Total fiber intake should be between 20 and 30 g/day. Oral supplements of calcium and folic acid have been shown to be safe measures that probably reduce the risk of colorectal cancer (Lee, 2005). And, of course, risk is lower for those who reduce their weight, stop smoking, minimize alcohol intake, and exercise regularly (Strohl, 2005).

Screening for colon cancer should be a part of routine care for all adults starting at age 50, especially for those with first-degree relatives with colorectal cancer. Screening is also important because of the frequency of the disease, the ability to identify high-risk groups, the demonstrated slow growth of primary lesions, the better survival of patients with early-stage lesions, and the relative simplicity and accuracy of screening tests (NCI, 2007).

Detection and screening have become the primary methods for reducing morbidity and mortality of colorectal cancer. Nevertheless, epidemiological data show that many patients do not report colorectal cancer symptoms until the disease has advanced.

Screening Modalities

There are several modalities of screening for colon cancer, but few patients choose them.

Fecal occult blood testing (FOBT) is a test for blood in the stool. Critics cite that this test looks only for cancer and not precancerous lesions. By the time the patient is bleeding, he or she is likely to already have a malignancy. Although the test is painless, its sensitivity and specificity are quite low, diminishing its utility as a screening tool.

A flexible sigmoidoscopy has the disadvantage of only examining the lower colon and rectum. In 2000, an influential and disparaging editorial in the *New England Journal of Medicine* was published that made this option less attractive to most patients and referring physicians (Podolsky, 2000).

A double-contrast barium enema (DCBE) is an unpleasant, time-consuming test whose sensitivity, according to most studies, does not exceed 50% (NCI, 2007).

Colonoscopy has become the most demanded test for colorectal screening. (During a colonoscopy, a physician inserts a special scope in the colon so that the internal lining of the lower colon can be viewed.) Most attribute the growing demand for colonoscopies to the attention focused on the procedure by "Today" show host Katie Couric and her televised procedure in 2000. A national study completed by researchers at the Universities of Michigan and Iowa noted that Couric's efforts led to a 20% increase in colonoscopies nationwide in the months following the airing of the show.

Since then, the rate of colonoscopies has continued to increase; the number of people experiencing at-risk symptoms—who go on to be checked by colonoscopy—has also increased due to Couric increasing the visibility of colorectal cancer (Maltzman, 2004b).

Another factor that has increased demand for colonoscopies is Medicare's decision in 2001 to pay for them—once every 2 years for high-risk patients and once every 10 years for low-risk individuals.

A newer screening and detection method for colorectal cancer is called the *virtual colonoscopy*. Although promising, it is not yet universally available (Maltzman, 2004a). A virtual colonoscopy uses computer and X-ray imaging to scan the colon, creating two- and three-dimensional images of the colon on a computer screen. The procedure avoids use of a colonoscope, the instrument used for standard colonoscopies.

The ACS screening recommendations for average- and increased-risk individuals are shown in Table 15-1.

TABLE 15-1: AMERICAN CANCER SOCIETY GUIDELINES ON SCREENING AND SURVEILLANCE FOR THE EARLY DETECTION OF COLORECTAL ADENOMAS AND CANCER (AVERAGE-RISK WOMEN AND MEN AGES 50 AND OLDER)

Test	Interval (beginning at age 50)	Comment
FOBT and flexible sigmoidoscopy	FOBT annually and flexible sigmoidoscopy every 5 years	Combined flexible sigmoidoscopy and FOBT is preferred over FOBT or flexible sigmoidoscopy alone. All positive tests should be followed up with colonoscopy.
Flexible sigmoidoscopy	Every 5 years	All positive tests should be followed up with colonoscopy.
FOBT	Annually	The recommended take-home multiple sample method should be used. All positive tests should be followed up with colonoscopy.
Colonoscopy	Every 10 years	Colonoscopy provides an opportunity to visualize, sample, and remove significant lesions.
DCBE	Every 5 years	All positive tests should be followed up with colonoscopy.

If colonoscopy is unavailable, not feasible, or not desired by the patient, DCBE alone or a combination of flexible sigmoidoscopy and DCBE are acceptable alternatives. Adding flexible sigmoidoscopy to DCBE may provide a more comprehensive diagnostic evaluation than DCBE alone in finding significant lesions. A supplementary DCBE may be needed if a colonoscopic exam fails to reach the cecum, and a supplementary colonoscopy may be needed if a DCBE identifies a possible lesion or does not adequately visualize the entire colorectal area.

(ACS, 2006)

In summary, colonoscopy—as the main screening and detection tool available for colorectal cancer—can detect the need to remove adenomatous polyps. This strategy can reduce the risk of colorectal cancer.

SYMPTOMS OF ADVANCING DISEASE

Symptoms of advancing colorectal disease are abdominal pain, blood in the stool, changes in bowel habits, jaundice, pruritus, weight loss, and anorexia. Unfortunately, the first symptoms arising from colorectal carcinoma may be from metastatic disease. Jaundice, pruritus, and ascites could indicate metastatic liver involvement. As cancer of the colon and rectum progresses, obstruction and perforation of the bowel become more likely. Figure 15-1 shows the colorectal anatomy.

FIGURE 15-1: COLORECTAL ANATOMY

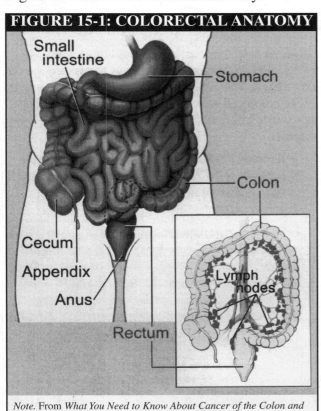

Note. From *What You Need to Know About Cancer of the Colon and Rectum,* by National Cancer Institute, 2006. Retrieved October 31, 2006, from http://cancer.gov/cancertopics/wyntk/colon-and-rectal/page2

STAGING SCHEMA, TUMOR MARKERS

Table 15-2 provides an overview of staging for colorectal cancer.

Tumor Markers

Carcionembryonic antigen (CEA) is a tumor marker in the blood that is followed during treatment to assess treatment effectiveness. During treatment, the monitoring of CEA level is used in concert with clinical assessments and imaging scans. Normal CEA range for nonsmokers is less than 3 mcg/L; for smokers, it is less than 5 mcg/L. For those not diagnosed with colorectal cancer, CEA is not valuable as a screening test. Studies of its use as a screening tool showed a large number of false-positive and false-negative reports (NCI, 2005c).

TREATMENT STRATEGIES

Primary Surgical Therapy

Surgery is the treatment of choice for early-stage, localized disease. When treated early, colorectal cancer is often curable. Approximately 50% of cancers localized to the bowel are curable. (NCI, 2005b). Surgical procedures that have improved outcomes and that have improved the patient's experience during surgery include anastomosis devices, bowel stapling, and laparoscopic techniques. These methods are also used as palliative measures to prevent or bypass obstruction.

Surgery is curative in 25% to 40% of highly selected patients who develop resectable metastases in the liver and lung. Improved surgical techniques and advances in preoperative imaging have allowed better patient selection for resection.

The role of sentinel lymph node mapping is being clinically evaluated to determine if it can spare complete lymph node dissection during surgery (NCI, 2005b).

TABLE 15-2: STAGING OF COLORECTAL CANCER

Cancer of the colon and rectum is the second most common type of cancer in the general population, but the incidence may be slowly decreasing. In 2006, an estimated 106,680 new cases were diagnosed, accounting for 56,000 deaths (NCI, 2006). Surgery remains the primary mode of therapy. Current clinical data have been more persuasive than ever for the use of adjuvant radiation and chemotherapy. Not all subsets of patients with this disease, however, have demonstrated equal benefit from adjuvant treatment. Therefore, the responsibility for careful staging remains paramount. This responsibility includes complete resection of the primary tumor associated with wide lymphadenectomy and careful inspection of peritoneal surfaces and intra-abdominal organs for evidence of metastatic disease.

For decades, classification of colorectal cancer has followed Dukes' system. Physicians are encouraged now to change to the TNM classification system outlined below. The unmodified Dukes' classification is also shown for comparison. Dukes' B2 (T4) lesions are considered for adjuvant chemotherapy.

Primary Tumor (T)

TX Unable to evaluate tumor
T0 Primary tumor cannot be found
Tis Carcinoma in situ, intraepithelial, or invasion of lamina propria
T1 Invasion of submucosa
T2 Invasion of muscularis propria
T3 Invasion into subserosa (or into perirectal tissues in the case of rectal cancer)
T4 Perforation of visceral peritoneum or direct invasion into adjacent structures

Regional Lymph Nodes (N)

NX Unable to evaluate regional lymph nodes
N0 No regional lymph node metastasis
N1 One to three regional lymph nodes involved
N2 Four regional lymph nodes involved

Distant Metastasis (M)

MX Unable to evaluate distant metastasis
M0 No evidence of distant metastasis
Ml Presence of any distant metastasis

Stage Grouping

				Dukes'
Stage 0	Tis	N0	M0	—
Stage I	T1	N0	M0	A
	T2	N0	M0	A
Stage IIA	T3	N0	M0	B
Stage IIB	T4	N0	M0	B
Stage IIIA	T1-T2	N1	M0	C
Stage IIIB	T3-T4	N1	M0	C
Stage IIIC	Any T	N2	M0	C
Stage IV	Any T	Any N	Ml	—

Note. Used with the permission of the American Join Committee on Cancer (AJCC), New York. The original source for this material is the *AJCC Cancer Staging Manual*, Sixth Edition (2002) published by Springer-Verlag, www.springeronline.com.

Adjuvant Radiation Therapy

Radiation therapy (RT) is a treatment option for localized disease, usually as an adjunct therapy after surgery.

Although combined chemotherapy and RT has a significant role in the management of patients with rectal cancer (below the peritoneal reflection), the role of adjuvant RT for patients with colon cancer (above the peritoneal reflection) is limited to those with residual disease. Metastasis to adjacent organs or lymph nodes reduces the 5-year survival rate to approximately 67% (ACS, 2006). If the cancer has spread to distant sites, survival becomes much less.

Adjuvant Chemotherapy

Adjuvant, postoperative chemotherapy treatment of patients with stage III colon cancer includes:

- fluorouracil (5-FU) and low-dose leucovorin for 6 months

- 5-FU and high-dose leucovorin for 7 to 8 months

- oxaliplatin (Eloxatin) combined with 5-FU-leucovorin (FOLFOX4*) for approximately 6 months

- irinotecan (Camptosar) combined with 5-FU and leucovorin

- capecitabine (Xeloda) daily for 2 weeks

Note: FOLFOX regimens include leucovorin (folinic acid) (FOL), 5-fluorouracil (F) and oxaliplatin (OX). Variations of FOLFOX (e.g., FOLFOX4, FOLFOX6, and FOLFOX7) alter dosing and schedules of the three chemotherapy agents.

Randomized trials indicate that elderly patients (older than 70 years) derive the same benefit from adjuvant treatment as younger individuals and, therefore, should not be excluded from these treatments based solely on age (NCI, 2005b).

Chemotherapy and Targeted Therapies for Recurrent and Metastatic Disease

Chemotherapy options for treatment of colorectal cancer remained relatively stagnant until the approval of irinotecan in 1996, followed by capecitabine (Xeloda), oxaliplatin, and the new targeted agents. The introduction of irinotecan in 1996, followed by the first new platinum analog agent, oxaliplatin, in 2002, offered considerable advances in chemotherapy for advanced and metastatic colorectal cancer.

Chemotherapy treatment for recurrent and advanced metastatic disease includes combinations of chemotherapies—and new novel agents—at various doses and schedules. Accepted first-line regimens are either irinotecan-based (protocol acronyms: IFL, FOLFIRI, AIO) or oxaliplatin-based (protocol acronyms: FOLFOX4, FOLFOX6).

The latest agents included in these regimens include:

- irinotecan combined with 5-FU and leucovorin

- irinotecan combined with 5-FU, leucovorin, and bevacizumab (Avastin)

- oxaliplatin combined with 5-FU and leucovorin (FOLFOX4, FOLFOX6, FOLFOX7)

- cetuximab (Erbitux) and irinotecan

- cetuximab and oxaliplatin

- capecitabine and oxaliplatin

- capecitabine and irinotecan.

These regimens have improved the response rate, time-to-tumor progression, and median survival of patients with advanced disease—and with tolerable side effects. Studies continue to show that these regimens can add months to survival for patients, doubling life expectancy in advanced disease to 24 months and longer (NCI, 2005b, 2007).

The oral fluorouracil agent capecitabine was released in 1998 and has been shown to have activity in colorectal cancer. Capecitabine is converted to 5-FU by thymidine synthase, which is more highly expressed in tumor cells than in normal tissue. Because capecitabine demonstrated efficacy equivalent to a 5-FU/leucovorin bolus or infusion, it received first-line indication in 2001 (Wilkes, 2005). It has also been a welcome treatment option for older patients and for those who, for various reasons, are not candidates for regular intravenously administered therapies.

Colorectal cancer chemotherapy schemas have developed as platforms for combined novel targeted agents, which are based on inhibiting epidermal growth factor receptor (EGFR) and vascular endothelial growth factor (VEGF). The newer targeted agents have improved efficacy of treatment for advanced colorectal cancer. Yet these new targeted therapies are expensive because they are new options in practice; the pharmaceutical companies that developed the agents will be recouping their development costs for many years.

In 2004, two new monoclonal antibody agents were approved for the treatment of patients with metastatic colorectal cancer:

- Cetuximab (Erbitux), a chimeric (a genetically fused product containing mouse and human antibodies) monoclonal antibody, binds to EGFRs that are overexpressed on tumor cells. The binding blocks the ability of epidermal growth factor to initiate receptor activation and signaling to the tumor. Cetuximab is approved as second-line treatment in combination with irinotecan or as a single agent in patients with EGFR-positive, metastatic, irinotecan-refractory colorectal cancer (Viale et al., 2005; Wilkes, 2005).

- Bevacizumab (Avastin) is a recombinant humanized monoclonal antibody that targets the VEGF molecule. It is 93% human and 7% murine and is thought to be less likely to cause an immune response. The antibody prevents VEGF from binding to its natural receptors on the vascular endothelium, which then inhibits VEGF-induced angiogenesis. Bevacizumab is approved as first-line therapy in combination with 5-FU-based chemotherapy for the treatment of metastatic colorectal cancer (Viale et al., 2005).

SUMMARY

More prevalent screening for colorectal cancer has allowed earlier and more effective treatments for this malignancy. Along with surgery and RT, chemotherapy and targeted therapies have increased the response of patients to treatment. Continued breakthroughs in colorectal cancer treatment are anticipated in the next few years.

EXAM QUESTIONS

CHAPTER 15
Questions 60-63

Note: Choose the option that BEST answers each question.

60. Among men and women with cancer, the death rate due to colorectal cancer is

    a. first of all cancers.
    b. second of all cancers.
    c. third of all cancers.
    d. fourth of all cancers.

61. A risk factor for colorectal cancer is

    a. sun exposure.
    b. viruses.
    c. exposure to benzene.
    d. diet.

62. A early symptom of colorectal cancer is

    a. anemia.
    b. blood in stool.
    c. cough.
    d. weakness.

63. A chemotherapy used in treating colorectal cancer is

    a. 5-FU.
    b. doxorubicin.
    c. letrozole.
    d. methotrexate.

REFERENCES

American Cancer Society. (2006). *Cancer facts & figures 2006.* Atlanta: Author.

American Joint Committee on Cancer. (2002). *AJCC cancer staging manual* (6th ed.). New York: Springer-Verlag.

Lee, D. (2005). *Colon cancer: The genetic factor.* Retrieved October 31, 2006, from http://www .medicinenet.com/script/main/art.asp?article key=46105

Maltzman, J. (2004a). *Hereditary syndromes in colorectal cancer.* Available from www.oncolink.upenn.edu

Maltzman, J. (2004b). *The Couric effect.* Available from www.oncollink.upenn.edu

National Cancer Institute. (2005a). *Cancer trends progress report—2005 update. Colorectal cancer screening.* Retrieved October 31, 2006, from http://progressreport.cancer.gov/doc _detail.asp?pid=1&did=2005&chid=22&coid= 218&mid=

National Cancer Institute. (2005b). *Cancer trends progress report—2005 update. Colorectal cancer treatment.* Retrieved October 31, 2006, from http://progressreport.cancer.gov/doc _detail.asp?pid=1&did=2005&chid=24&coid= 224&mid=

National Cancer Institute. (2005c). *Tumor markers: Questions and answers.* Retrieved April 17, 2007, from http://cancer.gov/cancertopics/fact sheet/detection/tumor-markers

National Cancer Institute. (2006). *What you need to know about cancer of the colon and rectum.* Retrieved October 31, 2006, from http://cancer .gov/cancertopics/wyntk/colon-and-rectal/

National Cancer Institute. (2007). *Colon and rectal cancer.* Retrieved October 31, 2006, from http:// cancer.gov/cancertopics/types/colon-and-rectal

Podolsky, D.K. (2000). Going the distance – The case for true colorectal-cancer screening. *New England Journal of Medicine,* July 20, 2000; *343*(3): 207-208.

Strohl, R. (2005). Nursing care of the client with cancers of the gastrointestinal tract. In J. K. Itano & K. N. Taoka (Eds.), *Core curriculum for oncology nursing* (4th ed., pp. 537–548). St. Louis: Elsevier.

Viale, P., Fung, A., & Zitella, L. (2005). Advanced colorectal cancer: Current treatment and nursing management with economic considerations. *Clinical Journal of Oncology Nursing, 9*(5), 541–552.

Wilkes, G. (2005). Therapeutic options in the management of colon cancer: 2005 update. *Clinical Journal of Oncology Nursing, 9*(1), 31–44.

CHAPTER 16

PROSTATE CANCER

CHAPTER OBJECTIVE

After completing this chapter, the reader will be able to describe the screening methods and treatment strategies for prostate cancer.

LEARNING OBJECTIVES

After studying this chapter, the reader will be able to

1. identify two early warning signs of prostate cancer.

2. recognize normal limits for prostate-specific antigen.

3. name two treatment strategies for early-stage prostate cancer.

4. recognize a hormonal treatment for metastatic prostate cancer.

INTRODUCTION

Prostate cancer, one of the most common cancers in men, is very treatable when detected early. Early detection is largely due to the prostate-specific antigen (PSA) test being used in men. The PSA test has also been used as a marker to help determine the effectiveness of treatment. This chapter reviews the incidence of and death rates for prostate cancer, risk factors, early warning signs, screening methods, and diagnostic workup and treatment strategies.

EPIDEMIOLOGICAL TRENDS

Prostate cancer is the most commonly diagnosed cancer among American men. One out of every six men will be diagnosed with prostate cancer during their lifetime. In 2006, approximately 234,460 new cases were diagnosed, with 27,350 deaths. The incidence of prostate cancer is higher among African American men than among Caucasian men and death rates for African American men are more than twice as high as those for Caucasian men. Japanese males have the lowest incidence and mortality rates from prostate cancer (American Cancer Society [ACS], 2006; Jemal et al., 2006).

Incidence rates have substantially changed over the last 20 years, with an initial rise from 1988 to 1992, then a sharp decline from 1992 to 1995, with a slight increase again since 1995. The sharp decline is thought to be due to the development of PSA blood test screening, especially among men younger than age 65 (ACS, 2006).

According to the National Cancer Institute's (NCI's) Surveillance Program, more than 90% of prostate cancers are discovered when they are in local or regional locations. The 5-year survival rate with early detection is almost 100%. Relative 10-

year survival for all stages is 93%; 15-year survival is 77% (ACS, 2006; Jemal et al., 2006).

Clinically diagnosable prostate cancer—if left untreated—continues to grow and threaten the life of the patient. Latent or clinically unimportant cancers do not threaten the patient's life. Of men age 50 and older, approximately one-third have malignant cells in their prostates. On autopsy, 75% of men older than 65 years have a prostate tumor (O'Rourke, 2005).

Testing and new diagnostic tools have affected prostate cancer incidence. PSA screening over the past 20 years is largely responsible for the initial increase and eventual decline in the number of newly diagnosed patients, causing the number of new cases diagnosed each year to stabilize (O'Rourke, 2005).

BACKGROUND

Prostate cancer grows relatively slowly compared with other types of cancer. The prostate gland, which is approximately the size of an inverted, triangularly shaped walnut, sits beneath the bladder and lies anterior to the rectum. The prostate gland is one of three primary sex glands in men (the other two are the testicles and the seminal vesicles). Together, these three glands produce fluids that make up semen. Figure 16-1 shows the anatomy of the prostate.

As one of the male sex glands, the prostate is affected by male sex hormones. These hormones stimulate the activity of the prostate and the replacement of prostate cells as they wear out. The chief male hormone is testosterone, which is produced almost entirely by the testicles (NCI, 2006).

Premalignant changes in the prostate can occur. Called *prostatic intraepithelial neoplasia* (PIN), these changes are categorized as low- or high-grade. They can be the first sign that a patient will develop prostate cancer within the next 10 years. On biopsy,

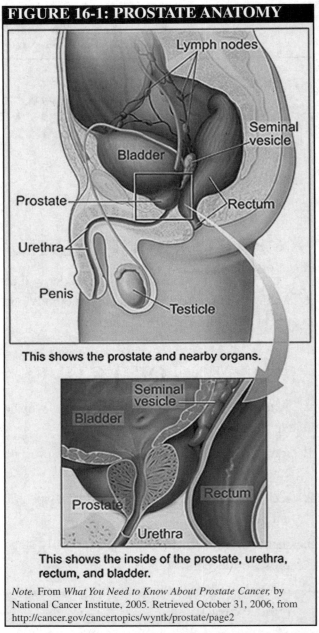

FIGURE 16-1: PROSTATE ANATOMY

This shows the prostate and nearby organs.

This shows the inside of the prostate, urethra, rectum, and bladder.

Note. From *What You Need to Know About Prostate Cancer,* by National Cancer Institute, 2005. Retrieved October 31, 2006, from http://cancer.gov/cancertopics/wyntk/prostate/page2

if PIN is established, the patient should have regular follow-up PSA testing and regular repeat biopsies (Brosman, 2005).

The vast majority of prostate cancers (95%) are adenocarcinomas, which start with epithelial cells proceeding through a variety of stages until they become malignant (O'Rourke, 2005).

When tumor cells travel outside the boundaries of the prostate, they spread to lymph nodes. The next most commonly involved metastatic site of prostate cancer is bone, especially the lumbar spine, pelvis, femur, and skull. Other sites of distant metastases include the lungs, bladder, and liver.

PRIMARY RISK FACTORS

The cause of prostate cancer is unknown. However, based on epidemiological data, several factors appear to increase the risk of prostate cancer, including age, race (highest in African Americans), family history, a high-fat diet, and environmental exposures (O'Rourke, 2005).

African American men have a 30% higher incidence of prostate cancer than Caucasian men—the highest incidence of prostate cancer in the world. Studies suggest that biologic factors in African American men need to be explored for their potential role in this disease. High levels of testosterone are thought to play a role. Serum testosterone levels are, on average, 15% higher in African American men than in white men (ACS, 2006).

Studies also suggest a familial risk of prostate cancer. One study reports that relatives of men with prostate cancer diagnosed before age 53 had a greater lifetime risk of developing the disease (NCI, 2006).

Asian males have the lowest prostate cancer incidence and mortality rates. A mostly vegetarian diet, which reduces serum testosterone levels, is suggested as a protective factor.

SCREENING AND DETECTION

Early warning signs of clinical prostate problems include dysuria, urinary frequency, nocturia, hematuria, weak or interrupted urine stream, pain on urination or ejaculation, and other signs of bladder outlet obstruction. Other reported symptoms include discomfort in the lower back, pelvis, or upper thighs (NCI, 2006).

When a cancerous prostate tumor is small and located only within the prostate itself, it may not cause any symptoms. In fact, a man may live many years with prostate cancer and never know he has it.

Screening for prostate cancer involves digital rectal examination (DRE), analysis of PSA level and, if appropriate, evaluation of the gland using transrectal ultrasound. The ACS recommends that regular prostate cancer screening (DRE and PSA analysis) begin for asymptomatic men at age 50. Men at high risk should begin screening earlier (at approximately age 45) (ACS, 2006).

Digital Rectal Examination

During a physical exam, the clinician can perform a DRE. DRE is useful for detecting abnormalities in the posterior and lateral aspects of the prostate gland but is limited in its sensitivity because up to 40% of tumors occur anterior to the midline and are undetectable by DRE (NCI, 2006). When used alone, DRE has been shown to have missed approximately 40% of cancers detected during initial screenings, because the tumor may also be too small for a clinician to feel during DRE (NCI, 2006).

Prostate-Specific Antigen

PSA levels reflect the severity of the patient's disease and are monitored during and after therapy, indicating treatment effectiveness. The normal reference range for PSA is 0.0 to 4.0 ng/ml; the normal range varies, however, based on age and race. Two factors that can affect a normal PSA range are prostatic growth (variation in PSA production and secretion) and racial differences (Balmer & Greco, 2004).

Worth noting, a man can have prostate cancer and still have a low level of PSA in his blood; conversely, a man can have a high PSA level and not have prostate cancer, because other prostate conditions can also cause elevated PSA levels. The prostate gland continues to grow in the adult male after the completion of puberty. As the prostate increases in size, PSA also increases. Benign prostatic hyperplasia (BPH) can produce a high serum concentration of PSA in both the absence and presence of prostate cancer.

Other factors can also affect PSA levels. For example, in a prostate cancer prevention trial over a period of 7 years, men receiving finasteride (Propecia), a 5-alpha-reductase inhibitor used to treat BPH, had a 24.8% lower risk of prostate cancer than men receiving a placebo but had a higher risk of high-grade cancer (Thompson et al., 2006).

Additional blood tests to diagnose and monitor prostate cancer include serum calcium, liver function tests, blood urea nitrogen, creatinine, and complete blood count. Not all prostate cancers produce PSA, so other diagnostic studies—such as magnetic resonance imaging (MRI), computed tomography scans, and other scans—may be needed to monitor the disease.

A bone scan is frequently performed to evaluate bone pain and may be performed as part of the staging workup. Bone scans are usually negative in patients with a PSA of less than 20 ng/ml.

The Merits of Universal Screening

Since the late 1980s and the widespread adoption of PSA screening, prostate cancer has become the most commonly diagnosed cancer in men in the United States. Despite screening recommendations, barriers to universal screening for prostate cancer exist and are based on cultural beliefs, fear of DRE, and the diagnosis of cancer and treatment (i.e., loss of continence and potency).

Disagreements continue about whether all men should be screened. Some experts advocate screening all men; others believe that only those at high risk should be screened. The ACS, American Urological Association, American College of Radiology, and Prostate Education Council recommend universal screening for prostate cancer. Proponents of screening suggest screening criteria that target annual DRE and PSA levels for men over age 50 (ACS, 2006).

Until there is clear proof that universal screening actually improves survival and outweighs the harm of unnecessary therapy, consensus on screening will remain illusive.

STAGING AND TREATMENT

Staging is key in determining treatment options. Prostate cancer in early stages is not necessarily treated. (No treatment, or watchful waiting, is based on the goal of increasing longevity and preserving quality of life.) But early-stage treatment can cure the disease in some men or control the disease for many years with few side effects.

Table 16-1 shows the American Joint Committee on Cancer staging for prostate cancer. Table 16-2 provides a guide to PSA levels in advanced disease (Wallace, Bailey, O'Rourke, & Galbraith, 2004).

PSA levels should be normal 3 to 18 months after completion of therapy. If PSA does not normalize after three consecutive readings, localized disease recurrence is suspected. Because results can vary slightly, men should have their PSA specimens processed by the same laboratory each year.

Treatments

Current treatment options include watchful waiting (periodic observation), surgery, radiation therapy (RT), hormonal manipulation, chemotherapy, and investigational drugs (NCI, 2006; O'Rourke, 2005).

Watchful Waiting

"Watchful waiting" (or periodic observation by the physician and clinical team) is a form of treatment. During watchful waiting, the clinician actively observes the indicators of disease progression. When the patient is older or has other health problems, monitoring disease progression for a period of time can offer less risk than initiating treatment. Especially for patients over age 70, watchful waiting may be an appropriate option (Wallace et al., 2004).

TABLE 16-1: STAGING OF PROSTATE CANCER

The incidence of prostate cancer has increased to the level where it is the most common cause of noncutaneous malignancy in men, accounting for 33% of all cancers in men (ACS, 2006). An estimated 234,460 cases occurred in 2006, with an estimated 27,350 deaths. The 5-year survival rate, with early detection, is almost 100% (ACS, 2006; Jemal et al., 2006).

Prostate cancer is distinct from other types of cancer in that the histologic grade of the tumor is important prognostic information. For this reason, grading classifications are included in the stage grouping. Prostate cancer is frequently diagnosed as an incidental finding after transurethral resection of the prostate gland (TURP) for hypertrophy. For this reason, the T1 category is subdivided as shown.

Primary Tumor (T)

TX	Primary tumor cannot be assessed
T0	No evidence of primary tumor
T1	Tumor is incidental histologic finding
T1A	$\leq 5\%$ of TURP specimen
T1B	$\geq 5\%$ of TURP specimen
T1C	Tumor on needle biopsy of nonpalpable mass
T2	Tumor presents grossly, confined to the gland
T2A	Tumor involves ½ of one lobe or less
T2B	Tumor involves > ½ of one lobe but not both lobes
T2C	Tumor involves both lobes
T3	Tumor invades
T3A	Extracapsular extension
T3B	Tumor invades seminal vesicles
T4	Tumor is fixed or invades adjacent structures other than those listed in T3

Regional Lymph Nodes (N)

NX	Regional lymph nodes not assessed
N0	No regional lymph node metastasis
N1	Metastasis in regional lymph node(s)

Distant Metastasis (M)

MX	Distant metastasis cannot be assessed
M0	No distant metastasis
Ml	Distant metastasis

Histopathologic Grade (G)

GX	Grade cannot be assessed
G1	Well differentiated, slight anaplasia
G2	Moderately differentiated, moderate anaplasia
G3–4	Poorly differentiated or undifferentiated, marked anaplasia

Stage Grouping

Stage I	T1A	N0	M0	G1
Stage II	T1A	N0	M0	G2, G3–4
	T1B	N0	M0	Any G
	T1C	N0	M0	Any G
	T1	N0	M0	Any G
	T2	N0	M0	Any G
Stage III	T3	N0	M0	Any G
Stage IV	T4	N0	M0	Any G
	Any T	N1	M0	Any G
	Any T	Any N	Ml	Any G

Note. Used with the permission of the American Join Committee on Cancer (AJCC), Chicago, Illinois. The original source for this material is the *AJCC Cancer Staging Manual,* Sixth Edition (2002) published by Springer-New York, www.springeronline.com.

TABLE 16-2: GENERAL RANGES FOR PSA LEVELS AS DISEASE ADVANCES

Stage I: 3.1 ng/ml to 12.1 ng/ml

Stage II: 12.3 ng/ml to 40 ng/ml

Stage III: 41 ng/ml to 102 ng/ml

Stage IV: 103 mg/ml to 563 ng/ml

Surgery

Various surgical options are available. Surgery as a treatment option also can have various goals, depending on the tumor and patient. Surgery is commonly used to remove cancer cells from the prostate and from nearby areas where it has spread. It is used primarily during the early stages, when the cancer is confined within the prostate or immediate areas.

Among surgery options are:

- **Transurethral resection of the prostate** (TURP) is used to treat symptoms of bladder outlet obstruction and, in some patients, provides pathological evidence that previously unsuspected cancer exists. (In suspected prostate cancer, this is usually a diagnostic procedure.)

- **Radical prostatectomy** is the procedure of choice for early-stage disease. A prostatectomy is a one-time procedure that may cure prostate cancer in its early stages and may help extend life in later stages.

Prostatectomy is a major operation and is usually an option for younger men (younger than 59 years.) It requires hospitalization and can cause side effects, including erectile dysfunction (loss of ability to have an erection), incontinence (loss of urinary control), and narrowing of the urethra, which can make urination difficult.

Up to 15% of men remain incontinent 6 months postoperatively. To address this problem, newer techniques, such as "nerve-sparing" surgery , are emerging to limit incontinence and erectile dysfunction (O'Rourke,

2005). Nursing care, in the form of education and support, is critical for a successful postoperative period and transition back to normal daily functioning (O'Rourke, 2005).

At some major cancer centers, laparoscopic prostatectomy, which is less invasive than radical prostatectomy, is a surgical option (O'Rourke, 2005). For patients with limited spread of disease, this technique can be less painful, cause less blood loss, and reduce the risk of impotence and incontinence (Held-Warmkessel, 2006).

- **Robotic prostatectomy** allows the surgeon to use a robot-assisted technique that is minimally invasive to perform radical prostatectomy. The robot, which has three multijoined arms, allows three-dimensional visualization via computer screen and a binocular endocope and scaling of movement and wristed instruments. Advantages of the technique include:

  – shorter procedure time (usually less than 2 hours)

  – minimal bleeding

  – minimal pain

  – reduced in-patient stay

  – earlier patient function and overall recovery.

(Tewari & Menon, 2004)

Radiation Therapy

For early-stage prostate cancer with cure as the goal, a viable treatment option is radiation via external beam. RT can be a choice for young men with early-stage cancer or for patients who are not surgical candidates.

Three-dimensional conformal radiotherapy delivers radiation doses directly to the prostate. The dose range—73 to 77 Gy over 7 to 8 weeks—depends on tumor size, PSA level, and core biopsies positive for cancer (Held-Warmkessel, 2006). Intensity-modulated radiation therapy (IMRT) is replacing three-dimensional treatments at major cancer centers (O'Rourke, 2005). An example of an IMRT dosing protocol is 81 Gy.

Side effects of RT can include urinary frequency, interrupted urine stream, urinary hesitancy, dysuria, urinary retention, impotence, rectal bleeding, fatigue, and gastrointestinal dysfunction, especially diarrhea (O'Rourke, 2005). Skin in the perineal area can also become thin and break down (Held-Warmkessel, 2006)

RT is also useful in managing complications of advanced prostate cancer, including hematuria, urinary obstruction, ureteral obstruction, and pain. RT can be used alone or in combination with hormone therapy (when cancer cells have spread beyond the prostate to the pelvic area) or for pain relief in advanced prostate cancer (NCI, 2006).

Another RT technique is brachytherapy, implanted seeds in the prostate gland. Implants can be temporary or permanent. Side effects can include pain, proctitis, dysuria, urinary retention, and (rarely) infection (Held-Warmkessel, 2006).

RT can also be used as palliative therapy for bone metastasis.

Hormone Therapy

Hormone therapy is most commonly used to treat cancer that has metastasized outside the pelvic area. Hormone therapy cannot cure prostate cancer but slows the cancer's growth and reduces the size of the tumor. Hormone therapy can also be used as neoadjuvant treatment for high-risk disease. In patients with early-stage cancer, hormone therapy may be used to compliment RT.

Among hormone therapy options are:

- removal of androgens, which are the hormone-dependent and hormone-sensitive cells. A surgical method to reduce testosterone is bilateral orchiectomy, or removal of the testicles.

- the administration of luteinizing hormone-releasing hormone (LHRH) agonists, which initially increases testosterone levels but, after several days of therapy, causes testosterone levels to fall to castration level. Flutamide (Drogenil) and bicalutamide (Casodex), which are antiandrogens, and megestrol acetate (Megace), a progestin, prevent the binding of testosterone to receptors on prostate cells.

- total androgen ablation combines antiandrogenic therapy with an LHRH agonist, such as leuprolide (Lupron) or goserelin (Zoladex) (NCI, 2006).

Chemotherapy

Chemotherapy has limitations as a prostate cancer treatment. It is reserved for metastatic disease and may be useful for palliation. Some agents, used in combination with other treatment modalities, include vinblastine (Velban), mitoxantrone (Novantrone), and estramustine (Emcyt). Docetaxel (Taxotere) is also being used in clinical trials and has shown effectiveness in treating metastatic prostate cancer (NCI, 2006).

Interventions for Treatment Side Effects

Sexual Dysfunction

Strategies to address sexual dysfunction caused by treatment start with providing information and creating an environment to discuss anatomical and functional changes. Several methods to reduce dysfunction are available, including medications, mechanical aids, and surgery.

Counseling can benefit the patient or the patient and his partner. Any counseling should take into account the patient's, and partner's pretreatment practices, cultural and religious beliefs, and intimacy issues (Krebs, 2006).

Urinary Incontinence

Interventions to address urinary incontinence may include a urinary catheter and perineal exercises to manage dribbling and urgency. Patients need to be aware of symptoms that need immediate medical attention, including fever; dysuria; urgency; hematuria; lymphedema of the legs, scrotum, or penis; cone pain; abdominal pain; neuritic pain; weight loss; and bowel dysfunction (O'Rourke, 2005).

SUMMARY

Early detection of prostate cancer has been largely due to the PSA test being conducted in middle-aged men. African American men have a 30% higher incidence of prostate cancer than Caucasian men, so are worthy of special screening and detection attention. In addition to surgery, effective treatment strategies for early prostate cancer include RT. Hormone therapy is a mainstay of metastatic disease, although some chemotherapy regimens are used for palliation.

CASE STUDY: PROSTATE CANCER

MT is a 59-year-old African American man who works as a mechanic. He sees his primary care physician (PCP), presenting with a history of dysuria for 6 months, continuing back pain, and problems with erection. In the last month, he has noticed blood in his urine.

At the encouragement of his wife, he agreed to an evaluation by his PCP although he has not had an annual physical for at least 8 years. On DRE, the PCP notes a left nodule on his prostate. PSA level from the blood draw is 15.55 ng/ml. Based on MT's clinical exam and PSA level, the PCP recommends a prostate biopsy.

Transrectal ultrasound-guided biopsy of the prostate shows a Gleason's 3 + 3 adenocarcinoma in the left apex of the gland. Clinically, the tumor is staged at T2A. After discussion with a urologic oncology surgeon and radiation oncologist, MT decides to proceed with robotic-assisted radical prostatectomy. He defers the decision about RT until after surgery.

His postoperative course was remarkable due to a slight fever on day 2. He was treated with ciprofloxacin 500 mg b.i.d. His JP (Jackson Pratt) drain and Foley catheter remained in place. On postop day 3, his JP drainage had decreased to 30 cc over 24 hours and the drain was removed. He was discharged to home with his Foley catheter in place.

Discharge instructions included 1) pain medication as needed (Vicodin 1 to 2 tablets every 4 to 6 hours, as needed), 2) medication for bladder spasms as needed (Detrol 2 mg b.i.d. prn), 3) no submerged bathing, 4) no sexual activity, 5) no heavy lifting, 6) report to physician or nurse fever, increased abdominal pain, nausea, vomiting, decreased urine output, blood or clots in the catheter, or purulent discharge at catheter site. The patient was instructed how to self-irrigate his Foley catheter with 120 ml of normal saline solution and how to troubleshoot the catheter if it became clogged. He returned for removal of the catheter 1 week postop.

MT's consult with the radiation oncologist reviewed the standard post-prostatectomy treatment radiation plan, using IMRT at a total dose of 70 Gy. (MT's PSA had fallen after surgery to 0.2 ng/ml.)

Additional Information

MT's family history is significant because his father was diagnosed with prostate cancer and died at age 70. His older brother, now 64, was diagnosed with early-stage prostate cancer last year and was treated with external beam radiation followed by monthly hormonal injections of goserelin (Zoladex).

MT is married with three stepchildren, one stepson in his mid-twenties still lives with him and his wife.

MT quit smoking 5 years ago after a 30 pack-year history of smoking cigarettes. He has one beer in the evening.

Since diagnosis, MT has become more sullen at home. He has no interest in social activities away from home because he is still anxious about incontinence (although his postop incontinence has lessened). Since his surgery, he has lost 20 lb; he states he has no interest in food. He also has lost interest in sexual relations with his wife. MT opted to not have adjuvant RT for now.

Six months post surgery, MT returned for follow-up evaluation. His PSA level had risen to 10.9 ng/ml. MT also reported back pain, which had progressed to numbness bilaterally in his legs. An MRI was ordered; it noted a 2.0 cm prostate nodule.

After RT, MT received hormonal treatment, leuprolide (Lupron), every 3 months. His physicians followed his progress, noting changes in his PSA level. The level fluctuated but steadily increased over the following 2 years.

Ultimately, MT died of advanced prostate cancer. His pain in his final month was managed with fentanyl patches, accompanied by adjuvant morphine sulfate (roxanol) dosing. During the final 2 months of his life, his care was managed by hospice, with a focus on palliative care.

Questions

1. What is the normal range for PSA?

2. What are treatment options for a stage T2A prostate tumor?

3. On discharge, how long does MT's Foley catheter need to be in place?

4. What were MT's risk factors for prostate cancer?

5. What are the most common side effects of leuprolide?

Answers

1. The normal reference range for PSA is 0.0 to 4.0 ng/ml. MT's first initial PSA level was 15.55 ng/ml. MT's PSA level contributed to his tumor staging.

2. Standard treatment for stage T2A prostate cancer includes surgery (prostatectomy and lymph node dissection), radiotherapy, or brachytherapy.

3. After a prostatectomy and discharge from the hospital, the Foley catheter should stay in place for approximately 1 to 3 weeks.

4. MT's risk factors for prostate cancer were his age (75% of prostate cancers are diagnosed in men over 65 years old), family history (a first-degree relative with prostate cancer increases MT's risk two- to three-fold), and ethnicity (African Americans have the highest incidence and mortality rates for prostate cancer).

5. The most common side effects of leuprolide include nausea, vomiting, hot flashes, night sweats, bone pain, swelling of the feet and ankles, headache and difficulty urinating the first few days after treatment begins, osteopenia or osteoporosis, anemia, weight gain, and muscle atrophy. Leuprolide may also reduce sexual desire.

EXAM QUESTIONS

CHAPTER 16
Questions 64-67

Note: Choose the option that BEST answers each question.

64. An early warning sign of prostate cancer is

    a. nervousness.

    b. hematuria.

    c. night sweats.

    d. fatigue.

65. A normal reading for PSA is

    a. 2.0 ng/ml.

    b. 5.1 ng/ml.

    c. 41.0 ng/ml.

    d. 100.0 ng/ml.

66. A treatment strategy for early-stage prostate cancer is

    a. colectomy.

    b. tamoxifen.

    c. enema.

    d. watchful waiting.

67. A hormonal treatment for metastatic prostate cancer is

    a. leuprolide.

    b. bevacizumab.

    c. anastrozole.

    d. pamidronate.

REFERENCES

American Cancer Society. (2006). *Cancer facts & figures 2006*. Atlanta: Author.

American Joint Committee on Cancer. (2002). *AJCC cancer staging manual* (6th ed.). New York: Springer-Verlag.

Balmer, L., & Greco, K. (2004). Prostate cancer recurrence fear: The prostate-specific antigen bounce. *Clinical Journal of Oncology Nursing, 8(4)*, 361-366.

Brosman, S. (2005). *Prostatic intraepithelial neoplasia (PIN)*. Retrieved October 31, 2006, from http://www.emedicine.com/med/topic 3056.htm

Held-Warmkessel, J. (2006). Prostate cancer. In C. Yarbro, M. Frogge, & M. Goodman (Eds.), *Cancer nursing: Principles and practice* (6th ed., pp. 1552-1580). Sudbury, MA: Jones & Bartlett.

Jemal, A., Siegel, R., Ward, E., Murray, T., Xu, J., Smigal, C., et al. (2006). Cancer statistics, 2006. *CA: Cancer Journal for Clinicians, 56(2)*, 106-130.

Krebs, L. (2006). Sexual and reproductive dysfunction. In C. Yarbro, M. Frogge, & M. Goodman (Eds.), *Cancer nursing: Principles and practice* (6th ed., pp. 841-869). Sudbury, MA: Jones & Bartlett.

National Cancer Institute. (2005). *What you need to know about prostate cancer.* Retrieved October 31, 2006, from http://cancer.gov/cancertopics/wyntk/prostate/

National Cancer Institute. (2006). *Prostate cancer.* Retrieved October 31, 2006, from http://cancer.gov/cancertopics/types/prostate

O'Rourke, M. (2005). Nursing care of the client with cancers of the urinary system. In J. K. Itano & K. N. Taoka (Eds.), *Core curriculum for oncology nursing* (4th ed., pp. 604-614). St. Louis: Elsevier.

Tewari, A., & Menon, M. (2004) Nerve sparing robotic prostatectomy: A novel and minimally invasive treatment of prostate cancer [Electronic version]. *PCRI Insights, 7(4)*. Retrieved October 31, 2006, from http://www.prostate-cancer.org/education/localdis/Tewari_NerveSparingRP.html

Thompson, I., Chi, C., Ankerst, D., Goodman, P., Tangen, C., Lippman, S., et al. (2006). Effect of finasteride on the sensitivity of PSA for detecting prostate cancer. *Journal of the National Cancer Institute, 98(16)*, 1128-33.

Wallace, M., Bailey, D., Jr., O'Rourke, M., & Galbraith, M. (2004). The watchful waiting management option for older men with prostate cancer: State of the science. *Oncology Nursing Forum, 31(6)*, 1057-1066.

CHAPTER 17

HEMATOLOGIC MALIGNANCIES: LYMPHOMA, MULTIPLE MYELOMA, AND LEUKEMIA

CHAPTER OBJECTIVE

After completing this chapter, the reader will be able to describe how lymphoma, multiple myeloma, and leukemia are diagnosed and how each of these hematologic malignancies is treated.

LEARNING OBJECTIVES

After studying this chapter, the reader will be able to

1. identify the presenting symptoms for non-Hodgkin's lymphoma.

2. list the presenting symptoms for acute lymphocytic leukemia.

3. recognize treatment strategies for specific malignancies.

4. list one of the targeted therapies for chronic myelogenous leukemia.

INTRODUCTION

Lymphoma, multiple myeloma, and leukemia are hematologic malignancies that are mainly treated with chemotherapy and targeted and biologic therapy protocols. This chapter reviews non-Hodgkin's and Hodgkin's lymphoma, multiple myeloma, and the five main categories of leukemia, focusing on their diagnostic workup and treatment strategies.

LYMPHOMA

Epidemiological Trends

In 2006, more than 66,690 new cases of lymphoma were diagnosed in the United States. Of those cases, 58,870 new cases were non-Hodgkin's lymphoma (NHL) and 7,800 were Hodgkin's disease (American Cancer Society [ACS], 2006; Jemal et al., 2006). Relative survival for NHL at 1 year is 93% and for Hodgkin's disease is 78%. Five-year survival for NHL is 85% and for Hodgkin's disease is 60% (ACS, 2006).

Lymphoma starts in the lymphatic system, a key component of the immune system that helps the body fight infections. Lymphocytes of the lymph system protect the body against infection and against the growth of tumors. These lymphocytes form lymph nodes in different places in the body, especially the axilla, groin, and neck area.

In the immune system, there are two main kinds of lymphocytes: B lymphocytes (B cells) and T lymphocytes (T cells). B cells fight foreign substances by making antibodies. These antibodies attach to bacteria and attract cells that eat the bacteria cells. The antibodies also attract proteins from the blood to help kill bacteria.

T cells protect the body from fungi, viruses, and some bacteria. They are able to recognize viral proteins in a virus-infected cell and then destroy the infected cell. They also release special proteins called *cytokines*, which bring white blood cells (WBCs) to the area of the infection. T cells can kill cancer cells (Iwamoto, 2005). Figure 17-1 shows the hematopoiesis cell lines.

The two main types of lymphatic system cancer are Hodgkin's disease and NHL. The difference between these two diseases is the way the cancer cells appear under a microscope (Iwamoto, 2005; National Cancer Institute [NCI], 2007c).

Non-Hodgkin's Lymphoma

NHL includes a diverse group of malignancies that originate from the lymphopoietic system. In NHL, cells in the lymphatic system grow out of control, causing the lymph glands to grow. In the last 15 years, the incidence of NHL has increased by almost 50%. More than 95% of all cases of NHL occur in adults (Iwamoto, 2005).

Risk factors for and origins of NHL include genetic abnormalities, viral infection, and immune system damage. B-cell lymphomas develop because of genetic abnormalities. The Epstein-Barr virus and human immunodeficiency virus (HIV) have been identified as possible origins of NHL (Iwamoto, 2005; NCI, 2007c).

Clinical Staging and Diagnosis

Classification of NHL can be very confusing because there are so many different types and classifications. One type of classification system divides NHL into grades (see Table 17-1).

NHL patients usually present with localized or generalized lymphadenopathy. Most present with advanced disease. Other symptoms may be vague,

FIGURE 17-1: HEMATOPOIESIS CHART

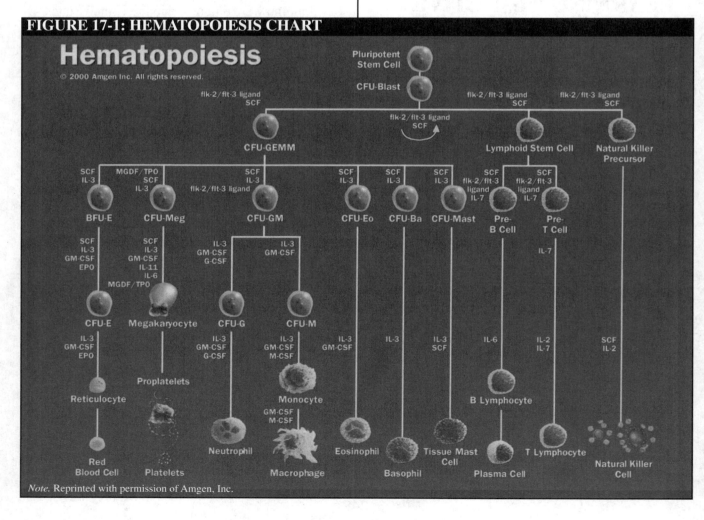

Note. Reprinted with permission of Amgen, Inc.

TABLE 17-1: NON-HODGKIN'S LYMPHOMA STAGING BY GRADES (RAPPAPORT STAGING CLASSIFICATION)

Grades	Presenting Symptoms
Low grade	Diffuse, lymphocytic, well-differentiated
	Nodular, lymphocytic, poorly differentiated
	Nodular, mixed lymphocytic and histiocytic
Intermediate grade	Nodular, histiocytic
	Diffuse, poorly differentiated lymphocytic
	Diffuse, mixed, lymphocytic and histiocytic
High grade	Diffuse, histiocytic
	Diffuse, lymphoblastic
	Undifferentiated

(Manson & Porter, 2006)

including back pain, abdominal discomfort, fever, sweats, and weight loss.

Approximately 90% of lymphomas worldwide are of B-cell origin. Patients present with disease involving the lymph nodes or bone marrow. Sometimes, B-cell lymphomas present with involvement in the liver and spleen (Manson & Porter, 2006).

So-called "B symptoms" include:

* fever (e.g., temperature > 38° C [100.4° F]) for 3 consecutive days

* weight loss exceeding 10% of body weight in 6 months

* drenching night sweats.

When the patient has one or more of these symptoms, the likelihood that the disease has spread to many areas of the body is increased (Manson & Porter, 2006).

Treatment

Treatment choices for NHL depend on the type and stage or extent of the disease and the grade of the lymphoma. The doctor also considers the person's age and general health. In some cases of early-stage low-grade disease, patients may go through a period of time without treatment.

In low-grade lymphomas, patients may be treated with radiation therapy (RT) and single-agent or combination chemotherapy. Low-grade lymphomas represent 20% to 30% of NHL cases, with a median survival of 7.5 to 9 years. Low-grade lymphomas include follicular center cell lymphoma, B-cell chronic lymphocytic leukemia (CLL) or small lymphocytic lymphoma, lymphoplasmacytoid lymphoma, mantle cell lymphoma, and marginal zone lymphoma (Estes & Clapp, 2004).

Intermediate- or high-grade lymphomas are treated with combination chemotherapy agents and stem cell transplants (SCTs; see Chapter 9). Table 17-2 highlights some of the chemotherapy protocols used in treatment.

Treatment strategies for NHL will continue to include chemotherapy, coupled with targeted therapies, other novel agents, and standard or revised SCT protocols:

* **Monoclonal antibodies** (MAbs) are proteins that target specific parts of the body. For NHL, one treatment uses a MAb called rituximab (Rituxan) against CD20, a protein on the

TABLE 17-2: SELECTED PROTOCOLS USED IN TREATMENT OF NON-HODGKIN'S LYMPHOMA (1 OF 2)

Combination Regimens

CHOP	**Cyclophosphamide** 750 mg/m² IV, day 1 **Doxorubicin** 50 mg/m² IV, day 1 **Vincristine** 1.4 mg/m² IV, day 1 **Prednisone** 100 mg/d PO, days 1 to 5 *Repeat cycle every 21 days*
CHOP-R	**Cyclophosphamide** 750 mg/m² IV, day 3 **Doxorubicin** 50 mg/m² IV, day 3 **Vincristine** 1.4 mg/m² day 3 (maximum 2 mg) **Prednisone** 100 mg PO, days 3 to 7 **Rituximab** 375 mg/m² IV, day 1 *Repeat cycle every 21 days*
CNOP	**Cyclophosphamide** 750 mg/m² IV, day 1 **Mitoxantrone** 10 mg/m² IV, day 1 **Vincristine** 1.4 mg/m² IV, day 1 **Prednisone** 50 mg/m² PO, days 1 to 5 *Repeat cycle every 21 days*
COP	**Cyclophosphamide** 800 mg/m² IV, day 1 **Vincristine** 1.4 mg/m² IV, day 1 **Prednisone** 60 mg/m² PO, days 1 to 5, then taper over 3 days *Repeat cycle every 14 days*
CVP	**Cyclophosphamide** 400 mg/m² PO, days 1 to 5 **Vincristine** 1.4 mg/m² IV, day 1 (max 2 mg) **Prednisone** 100 mg/m² PO, days 1 to 5 *Repeat every 21 days*
DHAP	**Dexamethasone** 40 mg PO or IV, days 1 to 4 **Cisplatin** 100 mg/m²/day CI, day 1 **Cytarabine** 2,000 mg/m² IV every 12 hours for 2 doses, day 2. Administer with saline, methylcellulose, or steroid eyedrops OU every 2 to 4 hours, beginning with cytarabine and continuing 48 to 72 hours after last cytarabine dose. *Repeat cycle every 21 to 28 days*

Table continued on next page.

surface of the cells of some lymphomas. Another treatment using a MAb strategy is radioimmunotherapy. Radionuclide-labeled MAbs that recognize tumor-associated antigens are administered systemically to selectively target radioactivity to tumor cells.

A radioimmunotherapy for low-grade NHL is tositumomab (Bexxar), a MAb combined with iodine-131. Ibritumomab tiuxetan (Zevalin), another MAb—combined with the MAb ritux-

imab, is a protocol that targets cells, incorporating RT and MAbs as treatment. It is indicated for relapsed or refractory low-grade, follicular, or transformed B-cell NHL, including rituximab-refractory follicular NHL. (For more on targeted therapies, see Chapter 7.)

- **Vaccines** currently under investigation are made from a patient's own tumor and can only modulate the immune system of the patient (Hohenstein, King, Fiore, O'Brien, & Blumel, 2005).

TABLE 17-2: SELECTED PROTOCOLS USED IN TREATMENT OF NON-HODGKIN'S LYMPHOMA (2 OF 2)

Combination Regimens (continued)

ESHAP	**Etoposide** 40 mg/m^2/day IV, days 1 to 4
	Methylprednisolone 500 mg IV, days 1 to 5
	Cytarabine 2 g/m^2 IV, day 5
	Cisplatin 25 mg/m^2, days 1 to 4 CI
	OR
	Etoposide 60 mg/m^2 IV, days 1 to 4
	Methylprednisolone 500 mg IV, days 1 to 4
	Cisplatin 25 mg/m^2/day CI, days 1 to 4
	Cytarabine 2,000 mg/m^2 IV, day 5, immediately following completion of etoposide and cisplatin. Administer with saline, methylcellulose, or steroid eyedrops OU every 2 to 4 hours, beginning with cytarabine and continuing 48 to 72 hours after last cytarabine dose.
	Repeat cycle every 21 to 28 days
	OR
	Mesna 1,330 mg/m^2 IV, administered at same time as ifosfamide, then 500 mg PO 4 hours after ifosfamide, days 1 to 3
	Ifosfamide 1,330 mg/m^2 IV over 1 hour, days 1 to 3
	Mitoxantrone 8 mg/m^2 IV, day 1
	Etoposide 65 mg/m^2 IV, days 1 to 3
	Repeat cycle every 21 days for 6 cycles, followed by 3 to 6 cycles of ESHAP
ProMACE/ cytaBOM	**Prednisone** 60 mg/m^2 PO, days 1 to 14
	Doxorubicin 25 mg/m^2 IV, day 1
	Cyclophosphamide 650 mg/m^2 IV, day 1
	Etoposide 120 mg/m^2 IV, day 1
	Cytarabine 300 mg/m^2 IV, day 8
	Bleomycin 5 units/m^2 IV, day 8
	Vincristine 1.4 mg/m^2 IV, day 8
	Methotrexate 120 mg/m^2 IV, day 8
	Leucovorin 25 mg/m^2 PO every 6 hours for 6 doses, beginning day 9
	Concomitant **trimethoprim/sulfamethoxazole** DS PO bid
	Repeat cycle every 21 to 28 days

Monoclonal Antibody Regimen

Rituximab	**Rituximab** 375 mg/m^2 IV, days 1, 8, 15, 22

Single-Agent Regimens

Bexarotene	300 mg/m^2/day PO until benefit is no longer derived
Cladribine	0.5 to 0.7 mg/kg/cycle SQ for 5 days or 0.1 mg/kg/day IV for 7 days
	Repeat cycle every 28 days
Denileukin diftitox	9 or 18 ug/kg/day IV, days 1 to 5
	Repeat every 21 days
Fludarabine	25 mg/m^2 IV, days 1 to 5
	Repeat cycle every 21 to 28 days

(Adams, Sheehan, & Holdsworth, 2001b)

- **SCT** is also used in the treatment of NHL. (See Chapter 9 for more information.)

Hodgkin's Disease

In 1832, Hodgkin's disease was named after the English physician Thomas Hodgkin, who first recognized the condition. The disease is identified by the appearance of a form of cancer cells called *Reed-Sternberg cells*. Many scientists believe that Reed-Sternberg cells are a type of B-cell cancer. Hodgkin's disease is most common in the third decade of life and after age 50 (Iwamoto, 2005).

Types of Hodgkin's Disease

Hodgkin's disease is categorized into these types:

- lymphocyte predominance nodular
- lymphocyte predominance diffuse
- nodular sclerosis (the most common form of Hodgkin's disease)
- mixed cellularity
- lymphocyte depletion.

Clinical Staging and Diagnosis

Patients may be asymptomatic except for lymphadenopathy, sometimes accompanied by flu-like symptoms. Diagnosis is confirmed by biopsy of the lymph nodes (Iwamoto, 2005).

Treatment

Regardless of type, Hodgkin's disease is malignant but has become one of the most curable malignancies. Each type is treated using similar treatment modalities. Specific treatments are based on the stage of disease. Localized disease is treated with RT. More advanced disease is treated with RT and chemotherapy, multiagent chemotherapy alone, or autologous bone marrow transplant (BMT) or peripheral SCT. The most frequently used chemotherapy protocols for Hodgkin's disease are:

- MOPP regimen: mechloramine (nitrogen mustard; Mustargen); vincristine (Oncovin), procarbazine (Mutalane), and prednisone.

- ABVD regimen: doxorubicin (Adriamycin), bleomycin (Blenoxane), vinblastine (Velban), and dacarbazine (DTIC-Dome) (Iwamoto, 2005).

MULTIPLE MYELOMA

Multiple myeloma, also called *myeloma* or *plasma cell myeloma*, is a cancer of the lymphoid line of the blood in which malignant plasma cells overproduce in the bone marrow. Plasma cells are a type of WBC that helps produce antibodies (immunoglobulins), which fight infection (Shinohara, 2006).

Epidemiological Trends

Multiple myeloma is thought to be triggered by environmental exposure to ionizing radiation, exposure to metals and chemicals, or genetic factors (Iwamoto, 2005).

In 2006, 15,270 new cases were diagnosed; 11,070 people died of the disease (ACS, 2006). The mean age at onset is 68 years. Mean survival time from diagnosis is 10 years, but most who are diagnosed with multiple myeloma die of the disease (Jemal et al., 2006).

Clinical Staging and Diagnosis

Patients with multiple myeloma produce a form of B-cell immunoglobulin called *paraprotein*—M (monoclonal) protein. These malignant cells replace normal plasma cells and other WBCs and can also proliferate in bone and other body organs.

Patients with multiple myeloma may present with bone pain symptoms. Routine laboratory values show elevated blood protein or anemia or signs of renal insufficiency or bone resorption (hypercalcemia, increased amyloid levels, increased immunoglobulin levels). The disease is highly treatable but is not yet curable (NCI, 2007b).

Diagnosis is based on bone marrow biopsy (showing greater than 10% plasma cells), serum protein electrophoresis (showing increased heavy-chain M protein levels), and urine protein immuno-electrophoresis (showing increased light-chain M proteins or Bence Jones proteins) (Iwamoto, 2005). In addition, skeletal bone scans showing "punched out" lesions contribute to the diagnosis.

Treatment

The most common chemotherapy and targeted therapy regimens for multiple myeloma include:

- melphalan (Alkeran) and prednisone

- VAD: vincristine, doxorubicin (Adriamycin), and dexamethasone

- bortezomib (Velcade) and dexamethasone (NCI, 2007b)

- thalidomide (Thalomid) and dexamethasone (Celegene Corporation, 2006)

- lenalidomide (Revlimid) and dexamethasone (Celegene Corporation, 2005)

Autologous or allogenic SCT (including a consolidation regimen) has been shown to produce a complete response half the time in patients with multiple myeloma (Iwamoto, 2005). RT is used to target bone lesions.

LEUKEMIA

Epidemiological Trends

Leukemia represents 3% of cancer incidence (ACS, 2006). In 2006, an estimated 35,070 new cases of leukemia (15,860 acute; 14,520 chronic) and 22,280 deaths due to leukemia were diagnosed. Since 1992, death rates have decreased about 1.9% per year. Leukemia is diagnosed 10 times more often in adults than in children (ACS, 2006; Jemal et al., 2006).

Background

In leukemia, cell control is missing or abnormal. This causes cells to appear in the early phase of their maturation process, causing the accumulation of immature cells that can crowd the bone marrow and other organs with leukemic cells.

The cause of leukemia is not known. In general, the etiology of leukemia is thought to be genetic predisposition or exposure to radiation chemicals, drugs, or viruses. In chronic leukemias, the predominant cell appears mature but does not function normally. In acute leukemias, the predominant cell is immature (NCI, 2007a).

Classifications

Leukemias are classified into two types: acute or chronic. Then they are further differentiated by the predominant cell affected—either lymphocytic or myelocytic. Thus, the main classifications for leukemia are acute lymphocytic leukemia (ALL), acute myelogenous leukemia (AML), chronic myelogenous leukemia (CML), and CLL. Hairy cell leukemia (HCL) is an additional type of chronic leukemia. Table 17-3 reviews signs and symptoms of the five types of leukemia (Adams et al., 2001a).

Initial diagnosis is confirmed by hematologic laboratory values—including complete blood count and flow cytometry—and bone marrow biopsy. (Flow cytometry is a method of measuring physical and chemical characteristics of cells—size, shape, internal complexity, and function—as the cells travel in suspension past a sensing point.)

Acute Lymphocytic (Lymphoblastic) Leukemia

Between 60% and 80% of patients (especially children) with ALL can be expected to attain complete remission status following appropriate induction therapy. Approximately 35% to 40% of adults with ALL can be expected to survive 2 years with aggressive induction combination chemotherapy and effective supportive care during induction therapy.

Presenting Symptoms

ALL typically presents with a characteristic abnormal proliferation of immature blood cells.

TABLE 17-3: LEUKEMIA: SIGNS, SYMPTOMS, AND WBC PRESENTATIONS

	Signs	Symptoms	WBC
ALL	Sudden onset Rapid deterioration Organ infiltration Neutropenia, thrombocy-topenia, and anemia Splenomegaly Lymphadenopathy	Fatigue Weight loss Fever Recurrent infections Unexplained bleeding and bruising Bone pain Headache Cranial nerve palsies (10% on presentation) Vomiting Vision changes Dyspnea	Low, normal, or high (85% normal to high) All patients have blasts (>two thirds of patients have >50% blasts)
AML	Same as ALL	Same as ALL	Low, normal, or high levels: 30% decreased, 30% normal, 30% increased
CLL	Gradual onset Splenomegaly Hepatomegaly Lymphadenopathy Neutropenia, thrombo-cytopenia, and anemia Bleeding disorders	None in early stages Recurrent infections Malaise Anorexia Fatigue Bleeding	Low Small mature or imma-ture lymphocytes > 20,000 cells/mm^3 early, then advances to > 100,000 cells/mm^3
CML	Splenomegaly Hepatomegaly Lymphadenopathy Neutropenia, thrombo-cytopenia, and anemia Rashes Philadelphia chromosome abnormality	Malaise Anorexia Weight loss Left upper quadrant pain Abdominal fullness Fever	Normal or high: > 100,000 cells/mm^3 in early stage; then, as disease progresses, becomes erratic In blast crisis, elevated or decreased
HCL	Splenomegaly Neutropenia, thrombocy-topenia, and anemia Under microscope, hairy cells	Malaise Left upper quadrant pain Abdominal fullness Fever	Elevated

With developing ALL, the effects of pancytopenia—a shortage of red and white cells and platelets—appear early in the course of the disease. Patients present with nonspecific symptoms, such as fever, tachycardia, and tachypnea. The skin and mucous membranes generally appear pale, with readily apparent ecchymoses or petechiae. Generalized or localized adenopathy may be present due to leukemic infiltration or infection.

To establish a definitive diagnosis for the specific type of leukemia, the patient goes through a complete workup, including history, physical exam, and detailed laboratory and blood studies. To correctly diagnose the type of leukemia, the origin of the leukemic cells needs to be established—from the B lymphocytes or T lymphocytes. For ALL, peripheral blasts are present in 90% of patients (Moran & Ezzone, 2005).

Treatment

ALL treatment differs from AML treatment as to:

- the length of treatment
- the inclusion of a central nervous system (CNS) prophylaxis protocol.

Initial treatment includes a combination of vincristine, prednisone, and an anthracycline chemotherapy, with or without asparaginase. This treatment results in complete remission in up to 80% of patients. Median remission duration for the complete responders is approximately 15 months (NCI, 2007a).

ALL treatment is scheduled in two phases: induction and postremission consolidation (which maintains remission). Among agents used in ALL induction protocols are anthracyclines, such as doxorubicin (Adriamycin); vincristine (Oncovin); prednisone; L-asparaginase (Elspar); methotrexate (Mexate); cyclophosphamide (Cytoxan); cytarabine (Cytosar-U, Ara-C); and thioguanine (Tioguanine). In general, the induction phase of treatment is less toxic in ALL than in AML.

During the consolidation phase, chemotherapy agents continue to be administered. In addition, CNS prophylaxis is given and includes RT or intrathecal chemotherapy to bypass the blood-brain barrier. Agents administered intrathecally include methotrexate and cytarabine.

An additional stage of the consolidation phase of treatment is called *maintenance therapy*. This therapy provides the patient with lower dose treatments that include the administration of agents such as methotrexate, mercaptopurine (Purinethol), vincristine, and prednisone. Maintenance therapy can continue for 2 to 3 years (Moran & Ezzone, 2005).

For high-risk ALL patients, BMT is an option to establish a first complete remission (see Chapter 9).

Acute Myelogenous Leukemia

AML is a disease that increases in incidence with age (median age of an AML patient is 55 to 60 years). Risk factors include congenital chromosomal abnormalities, such as Down syndrome, or other acquired disorders, such as myelodysplastic syndromes. Exposure to ionizing radiation, chemicals, and selected chemotherapies (e.g., alkylating agents) are also risk factors (NCI, 2007a).

Presenting Symptoms

Presenting signs and symptoms of AML are similar to those of ALL. They include fever, weight loss, fatigue, bleeding, and joint pain. With AML, additional symptoms may include headache, vomiting, and clouded vision.

Treatment

As with ALL, treatment for AML is in two phases: induction and postremission or consolidation therapy. Induction protocols can include cytarabine and anthracyclines, such as daunorubicin (Cerubidine) or doxorubicin. Table 17-4 lists common AML protocols.

Gemtuzumab ozogamicin (Mylotarg), an MAb, is a U.S. Food and Drug Adminstration (FDA)–approved treatment option for patients age

60 years and older who have a first relapse with CD33+ AML (Wyeth Pharmaceuticals, Inc., 2007).

After successful completion of an induction protocol in which the patient has established complete remission, allogenic or autologous BMT can be a treatment option.

Myelodysplastic Syndromes

Myelodysplastic syndromes (MDSs) are a group of hematologic disorders that increase the risk of transforming to AML. MDS, a preleukemic stage of blood abnormalities, is characterized by a change of quality and quantity of specific stem cells in the bone marrow, indicating various subtypes of refractory anemia. The cause for the change of the stem cells is unknown, but chromosomal abnormalities are linked to MDS origin.

Most patients diagnosed with MDS are younger than 50 years old. Diagnosis is by bone marrow biopsy, with treatment based on the aggressiveness of the disease progression. When warranted, aggressive treatment for MDS can include high-dose chemotherapy or BMT. For low-risk MDS, treatment can include blood transfusions and other supportive strategies (e.g., antibiotics for infections, administration of growth factors, and administration of chemoprotective agents, such as amifostine, to help promote and mobilize progenitor cells) (Wujcik, 2006).

Chronic Leukemias

Chronic leukemias represent about 14% of all leukemias and occurs with a frequency of about 1 in 100,000. It is rare in children (D'Antonio, 2005). The characteristics of chronic leukemias differ from those of acute leukemias because of their accumulation of more mature-appearing cells at a slower, progressive course (2 to 5 years).

Initial symptoms include abdominal pain, resulting from splenomegaly due to infiltration of the spleen by leukemic cells. Patients can also present with a history of malaise, fatigue, weight loss, and fever.

To establish a clear diagnosis of chronic leukemia, past medical history, physical exam data, and laboratory data are reviewed. Chromosomal aberrations may be significant in the initial diagnosis of the chronic leukemia type and in establishing treatment options (D'Antonio, 2005; NCI, 2007a).

Chronic Myelogenous Leukemia

CML can affect all age-groups, although it is rare in children and adolescents. A chromosomal abnormality known as the *Philadelphia chromosome* is a diagnostic marker found in about 90% of patients with CML. Ionizing radiation exposure is thought to be one of the main risk factors for CML. Other risk factors include exposure to benzene and selected other chemicals (D'Antonio, 2005).

Presenting Symptoms

CML presents in three general phases:

1. A mild, stable, chronic phase, which prompts changes in laboratory values (anemia, neutropenia, and thrombocytopenia) and subtle symptoms (fatigue, fever, malaise, weight loss, night sweats, and left upper quadrant fullness and pain)

2. Accelerated phase that leads to symptoms that have progressed, with more pronounced fevers, bone pain, and weight loss

3. Blast crisis, when the spleen dramatically enlarges and other signs and symptoms include infection, bleeding, and symptoms of immature pluripotent cells that crowd out the bone marrow and peripheral blood.

Treatment

Standard therapies for CML include hydroxyurea (Hydrea), busulfan (Myleran), and interferon and low-dose cytarabine (Cytosar-U, Ara-C). (See Table 17-4.) Allogenic bone marrow transplant has been a treatment option for younger patients. Autologous and peripheral SCTs for CML are controversial treatment options (Moran & Ezzone, 2005). As long as the Philadelphia chromosome is present, the patient is not considered cured (D'Antonio, 2005).

Patients in blast crisis have a poor prognosis. As the crisis advances, patients may develop myeloid blast crisis and may respond to therapies for AML,

or they may develop lymphoid blast crisis and may respond to ALL therapies (Moran & Ezzone, 2005).

In 2001, the agent imatinib mesylate (Gleevec) was approved by the FDA as a treatment for adult patients with Philadelphia chromosome (bcr-abl)-

TABLE 17-4: SAMPLE PROTOCOLS (1 OF 2)

Acute Myelogenous Leukemia

Combination Regimens (Induction)

7+3+7	**Cytarabine** 100 mg/m²/day CI, days 1 to 7
	Daunorubicin 50 mg/m²/day IV, days 1 to 3
	Etoposide 75 mg/m²/day I.V. over 1 hour, days 1 to 7
Idarubicin	**Idarubicin** 5 mg/m² slow IV push, days 1 to 5
Cytarabine	**Cytarabine** 2 g/m² every 12 hours as 3-hour infusion, days 1 to 5
Etoposide	**Etoposide** 100 mg/m² as 1-hour infusion, days 1 to 5
	OR
	Idarubicin 6 mg/m² IV bolus, days 1 to 5
	Cytarabine 600 mg/m² IV over 2 hours, days 1 to 5
	Etoposide 150 mg/m² over 2 hours, days 1 to 3
7+3	**Cytarabine** 100 mg/m²/day CI, days 1 to 7
	WITH
	Daunorubicin 45 mg/m² IV, days 1 to 3
	OR
	Idarubicin 12 mg/m² I. days 1 to 3
	OR
	Mitoxantrone 12 mg/m² IV days 1 to 3
5+2	**Cytarabine** 100 mg/m²/day CI, days 1 to 5
	WITH
	Daunorubicin 45 mg/m² IV, days 1 to 2
	OR
	Mitoxantrone 12 mg/m² IV days 1 to 2
	For reinduction

Single-Agent Regimens (Induction)

Arsenic	**Arsenic trioxide** 0.15 mg/kg IV daily until remission, not to exceed 60 doses
ATRA	**All transretinoic acid (ATRA)** 45 mg/m²/day PO (1 or 2 divided doses)
	Starts 2 days before induction

Monoclonal Antibody Regimen

Gemtazumab	**Gemtazumab** Two doses of 9 mg protein/m² IV, separated by 2 weeks

Single-Agent Regimens (Postremission)

Arsenic	**Arsenic trioxide** 0.15 mg/kg IV daily for 25 doses over a period of up to 5 weeks
Cytarabine	**Cytarabine** 100 mg/m²/day CI, days 1 to 5, for patients > 60 years of age
	Repeat cycle every 28 days

TABLE 17-4: SAMPLE PROTOCOLS (2 OF 2)

Acute Myelogenous Leukemia (continued)

Single-Agent Regimens (Postremission)

HiDAC	**Cytarabine** 3000 mg/m² IV over 1 to 3 hours, every 12 hours, days 1 to 6
	OR
	Cytarabine 3000 mg/m² IV over 1 to 3 hours, every 12 hours, days 1, 3, 5. Administer with saline, methylcellulose, or steroid eyedrops OU every 2 to 4 hours, beginning with cytarabine and continuing 48 to 72 hours after last cytarabine dose.
	Repeat cycle every 28 days

Chronic Lymphocytic Leukemia (CLL)

Chlorambucil	**Chlorambucil** 6 to 14 mg/day until signs and symptoms diminish
	THEN (as intermittent therapy)
	Chlorambucil 0.7 mg/kg PO over 2 to 4 days
	Repeat every 3 weeks until disease stabilizes
Cladribine	**Cladribine** 0.1 mg/kg/day CI, days 1 to 5 or 1 to 7
	Repeat cycle every 28 to 35 days
Cyclophosphamide	**Cyclophosphamide** 2 to 3 mg/kg PO, days 1 to 10, every 21 to 28 days
	OR
	Cyclophosphamide 20 mg/kg IV every 2 to 3 weeks
Fludarabine	**Fludarabine** 25 mg/m²/day IV over 30 minutes, days 1 to 5
	Repeat cycle every 28 days
Prednisone	**Prednisone** 20 to 40 mg/m²/day PO for 1 to 3 weeks
	Use if patient is symptomatic with autoimmune thrombocytopenia or hemolytic anemia

Chronic Myelogenous Leukemia

Interferon alfa-2b/ Cytarabine	**Interferon alfa-2b** 5 million IU/m² SQ qd for the duration of treatment period
	Hydroxyurea 50 mg/kg qd for duration of treatment period
	Cytarabine 20 mg/m² SQ for 10 days starting 2 weeks after initiation of induction therapy
	Repeat every month
Hydroxyurea	**Hydroxyurea** 1 to 5 g/day PO
Interferon alfa-2a	**Interferon alfa-2a** 9 million IU/d SQ. Tolerance dose: 3 million IU/day for 3 days, then 6 million IU/day SQ, to a target dose of 9 million IU/day SQ for the duration of the treatment period.

Hairy Cell Leukemia

Cladribine	**Cladribine** 0.09 mg/kg/dy CI, days 1 to 7
	Administer 1 cycle
Interferon alfa-2a	**Interferon alfa-2a** 3 million IU SQ three times a week
Pentosatin	**Pentosatin** 4 mg/m² IV, day 1
	Repeat cycle every 14 days

(Adams, Sheehan, & Holdsworth, 2001a; NCI 2007a)

positive CML in chronic phase after failure of interferon-alpha therapy. Imatinib mesylate is one of the first molecular agents approved for cancer treatment. This oral agent blocks the rapid growth of WBCs by targeting the protein that results from the genetic defect found in CML.

Chronic Lymphocytic Leukemia

CLL is the most common form of leukemia in the Western hemisphere. It is characterized by the accumulation of mature-looking lymphocytes, most frequently B cells (NCI, 2007a).

Unlike other leukemias, radiation exposure and chemicals do not appear to be risk factors for CLL. It is a disease of age, occurring primarily in the elderly and thought to be associated with a patient's impaired immune system (NCI, 2007a).

Presenting Symptoms

Patients may have CLL and present with no symptoms or only occasional mild symptoms. More advanced stages of CLL cause patients to present with fatigue, shortness of breath, night sweats, and bleeding. As the disease progresses, the patient has more serious symptoms, including fever, lymph node swelling, weight loss, and abdominal pain (NCI, 2007a).

Treatment

Until symptoms progress, CLL might not be treated. Then treatment options include chlorambucil (Leukeran) with and without steroids. Other agents used in treatment include fludarabine (Fludara) and cladribine (Leustatin), accompanied by antibiotics. Standard chemotherapy protocols, such as CVP (cyclophosphamide [Cytoxan], vincristine [Oncovin], and prednisone) or CHOP (cyclophosphamide [Cytoxan], doxorubicin [Adriamycin], vincristine [Oncovin], and prednisone) also may be treatment options (NCI, 2007a). Table 17-4 highlights some protocols used to treat chronic leukemia.

Hairy Cell Leukemia

HCL accounts for about 1% to 2% of all adult leukemias. It is more prevalent in males (4:1).

Presenting symptoms of HCL

The presenting symptoms of HCL, like the other leukemias, are weakness, fatigue, and abdominal pain.

Treatment

Sometimes, HCL is not treated in its early stages. However, treatment usually begins when symptoms progress. Those progressing signs and symptoms are anemia, neutropenia, thrombocytopenia, abdominal pain, infection, and swollen lymph nodes.

A mainstay of treatment for HCL has been splenectomy. Now, more-durable responses are possible, with treatments including alpha interferon, pentostatin (Nipent), and cladribine (Leustatin). The agent cladribine has been shown to be such an effective treatment that it is used as a first-line therapy. Table 17-4 lists common HCL protocols.

Myelosuppression

For patients diagnosed with any of the leukemias, a toxicity or side effect of particular importance in their care is myelosuppression, which can be caused by the disease or its treatments. Nursing support of the patient includes the administration and monitoring of transfusions, administration of antibiotic therapies, and other methods to manage and monitor neutropenia, anemia, and thrombocytopenia. (See Chapter 11 for a more detailed review of myelosuppression and neutropenia.)

SUMMARY

Lymphoma, multiple myeloma, and leukemia are hematologic malignancies that are primarily treated with chemotherapy and targeted or biologic therapy protocols. This chapter reviewed NHL and Hodgkin's disease, multiple myeloma, and the main classifications of leukemia. Treatment protocols were reviewed.

CASE STUDY: T-CELL NHL

GG is a 55-year-old Caucasian woman who developed a pruritic, erythematous rash, which appears on her thighs, torso, and back. She originally thought it was a drug allergy. She was treated with corticosteroids and antihistamine medication, but the rash did not improve. By then, she had developed joint pain and lymphadenopathy in the neck.

She was referred to a medical oncologist for evaluation. In the meantime, she had developed lymphadenopathy in her axillae and inguinal region. On computed tomography (CT) of the thorax and abdomen, multiple nodes were noted.

Excision biopsy of the inguinal lymph nodes and further bone marrow biopsy confirmed a diagnosis of peripheral T-cell non-Hodgkin's lymphoma. Immunophenotyping indicated that the cells were positive for CD3, CD5, and CD43 and negative for CD10, CD19, CD20, CD30, and CD56. She was staged as stage III at presentation due to extensive skin involvement and involvement of the inguinal lymph nodes.

Before proceeding with chemotherapy treatment, a Port-a-Cath vascular access device was placed to allow administration of chemotherapy. GG was treated with six cycles of CHOP-R therapy, which put her lymphoma into remission.

GG was restaged and underwent further work-up for an autologous SCT. (Work-up included baseline CTs of the chest, abdomen, and pelvis; a bone scan; and laboratory testing.)

In educating GG on the risks associated with autologous SCT, her physician reviewed the risk of infection during neutropenic periods, mucositis, and organ-related toxicities. GG decided to proceed with the SCT.

On hospital admission 7 days before her SCT, GG's high-dose chemotherapy began, which included the regimen BCNU (etoposide, cytara-bine, and melphalan). Her Port-a-Cath, still in place from her previous CHOP-R therapy, allowed IV access. Filgrastim (Neupogen) injections were also given to minimize the neutropenic period.

Once her stem cells were transplanted, GG experienced mucositis on day +4, which was treated with morphine via a patient-controlled analgesia pump and mucositis mix (lidocaine based). By day +11, her mucositis was well healed. On day +14, GG had a fever of 102° F, which was treated with antibiotics. She was afebrile again on day +15. She also had periods of diarrhea on days +10 to +13, which were treated with diphenoxylate hydrochloride (Lomotil) and a blander diet.

Engraftment began on day +12. She was discharged to home on day +19 and instructed to have regular (twice per week) blood draws. Blood transfusion parameters were in place: two units of packed red blood cells if hemoglobin < 8 mg/dl; one bag single-donor platelet if platelet count < 20,000/mm³.

After high-dose chemotherapy and autologous SCT, GG was admitted to the hospital again when she spiked a temp to 103° F. She was treated with antibiotics and was discharged home on day +3.

On day +34 after SCT, GG's selected laboratory studies were:

- WBC   5.5 (x 10³/μL)
- HG   9.5 g/dL
- HCT   28.5%
- MCV   94.4 μm³
- Platelets   77,000/mm³
- WBC diff
    - Segs   49%
    - Monocytes   16%
    - Eosinophils 4%
    - Lymphocytes 29%
- BUN   6 mg/dL
- Creatinine   0.6 mg/dL
- Na   139 mEq/L
- K   3.8 mEq/L
- Cal   9.1 mg/dL

– Total protein   6.3 g/dL
– Albumin   3.6 g/dL
– AST   26 U/L
– ALT   32 U/L
– LDH   154 U/L
– Alk phos   95 U/L
– Tot Bilirubin   1.0 mg/dL

GG continues to gain strength and stamina. She is seen every month in the clinic for a clinical exam and laboratory tests. Imaging scans are ordered every 3 to 6 months.

At 1 year post-transplant, GG continues to be in remission.

Additional Information

GG has been married for 39 years. Her husband, who is retired from the military, keeps a detailed journal of her health history, reports of labs and procedures, and clinic visits.

GG was an office manager before her illness; she decided to take an early retirement to focus on her treatment and returning to health. She was also a 20 pack-year smoker. (GG quit smoking when her friend was diagnosed with breast cancer 10 years ago.)

From the time she was diagnosed, GG attempted to use complementary and alternative medicines to help her keep a sense of control and help with side effects. She participates in yoga classes weekly, when she can, and enjoys massages every 2 weeks. She treats herself occasionally to aromatherapy to help her with her anxiety and nausea.

Throughout her illness and treatment, she was able to journal and practice meditation, which strengthened her spiritually. She was also a member of a cancer support group, which met biweekly at a local community center.

She and her husband plan to travel when her health has further stabilized. Travel has been their dream in retirement. Long-term survivor issues continue to challenge GG after her treatment. They include the practical problems of finances and continued health and life insurance.

Questions

1. What were GG's risk factors for NHL?

2. CHOP-R therapy includes what chemotherapy agents?

3. What side effects should GG anticipate during CHOP-R therapy?

4. After autologous transplant, when is engraftment expected?

5. What psychological and social challenges face long-term survivors of NHL.

Answers

1. The risk factors for NHL include genetic abnormalities, viral infections, and immune system damage. B-cell lymphomas develop because of genetic abnormalities. The Epstein-Barr virus and HIV have been identified as possible origins of NHL.

2. CHOP-R stands for the chemotherapy protocol cyclophosphamide, doxorubicin, vincristine, prednisone, and rituximab.

3. Those receiving CHOP-R therapy can anticipate these main side effects from treatment: 1) leukopenia and neutropenia, 2) alopecia, 3) nausea and vomiting. Reports of less common side effects of CHOP-R include fever, flu-like symptoms, infection, mucositis, cardiac toxicity, lung toxicity, neurologic toxicity, and liver toxicity.

4. The first signs of engraftment after autologous transplant usually occur 12 to 17 days after transplant. The cells that first show engraftment are monocytes and neutrophils.

5. Studies show that long-term survivors of cancer therapy face practical problems, which can include continuing meaningful work, obtaining health care and life insurance and having financial security.

EXAM QUESTIONS

CHAPTER 17
Questions 68-71

Note: Choose the option that BEST answers each question.

68. A presenting symptom for Non-Hodgkin's lymphoma (NHL) is

    a. lymphadenopathy.

    b. cough.

    c. dizziness.

    d. anemia.

69. A treatment strategy for localized Hodgkin's disease is

    a. chemotherapy.

    b. surgery.

    c. RT.

    d. tumor markers.

70. A presenting symptom for acute lymphocytic leukemia (ALL) is

    a. nausea.

    b. blood in stool.

    c. peripheral neuropathy.

    d. fever.

71. One of the approved targeted therapies for chronic myelogenous leukemia (CML) is

    a. rituximab.

    b. bevacizumab.

    c. imatinib mesylate.

    d. ibritumomab tiuxetan.

REFERENCES

Adams, V., Sheehan, & Holdsworth, M. (2001a). *Leukemia-AML, CLL, CML, HCL: Guide to cancer chemotherapeutic regimens.* Oncology Special Edition, (4)139-140. New York: McMahon.

Adams, V., Sheehan, & Holdsworth, M. (2001b). Lymphoma: Non-Hodgkin's: Guide to cancer chemotherapeutic regimens. Oncology Special Edition, (4)141. New York: McMahon.

American Cancer Society. (2006). *Cancer facts & figures 2006.* Atlanta: Author.

American Joint Committee on Cancer. (2002). *AJCC cancer staging manual* (6th ed.). New York: Springer-Verlag.

Celegene Corporation. (2005). *Revlimid.* Retrieved October 31, 2006, from http://revlimid.com

Celegene Corporation. (2006). *Thalomid® sNDA granted FDA approval for treatment of newly diagnosed multiple myeloma.* Available from http://www.multiplemyeloma.org/in_the_news/6.03.023.php

D'Antonio, J. (2005). Chronic myelogenous leukemia. *Clinical Journal of Oncology Nursing, 9*(6), 535–538.

Estes, J., & Clapp, K. (2004). Radioimmunotherapy with tositumomab and iodine-131 tositumomab for low-grade non-Hodgkin lymphoma: Nursing implications. *Oncology Nursing Forum, 31*(6), 1119–1126.

Hohenstein, M., King, S., Fiore, J., O'Brien, T., & Blumel, S. (2005). Patient-specific vaccine therapy for non-Hodgkin lymphoma. *Clinical Journal of Oncology Nursing, 9*(1), 85–90.

Iwamoto, R. (2005). Nursing care of the client with lymphoma and multiple myeloma. In J. K. Itano & K. N. Taoka (Eds.), *Core curriculum for oncology nursing* (4th ed., pp. 689–700). St. Louis: Elsevier.

Jemal, A., Siegel, R., Ward, E., Murray, T., Xu, J., Smigal, C., et al. (2006). Cancer statistics, 2006. *CA: Cancer Journal for Clinicians, 56(2),* 106–130.

Manson, S., & Porter, C. (2006). Lymphomas. In C. Yarbro, M. Frogge, & M. Goodman (Eds.), *Cancer nursing: Principles and practice* (6th ed., pp. 1414–1459). Sudbury, MA: Jones & Bartlett.

Moran, M., & Ezzone, S. (2005). Nursing care of the client with leukemia. In J. K. Itano & K. N. Taoka (Eds.), *Core curriculum for oncology nursing* (4th ed., pp. 676–688). St. Louis: Elsevier.

National Cancer Institute. (2007a). *Leukemia.* Available from http://www.cancer.gov/cancer topics/types/leukemia

National Cancer Institute. (2007b). *Multiple myeloma/Other plasma cell neoplasms.* Available from http://www.cancer.gov/cancer topics/types/myeloma/

National Cancer Institute. (2007c). *Non-Hodgkin's lymphoma.* Available from from http://www .cancer.gov/cancertopics/types/non-hodgkins-lymphoma

Shinohara, E. (2006). *Multiple myeloma.* Retrieved April 17, 2007, from http://www.oncolink.com//types/article.cfm?c=13&s=42&ss=836&id=9552

Wujcik, D. (2006). Leukemia. In C. Yarbro, M. Frogge, & M. Goodman (Eds.), *Cancer nursing: Principles and practice* (6th ed., pp. 1330–1354). Sudbury, MA: Jones & Bartlett.

Wyeth Pharmaceuticals, Inc. (2007). *Mylotarg.*
Retrieved April 17, 2007, from http://www
.wyeth.com/products?page=2&letters=all&from
Letters=all

CHAPTER 18

SKIN CANCER

COURSE OBJECTIVE

After completing this chapter, the reader will be able to describe the types of skin cancer and their treatments.

LEARNING OBJECTIVES

After studying this chapter, the reader will be able to

1. identify the incidence of and death rates for melanoma in the United States.

2. describe the ABCD assessment for skin moles.

3. recognize a staging workup for melanoma.

4. name two treatment strategies that are used in treating melanoma.

INTRODUCTION

Skin cancer has its origin in epidermal cells—the upper, outer lay of the skin. The epidermis is made of three types of cells:

Squamous cells: Thin, flat cells that form the top layer of the epidermis.

Basal cells: Round cells under the squamous cells.

Melanocytes: Cells found in the lower part of the epidermis that make melanin, the pigment that gives skin its natural color.

Skin cancer can occur anywhere but most commonly occurs in areas of the body exposed to sunlight, such as the face, neck, hands, and arms (National Cancer Institute [NCI], 2006a).

Prevention strategies for skin cancer are listed in Chapter 3, Table 3-5. According to the most recent estimates, skin cancer is the most common type of cancer diagnosed in the United States. At least 50% of all individuals age 65 or older have had at least one episode of skin cancer (Maltzman, 2004).

BASAL AND SQUAMOUS CELL CANCERS

Basal cell carcinoma is the most common form of skin cancer, and squamous cell carcinoma is the second most common type of skin malignancy (NCI, 2006a). These two types of skin cancer are relatively not deadly, accounting for less than 0.1% of deaths due to cancer. They both initiate in the epithelial cells.

Risk Factors

Risk factors for basal and squamous cell cancers include:

- being exposed to a lot of natural or artificial sunlight

- having a fair complexion (blond or red hair, fair skin, green or blue eyes, history of freckling)

- having scars or burns on the skin

- being exposed to arsenic
- having chronic skin inflammation or skin ulcers
- being treated with radiation
- taking immunosuppressive drugs (for example, after an organ transplant)
- having actinic keratosis.

(NCI, 2006a)

Other Malignant Skin Cancers

Malignant forms of skin cancer include malignant melanoma, cutaneous T-cell lymphomas (e.g., mycosis fungoides), Kaposi's sarcoma, Merkel cell carcinoma, extramammary Paget's disease, and apocrine carcinoma of the skin. These cancers are much more serious and difficult to treat. Cure rates for these cancers are based on the stage of the cancer at treatment (size of the tumor, depth, histopathology) and the types of treatment the patient undergoes.

Treatment

Standard treatment for skin cancer that has not spread is surgery, usually simple excision, Mohs micrographic surgery, electrodesiccation and curettage, or cryosurgery. Table 18-1 lists treatment strategies for basal and squamous cell cancers.

Radiation therapy (RT) is also a treatment for basal and squamous cell cancers. After treatment, clinical follow-up is usually scheduled every 6 months for 5 years. For squamous cell cancers, which have more metastatic potential, clinical follow-up is every 3 months for a few years (NCI, 2006a).

MELANOMA

Melanoma is a very serious cancer diagnosis with few effective treatments.

It is a disease of the skin in which malignant cells are found in melanocytes. Melanocytes, located in the epidermis, produce the pigment melanin, which generates the skin's color (see Figure 18-1). When melanocytes gather together, malignancies can sometimes develop. Melanoma can metastasize quickly, most commonly to the lungs and liver. Although most melanomas begin in the skin, 10% begin in the eye (Longman, 2005; NCI, 2006b).

In 2006, 62,190 individuals were diagnosed with melanoma. Approximately 83% were diagnosed at an early stage. The 5-year survival for melanoma is 64% if the disease is diagnosed at a regional level; the 5-year survival when diagnosed with distant metastasis is 16% (ACS, 2006).

Melanoma occurs predominantly in adults, and more than 50% of cases arise in previously normal-appearing areas of the skin. An early sign of melanoma is a nevus that suggests malignant changes—for example, darker or variable discoloration, itching, an increase in size, or the development of satellites. Ulceration or bleeding of the nevus are later signs. Melanoma occurs more commonly on the extremities in women. For men, melanoma most frequently appears on the trunk, head, and neck, but it can arise from any site on the skin surface (NCI, 2006b).

Malignant melanoma is the most life-threatening form of skin cancer. Although malignant melanoma accounts for only 3% of reported skin cancer cases, it causes over 79% of skin-cancer-related deaths (American Cancer Society [ACS], 2006).

Primary Risk Factors

Despite the universal understanding of sun exposure being a cardinal risk for melanoma, studies have shown that individuals do not avoid sun exposure to reduce their risk of melanoma (Guile & Nicholson, 2004). More sophisticated strategies need to be developed to address this disconnect in risk reduction and behavior.

Detection and Screening Strategies

Self-examination and examination by one's clinician are the first and foremost strategies for

TABLE 18-1: COMMON TREATMENT STRATEGIES FOR BASAL AND SQUAMOUS CELL CANCERS

Mohs micrographic surgery

Surgical treatment with the highest cure rate of all surgical treatments because the tumor is microscopically delineated until it is completely removed

Also indicated for:

- tumors with poorly defined clinical borders
- tumors with diameters greater than 2 cm
- tumors with histopathologic features showing sclerotic patterns
- tumors arising in regions where maximum preservation of uninvolved tissue is desirable, such as the eyelid, nose, finger, and genitalia

Simple excision with frozen or permanent sectioning for margin evaluation

Traditional surgical treatment that relies on surgical margins ranging from 3 mm to 10 mm, depending on the diameter of the tumor

Electrodesiccation and curettage

Most widely employed method for removing primary basal cell carcinomas

Cryosurgery

For small, clinically well-defined primary tumors in specific areas or for patients who may not be candidates for surgery

Contraindicated for patients with abnormal cold tolerance and platelet deficiencies

Radiation therapy

For patients with primary lesions requiring difficult or extensive surgery (e.g., eyelids, nose, or ears) or for recurring tumors after surgery

Carbon dioxide laser

For a superficial type of basal cell carcinoma

Photodynamic therapy

For tumors on or just under the skin or in the lining of internal organs, such as the lungs or esophagus

Starts with the infusion of a drug that is not active until it is exposed to light; fiberoptic tubes deliver laser light to the cancer cells, where the drug becomes active and kills the cells

(NCI, 2006a)

detection. Those susceptible to skin damage or with risk factors for skin cancer should be evaluated at regular periodic exams. In general, self-exam is recommended every 6 to 8 weeks. An exam includes inspection of the back and all hidden areas (including the scalp and between the toes).

During examination, the ABCD assessment is a guide to identify early signs of malignancy in a skin mole: A (Asymmetry in shape), B (uneven Border), C (many shades of Color), and D (Diameter greater than 6 mm—the size of a pencil eraser). Other signs of concern include an oozing or bleeding mole or a mole that becomes itchy, swollen, or sensitive (Longman, 2005; NCI, 2006b).

Prognosis worsens when there is lymph node involvement or systemic metastasis. Melanoma can spread by local extension (through lymphatics) or by hematogenous routes to distant sites. Any organ may be involved by metastasis, but the lungs and liver are common sites (NCI, 2006b).

Ocular Melanoma

When melanoma occurs in the eye, it is called *ocular melanoma.* Around 2,500 people in the

FIGURE 18-1: SKIN ANATOMY

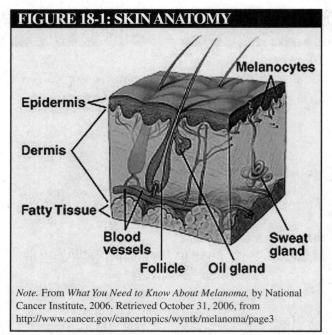

Note. From *What You Need to Know About Melanoma,* by National Cancer Institute, 2006. Retrieved October 31, 2006, from http://www.cancer.gov/cancertopics/wyntk/melanoma/page3

United States are diagnosed with ocular melanoma every year. Ocular melanoma is a lethal and very rare disease. Many people die from it, especially when it spreads to the liver, a common complication. Although there are other types of eye cancer, melanoma is the most common.

Ocular melanoma begins when the pigmented cells in the eye (melanocytes) grow uncontrollably. It occurs in five distinct sites around and in the eye: the eyelid, conjunctiva, iris, choroid, and optic nerve.

The main reasons for treating intraocular melanoma are to reduce the risk of tumor spread and to maintain the health and vision of the eye. If the tumor grows bigger than 10 mm in diameter or 2 to 3 mm in height (thickness), then treatment is considered. Treatment options include surgery (enucleation), external beam RT, and internal RT (brachytherapy), and laser therapy (Ocular Melanoma Foundation, 2004).

Treatments

Malignant melanoma has four stages in its staging system (see Table 18-2). Treatment depends on the patient's age and general health and the stage of the malignancy, especially the thickness of the lesion and whether it has invaded beyond the papillary dermis.

Treatment strategies include surgery, biological therapy (using interferons and interleukins), chemotherapy, and RT. Unfortunately, effective treatments for advanced melanomas have not been established (NCI, 2006b).

Depending on the malignancy stage, the focus of surgery may include excisional biopsy (removal of the mole), reexcision (removal of the mole and skin around the site to ensure clear margins), and lymph node biopsy and removal (to remove areas where the melanoma has spread). Punch biopsies are contraindicated.

After surgery, in order to slow the growth of the malignancy, biologic therapy attempts to stimulate the immune system. The two biologic therapies that appear most active against melanoma are interferon-alfa and interleukin-2 (IL-2). Response rates for interferon range from 8% to 22% (NCI, 2006b).

Temozolomide (Temodar), an approved treatment for brain cancer, alone or concomitant with thalidomide or IL-2, has shown promise in clinical trials as a treatment for advanced melanoma (cancerconsultants.org, 2006).

Other therapies being studied include vaccines. RT can also be an option incombined therapy and can be useful in palliation (NCI, 2006b).

SUMMARY

Melanoma remains a difficult cancer to treat. Surgery is the primary treatment modality, with few chemotherapies or biologic therapies showing activity against metastasis of the disease.

TABLE 18-2: STAGING OF MELANOMA

The incidence of melanoma is rising in the United States. In 2006, more than 62,000 melanoma cases and 7,910 deaths related to melanoma occurred (ACS, 2006). Surgical resection is the cornerstone of treatment for melanoma, as conventional forms of adjuvant chemotherapy have been ineffective. The efficacy of elective lymph node dissection continues to be controversial due to the results of a prospective series demonstrating that it has no benefit. The depth of primary tumor invasion has always been recognized as an important prognostic feature. The methods of Clark and Breslow have historically been the systems used for classification of these tumors. Surgical resection is the cornerstone of treatment for melanoma. Newer forms of adjuvant treatment (e.g., interferon) now have survival efficacy in stage III cases. Sentinel lymph node sampling is replacing elective lymph node dissection for node staging.

Primary Tumor (T)

TX   Unable to assess primary tumor
T0   Primary tumor cannot be found
Tis   Melanoma in situ, noninvasive lesions, or severe dysplastic nevi
T1 ≤ 1.0 mm thickness, with or without ulceration
T1a ≤ 1.0 mm thickness and level II or III, no ulceration
T1b ≤ 1.0 mm thickness and level IV or V or with ulceration
T2   Between 1.01 and 2 mm thickness, abutment of papillary-reticular dermal interface
T3   Between 2.01 and 4.0 mm thickness, with or without ulceration
T4 > 4.0 mm thickness, with or without ulceration

Regional Lymph Nodes (N)

NX   Unable to evaluate regional lymph nodes
N0   Regional lymph nodes negative for metastasis
N1   Positive regional lymph nodes ≤ 3 cm in size
N2   Positive regional lymph nodes, > 3 cm in size, presence of in-transit lesions

Distant Metastasis (M)

MX   Unable to evaluate distant metastasis
M0   No evidence of distant metastasis
M1A   Distant metastasis to skin or subcutaneous tissue
M1B   Visceral metastasis

Stage Grouping

Stage 0	Tis	N0	M0
Stage I	T1	N0	M0
	T2	N0	M0
Stage II	T3	N0	M0
	T4	N0	M0
Stage III	Any T	N1, N2	M0
Stage IV	Any T	Any N	M1

Note. Used with the permission of the American Joint Committee on Cancer (AJCC), Chicago, Illinois. The original source for this material is the *AJCC Cancer Staging Manual,* Sixth Edition (2002) published by Springer-New York, www.springeronline.com.

EXAM QUESTIONS

CHAPTER 18
Questions 72-75

Note: Choose the option that BEST answers each question.

72. In the United States, the 5-year survival rate for patients with metastatic melanoma with distant metastases is

    a. 36%.

    b. 26%.

    c. 16%.

    d. unknown.

73. Early signs of melanoma that require further evaluation are

    a. A (asymmetry), B (clear border), C (one color), D (small diameter).

    b. A (asymmetry), B (uneven border), C (one color), D (at least 2 mm diameter).

    c. A (asymmetry), B (uneven border), C (many shades of color), D (at least 6 mm diameter).

    d. A (asymmetry), B (clear border), C (one color), D (at least 6 mm diameter).

74. A staging workup for melanoma would include

    a. lymph node biopsy.

    b. brain scan.

    c. calcium levels.

    d. sestimibi scan.

75. An agent used in the treatment of malignant melanoma is

    a. ondansetron.

    b. interferon-alfa.

    c. tamoxifen.

    d. cladribine.

REFERENCES

American Cancer Society. (2006). *Cancer facts & figures 2006.* Atlanta: Author.

American Joint Committee on Cancer. (2002). *AJCC cancer staging manual* (6th ed.). New York: Springer-Verlag.

Cancerconsultants.org. (2006). *Temodar® and Peg-Intron® active in metastatic melanoma.* Retrieved April 17, 2007, from http://professional.cancerconsultants.com/oncology_melanoma_news.aspx?id=37702

Guile, K., & Nicholson, S. (2004). Does knowledge influence melanoma-prone behavior? Awareness, exposure, and sun protection among five social groups. *Oncology Nursing Forum, 31*(3), 641–646.

Longman, A. (2005). Nursing care of the client with skin cancer. In J. K. Itano & K. N. Taoka (Eds.), *Core curriculum for oncology nursing* (4th ed., pp. 615–623). St. Louis: Elsevier.

Maltzman, J. (2004). *Be sun-smart and be cancer smart.* Available from www.oncolink.upenn.edu

National Cancer Institute. (2006a). *What you need to know about melanoma.* Retrieved October 31, 2006, from http://www.cancer.gov/cancer topics/wyntk/melanoma/page3

National Cancer Institute. (2006b). *What you need to know about melanoma.* Retrieved April 17, 2007, from http://www.cancer.gov/cancer topics/types/melanoma

Ocular Melanoma Foundation. (2004). About ocular melanoma. Retrieved April 23, 2007, from http://www.ocularmelanoma.org/disease.htm

CHAPTER 19

COMPLEMENTARY THERAPIES

CHAPTER OBJECTIVE

After completing this chapter, the reader will be able to recognize complementary and alternative therapies that cancer patients can use during their treatments.

LEARNING OBJECTIVES

After studying this chapter, the reader will be able to

1. name a category of complementary and alternative therapy (CAM).

2. identify an herb that is popular among cancer patients.

3. list a question that a patient may want to ask before including a CAM in his or her diet.

4. name an herb that is contraindicated in patients receiving chemotherapy.

INTRODUCTION

Complementary and alternative therapies—commonly called CAMs—are popular with cancer patients. They can provide comfort, help patients feel better, and allow patients a sense of control over treatment and its many complexities. This chapter highlights what the nurse caring for cancer patients should know about CAMs. *Note:* The term CAMs—the original acronym for complementary and alternative medicines—now has expanded to include many types of therapies.

Among the many questions patients have during treatment are questions about so-called "complementary therapies." The definition or description of this therapy category is broad. In addition to the term *complementary therapies,* the National Center for Complementary and Alternative Medicine (NCCAM) of the National Institutes of Health (NIH) also calls these therapies *alternative medicine, alternative therapies, integrative medicine, integrative health care, holistic care, nonallopathic treatments, nonbiomedical therapies,* and *nontraditional care* (CancerSource, 2006; NCCAM, 2006a).

The term *complementary therapies* is preferred to *alternative therapies* because it conveys that these therapies are used in conjunction with—rather than as replacements for—biomedical treatment. Table 19-1 provides definitions for these therapies. Table 19-2 lists classifications.

HISTORY

So-called complementary therapies have been used for centuries. Hippocrates, Plato, and Aristotle made reference to the effectiveness of a number of therapies that are now called *complementary.* In nursing, Florence Nightingale described the use of a number of complementary

TABLE 19-1: COMPLEMENTARY AND ALTERNATIVE MEDICINE DEFINITIONS

CAM is any medical system, practice, or product that is not thought of as standard care. Standard medical care is care that is based on scientific evidence. For cancer, it includes chemotherapy, radiation therapy (RT), biological therapy, and surgery.

Complementary Medicine

- Complementary medicine is used along with standard medical treatments.

- One example is using acupuncture to help with side effects of cancer treatment.

Alternative Medicine

- Alternative medicine is used in place of standard medical treatments.

- One example is using a special diet to treat cancer instead of a method that a cancer specialist suggests.

Integrative Medicine

- Integrative medicine is a total approach to care that involves the patient's mind, body, and spirit. It combines standard medicine with the CAM practices that have shown the most promise.

- For example, some people learn to use relaxation as a way to reduce stress during chemotherapy.

Note. From *CAM Basics,* by National Center for Complementary and Alternative Medicine, 2007. Retrieved May 31, 2007, from http://nccam.nih.gov/health/whatiscam/

therapies—such as music—in the holistic care of patients (National Cancer Institute [NCI], 2006).

Until the last decade, complementary therapies had been more popular in Europe than in the United States. Herbs have long been an integral part of German health care and are the foundation of Far Eastern and Asian treatments. Much of the research on herbal preparations has been conducted in Germany. Therapies that Americans have labeled as "complementary" or "alternative" have often been one of the main modes of health care across the world. It is estimated that 70% to 90% of the world's population uses complementary therapies as a routine part of their health care (NCCAM, 2006a; NCI, 2006).

To establish the true clinical and economic value of these therapies and provide a better scientific basis for the use of complementary therapies, carefully designed research studies need to be performed. A 2002 survey determined that at least 36% of Americans use one or more complementary or alternative therapies (Wyatt & Post-White, 2005), with another estimate at 50% (Ross, 2005). Moreover, payment for these therapies was out-of-pocket, estimated at more than $22 billion. Unlike conventional treatments for cancer, most complementary and alternative therapies are not covered by insurance (Ross, 2005).

CANCER PATIENTS AND COMPLEMENTARY THERAPIES

Factors that motivate cancer patients to consider using CAMs vary by patient. Among the reasons are to find the right treatment to better fight their disease, to prevent illness, to reduce stress, and to prevent or reduce side effects and symptoms. In addition, CAMs are readily available. For many patients, the motivation to use them is that CAMs originate from a more supportive, natural source (Deng & Cassileth, 2005; Fellowes, Barnes, & Wilkinson, 2004).

The belief in and practice of complementary therapies is closely linked with cultural values. Many immigrants to the United States come without a tradition of Western medicine practice. Recent and first- or second-degree immigrants to the United States may use a therapy similar to one used in the United States, but the purpose may be significantly different.

Alternative therapies are used across cultures. For example, in addition to herbal remedies, Americans have become very familiar with such

TABLE 19-2: CLASSIFICATIONS OF COMPLEMENTARY AND ALTERNATIVE MEDICINE

Mind-Body Medicines

These are based on the belief that your mind is able to affect your body. Some examples are:

- **Meditation:** Focused breathing or repetition of words or phrases to quiet the mind
- **Biofeedback:** Using a simple machine to learn how to affect certain body functions that are normally out of one's awareness (such as heart rate)
- **Hypnosis:** A state of relaxed and focused attention in which the patient concentrates on a certain feeling, idea, or suggestion to aid in healing
- **Yoga:** Systems of stretches and poses, with special attention to breathing
- **Imagery:** Imagining scenes, pictures, or experiences to help the body heal
- **Creative outlets:** Such as art, music, or dance

Biologically Based Practices

This type of CAM uses things found in nature, including dietary supplements and herbal products. Some examples are:

- Vitamins
- Herbs
- Foods
- Special diets

Manipulative and Body-Based Practices

These are based on working with one or more parts of the body. Some examples are:

- **Massage:** Manipulation of tissues with hands or special tools
- **Chiropractic care:** Manipulation of the joints and skeletal system
- **Reflexology:** Using pressure points in the hands and feet to affect other parts of the body

Energy Medicine

Energy medicine involves the belief that the body has energy fields that can be used for healing and wellness. Therapists use pressure or move the body by placing their hands in or through these fields. Some examples are:

- **Tai Chi:** Involves slow, gentle movements with a focus on breathing and concentration
- **Reiki:** Balancing energy either from a distance or by placing hands on or near the patient
- **Therapeutic touch:** Moving hands over energy fields of the body

Note. From *Thinking About Complementary and Alternative Medicine, Types of Complementary and Alternative Medicine (CAM)*, by National Cancer Institute, 2005. Retrieved May 31, 2007, from http://www.cancer.gov/cancertopics/thinking-about-CAM/page5

therapies as acupuncture and meditation. Many view herbal supplements as "safe" and less toxic than chemotherapy. However, these perceptions are commonly based more on anecdotal evidence than on empirical research (Ross, 2005).

HERBAL SUPPLEMENT USE IS BOOMING BUSINESS

Americans paid more than $5 billion out-of-pocket for herbs and herbal supplements in 1997, the most recent estimate from national surveys (NCCAM, 2006b). In the United States, herbs are considered nutritional supplements. This billion-dollar supplement industry is essentially unregulated. This means that the safety and quality of supplements remain in question even after they are put on the market (Ross, 2005).

In 1998, in response to the need for clear information and standards, the NCI created the NCCAM, which is mandated to develop and support quality research on complementary therapies related to cancer. Studies show that patients may hide the fact they are taking CAMs from their (Western) health care providers (Laino, 2005; Smith, 2005).

The NCCAM follows other efforts to better understand complementary therapies and their merit. In 1994, Congress passed the Dietary Supplement Health and Education Act (DSHEA); among the law's provisions is that it allows the supplement industry to regulate itself. The DSHEA gives supplement manufacturers sole responsibility for ensuring that their products are safe for sale to the public. The U.S. Food and Drug Administration (FDA) does monitor products after they are marketed (Wyatt & Post-White, 2005).

One safeguard for consumers is that supplement labeling may include the initials for the United States Pharmacopeia (USP). The USP sets standards for more than 3,700 prescription and nonprescription medications as well as herbal and nonherbal supplements. It attempts to ensure the quality and purity of products. Participation in the program is strictly voluntary, so the USP tests only those supplements submitted by their manufacturers.

Table 19-3 provides guidelines for patients researching the benefits of supplements.

HERBALS AS TREATMENT

More than 30% of modern medicines are derived from plant sources. After all, many of the chemotherapy agents that are used to fight cancer are derived from plants. Some examples of these chemotherapy agents are the vinca alkaloids

TABLE 19-3: SUGGESTIONS FOR PATIENTS WHO WANT TO TAKE SUPPLEMENTS

- Research the supplement thoroughly. Encourage research from reputable web sites, such as NCI and NCCAM.

- Always inform the doctor or nurse about supplements you have taken or are considering taking.

- Seek new information on the supplement, preferably from clinical trials rather than anecdotal evidence or personal testimonials.

- Be selective if seeking the advice of a practitioner of CAM. Verify experience and credibility of the practitioner by confirming the practitioner's licensure, education, and any details about his or her practice, including any complaints on record.

Ask these questions:
- What are the possible benefits of the supplement?

- What are the known risks or negative side effects?

- Will the supplement interact with other cancer treatments?

- What is the recommended duration of use of the supplement?

- What are the anticipated results?

(CancerSource, 2006)

(from the periwinkle plant) and the taxanes (from the Pacific yew tree) (Treasure, 2005).

Patients may take nutritional supplements such as herbs to boost their immune systems to fight cancer as well as to minimize side effects of treatment. For example, the herb astragalus is used to strengthen and regulate the immune system and to increase red blood cell production. It is an antioxidant that inhibits free radical production and is believed to potentiate the effects of natural interferons. Because of its effects on blood, patients receiving chemotherapy should not use it (D'Andrea, 2005).

Glutamine, a naturally occurring amino acid, has been shown to decrease glutathione levels in tumor cells, making them more sensitive to RT and chemotherapy. It also has been shown to increase glutathione levels in nontumor tissues, thereby protecting them from the toxicities of RT and chemotherapy (Montbriand, 2004a).

Shitake and maitake mushrooms have shown activity in treatment of gastrointestinal, breast, lung, and ovarian cancers (Wyatt & Post-White, 2005).

Chinese herbs, called PC-SPES, have shown responses in pilot studies with prostate cancer patients; those taking the herbs were shown to have decreasing prostate-specific antigen levels (Lee, 2005c).

Electroacupuncture has shown early effectiveness in reducing symptoms of nausea and vomiting (NCCAM, 2006a).

CONTRAINDICATIONS: HERBS AND STANDARD CANCER THERAPIES

Despite the promise of some herbs, others are specifically contraindicated in patients receiving selected standard chemotherapy agents.

Echinacea (from the purple cone flower) has been popular in Germany and other Western European countries since the 1930s. It is thought to stimulate phagocytosis and increase leukocyte mobility, as well as boost T4 helper cells and interferon. Although usually taken to minimize symptoms of cold and flu, cancer patients may take it as an immune stimulant. However, for patients on chemotherapy, echinacea should be discontinued because it can interact with the chemotherapy, affecting metabolism and immunosuppression (Lee, 2005d; Ross, 2005).

Ginseng is contraindicated in patients with estrogen-sensitive cancers, such as breast cancer. Like many other herbs, it has anticoagulant properties and can potentiate the anticoagulant properties of aspirin and other nonsteroidal anti-inflammatory drugs. It also should not be used with phenelzine sulfate (Nardil), because this combination may cause headaches, tremors, and manic episodes (Montbriand, 2004b, 2004c, 2005).

Other contraindications of herbals and herbal supplements with chemotherapy are listed here:

- St. John's wort is contraindicated in patients taking etoposide (VePesid) or vincristine (Oncovin). Due to its mechanism of action and metabolic route, St. John's wort can prevent those chemotherapy drugs from entering the cancer cell (Montbriand, 2004b, 2004c).

- Numerous herbs can potentiate bleeding in patients who are on anticoagulant therapy. A few of these are garlic, ginger, gingko, red clover, and feverfew (Lee, 2005d; Montbriand, 2004b, 2004c, 2005).

- Black cohosh is a widely used herbal remedy for menopausal symptoms. Yet it is contraindicated for those diagnosed with breast cancer because some animal studies have shown that black cohosh can stimulate breast cancer cell spread. In another recent trial that enrolled women with breast cancer who had completed chemotherapy, black cohosh was not found to be any more effective in reducing hot flashes than the placebo (Lee, 2005b).

- High-dose vitamin C is considered a contraindication for patients in chemotherapy-based treatment because it is taken up by the cells in oxidized form and counteracts the effects of chemotherapy (Montbriand, 2004b).

- Regular high-level consumption of soy is controversial. Some studies suggest soy consumption protects against the development of breast cancer. Other studies suggest that soy consumption, especially when taken with tamoxifen, can increase breast cancer risk (Montbriand, 2004c).

Careful clinical trials must continue so that cytoprotectants—agents that claim to prevent malignancies from developing—are appropriately tested. The key in testing is to show that cytoprotectants are protecting only healthy tissue from the toxicities of cancer therapy and not protecting the tumor or malignant cells (Lee, 2005a; Ross, 2005).

RESEARCH

The NIH Center for Complementary and Alternative Research is coordinating various studies involving complementary therapies. A major focus of clinical trials is to observe the effects of herbal and nonherbal supplements on a tumor's response to chemotherapy or RT. Some of these interactions are thought to worsen the side effects of treatment. Antioxidation and "cleaning up" free radicals—the mechanisms of action of many herbals and supplements—may damage cell deoxyribonucleic acid even though cancer treatments, such as RT and chemotherapy, often work by creating those free radicals. It is not yet known if free radicals repair tumor cells in addition to healthy tissues (thus reducing side effects), which could defeat the purpose of primary cancer therapy (NCI, 2006; Ross, 2005).

One complementary therapy study evaluated the effects of a diet low in fat and high in soy, fruits, vegetables, green tea, vitamin E, and fiber in patients with prostate cancer. An additional example of an ongoing clinical trial is the use of oral cartilage for patients with unresectable stage IIIA or IIIB non-small-cell lung cancer. Also, selenium is being studied as a protective agent to reduce development of prostate and lung cancers.

Among early results published in peer-reviewed medical journals is the value of green tea in decreasing the risk of gastric cancers (FDA, 2005).

To date, studies focused on St. John's wort as an antidepressant have shown inconclusive results.

NURSING ROLE AND SUPPORT

The best way for nurses to help patients who are attracted to the promise of CAM, is to serve as reliable sources of information and support. A major focus of nursing is to help patients evaluate the therapy (CancerSource, 2006; Fouladbakhsh, Stommel, Given, & Given, 2005; Lee, 2004; Rosser, 2005; Wyatt & Post-White, 2005).

Nurses can support patients in the following ways:

1. **Encouraging patients to find reputable, credible information** about therapies. Nurses can pass on reputable web sites as resources, such as that of NCCAM (www.nccam.nih.gov).

2. **Providing information** about results of clinical trials rather than anecdotal evidence or personal testimonies.

3. **Encouraging patients to be selective** when seeking advice about CAMs.

4. **Encouraging patient full disclosure,** so that CAMs can be evaluated against chemotherapy agents and other prescribed therapies.

5. **Negotiating "reasonable" use** of supplements. For example, a common compromise is to allow patients to use higher-dose herbals or dietary antioxidants (e.g., vitamins C and E) between or after cancer treatments. However, 1 to 2 weeks before conventional cancer treatments, patients are advised to discontinue supplements entirely.

Another negotiating position concerns vitamin and mineral antioxidant supplements. Patients should be advised to use no more than the recommended dietary allowances during treatment (NCCAM, 2006a).

A common complaint from patients is that health professionals do not listen to them. They claim that professionals hurriedly make an assessment, prescribe treatment, and lack the interpersonal skills to support their beliefs in complementary treatments. Many patients long for a holistic, caring approach to their treatment, especially to maintain an environment that is conducive to open dialogue.

Patients seek a willingness on the part of clinicians to consider CAMs. Many want to include complementary therapies in their treatment plans, if those CAMs will not have a negative effect on standard therapy (Lee, 2004; NCI, 2006; Rosser, 2005).

It is worth remembering that patients still have the right to make treatment decisions. Thus, even more so with complementary therapies , it is the role of the nurse to contribute to a foundation of accurate information for the patient. This foundation can lead to sound, safe, patient-focused decisions (Wyatt & Post-White, 2005).

SUMMARY

Practitioners of complementary therapies state that their interventions seek to restore balance and facilitate the body's own healing responses. Their recommendations may include modification of lifestyle, dietary changes, and exercise as well as specific treatments. Nurses caring for cancer patients can support the use of complementary therapies that have been shown to provide benefit to the patient both physically and psychologically.

EXAM QUESTIONS

CHAPTER 19
Questions 76-79

Note: Choose the option that BEST answers each question.

76. A category of CAM is

    a. alkylating agents.
    b. radiotherapy.
    c. energy medicine.
    d. narcotics.

77. An herb that is popular among cancer patients is

    a. basil.
    b. oregano.
    c. pepper.
    d. echinacea.

78. To help patients assess a CAM before including it in their diet, encourage them to find out

    a. what the benefits are according to the manufacturer.
    b. what it costs.
    c. how it is supplied.
    d. who else is using it.

79. A CAM contraindicated during etoposide- or vincristine-based chemotherapy treatments is

    a. salmon cartilage.
    b. aromatherapy.
    c. St. John's wort.
    d. green tea.

REFERENCES

CancerSource. (2006). *Cancer and complementary care.* Available from http://www.cancersource.com/

D'Andrea, G. (2005). Use of antioxidants during chemotherapy and radiotherapy should be avoided. *CA: Cancer Journal for Clinicians, 55*(5), 319–321.

Deng, G., & Cassileth, B. (2005). Integrative oncology: Complementary therapies for pain, anxiety, and mood disturbance. *CA: Cancer Journal for Clinicians, 55(2),* 109–116

Fellowes, D., Barnes, K., & Wilkinson, S. (2004). Aromatherapy and massage for symptom relief in patients with cancer. *Cochrane Database of Systematic Reviews,* (2). Art No.: CD002287. DOI: 10.1002/14651858.CD002287.pub2.

Fouladbakhsh, J., Stommel, M., Given, B., & Given, C. (2005). Predictors of use of complementary and alternative therapies among patients with cancer. *Oncology Nursing Forum, 32*(6), 1115–1122.

Laino, C. (2005). People with cancer may hide supplement use. Retrieved October 31, 2006, from WebMD http://www.webmd.com/content/ARTICLE/113/110866.htm

Lee, C. (2004). Homeopathy in cancer care: Part II—Continuing the practice of "like curing like." *Clinical Journal of Oncology Nursing, 8*(3), 327–330.

Lee, C. (2005a). Clinical trials in cancer. Part 1, Biomedical, complementary, and alternative medicine: Finding active trials and results of closed trials. *Clinical Journal of Oncology Nursing, 8*(5), 531–535.

Lee, C. (2005b). Complementary and alternative medicine patients are talking about: Black cohosh. *Clinical Journal of Oncology Nursing, 9*(5), 628–629.

Lee, C. (2005c). Complementary and alternative medicine patients are talking about: PC-SPES. *Clinical Journal of Oncology Nursing, 9*(1), 113–114.

Lee, C. (2005d). Herbs and cytotoxic drugs: Recognizing and communicating potentially relevant interactions. *Clinical Journal of Oncology Nursing, 9*(4), 481–487.

Montbriand, M. (2004a). Herbs or natural products that decrease cancer growth: Part one of a four-part series. *Oncology Nursing Forum, 31*(4), E75–90.

Montbriand, M. (2004b). Herbs or natural products that increase cancer growth: Part two of a four-part series. *Oncology Nursing Forum, 31*(5), E99–115.

Montbriand, M. (2004c). Herbs or natural products that decrease cancer growth: Part three of a four-part series. *Oncology Nursing Forum, 31*(6), E127–146.

Montbriand, M. (2005). Herbs or natural products that may cause cancer and harm: Part four of a four-part series. *Oncology Nursing Forum, 32*(1), E20–9.

National Cancer Institute. (2005). *Thinking about complementary and alternative medicine, Types of complementary and alternative medicine (CAM).* Retrieved May 31, 2007, from http://www.cancer.gov/cancertopics/thinking-about-CAM/page5

National Cancer Institute. (2006). *Complementary and alternative medicine (CAM)*. Available from http://www.cancer.gov/cancertopics/treatment/cam

National Center for Complementary and Alternative Medicine. (2006a). *Health information.* Retrieved October 31, 2006, from http://nccam.nih.gov/health

National Center for Complementary and Alternative Medicine. (2006b). The use of complementary and alternative medicine in the United States. Retrieved October 31, 2006, from http://nccam.nih.gov/news/camsurvey_fs1.htm#spend

National Center for Complementary and Alternative Medicine. (2007). *CAM basics.* Retrieved May 31, 2007, from http://nccam.nih.gov/health/whatiscam/

Ross, P. (2005). Complementary and alternative medicine. In J. K. Itano & K. N. Taoka (Eds.), *Core curriculum for oncology nursing* (4th ed., pp. 828–838). St. Louis: Elsevier.

Rosser, C. (2005). Homeopathy in cancer care: Part I—An introduction to "like curing like." *Clinical Journal of Oncology Nursing, 8*(3), 324–326.

Smith, A. (2005). Opening the dialogue: Herbal supplementation and chemotherapy. *Clinical Journal of Oncology Nursing, 9*(4), 447–450.

Treasure, J. (2005). Herbal medicine and cancer: An introductory overview. *Seminars in Oncology Nursing, 21*(3), 177–183.

U.S. Food and Drug Administration. (2005). FDA issues information for consumers about claims for green tea and certain cancers. Retrieved October 31, 2006, from http://www.fda.gov/bbs/topics/NEWS/2005/NEW01197.html

Wyatt, G., & Post-White, J. (2005). Future direction of complementary and alternative medicine (CAM) education and research. *Seminars in Oncology Nursing, 21*(3), 215–224.

CHAPTER 20

PSYCHOSOCIAL DIMENSIONS OF CANCER CARE

CHAPTER OBJECTIVE

After completing this chapter, the reader will be able to identify psychosocial stressors and support strategies for cancer patients and families.

LEARNING OBJECTIVES

After studying this chapter, the reader will be able to

1. recognize how to assess for psychosocial stressors.

2. identify interventions to reduce anxiety.

3. identify signs of depression in cancer patients.

4. list interventions to reduce depression in cancer patients.

5. describe ways to provide psychosocial support to patients and families.

INTRODUCTION

The psychosocial aspect of a cancer diagnosis is one of the important domains of cancer nursing. Many emotions are involved in the trajectory of the cancer experience, both for the patient and the family. Moods can change in an instant or can set the overriding tone for the patient's entire cancer battle.

In addition to the patient, each member of the patient's immediate and extended family has psy-chosocial needs that affect the patient. To best address these psychosocial needs, nurses should establish a comprehensive approach that calls on appropriate psychological resources that best bene-fit the patient and family members.

The nurse should start with a thorough psy-chosocial assessment that addresses the patient's and family's previous coping strategies, levels of anxiety and depression, feelings of hopelessness, and "meaning making" about illness and health. Studies show that interventions—not only by the nurse but by the entire care team of social workers, chaplains, and other health care professionals—are integral to the cancer patient navigating through ill-ness, recurrence, recovery, and survivorship (Grimm, 2005).

COPING AND PSYCHOLOGICAL DISTRESS

Hearing the diagnosis of cancer can be one of the ultimate stressors in a person's life experi-ence. Not surprisingly, a patient and family respond to acute stress—such as the diagnosis of cancer—using coping skills developed over the years. They consciously and subconsciously mobilize coping skills that they have used when confronted with pre-vious life stressors.

By starting with a psychosocial assessment, the nurse can help support appropriate old coping strategies and cultivate new ones. Based on the assessment, the nurse and health care team can help equip the patient and family members with an understanding of coping mechanisms. This allows the team to better mobilize coping methods during the patient's experience of cancer, including the periods of treatment and recovery.

Figure 20-1 shows components of a screening tool for measuring distress. A tool such as this one can help the nurse identify the factors preventing or leading to coping by the patient and family. Included in any coping assessment are predictable areas of patient and family response toward grief, anxiety, depression, and hopelessness (Grimm, 2005).

The cancer diagnosis does not always provoke a severe stressful response from patients. Each patient has an individual response to the stress, which can vary hour-to-hour and day-to-day. A response to stress has at least two components: 1) the response to the stress and 2) the feelings associated with that response.

Communication

One important component of the psychosocial domain—and a means to support patient and family coping—is open and clear communication. Communication should include the communication styles that the patient and family use. The effects of stress can strain a family's preexisting communication styles. Moreover, a patient may be attempting to deal with all the new information he or she has received and may not be capable of meeting the family's needs for communication. That is when the nurse can step in to facilitate communication and support coping behaviors (Goodell & Nail, 2005; Grimm, 2005).

For example, a patient may digest information about his illness when given in great detail. Yet a family member may better understand—and better cope with—the facts of the illness when the information presented is more general. The nurse can tai-

lor the information to meet the needs of each member of the family; the ability to do this is a key component in supporting the family's psychosocial needs (Grimm, 2005).

Another situation that requires the nurse to have excellent communication skills can arise during the course of treatment if the patient experiences anxiety, depression, or hopelessness and is unable to interact with family members. Family members may feel hurt and, in turn, be unable to help their loved one. A nurse who is acutely aware of communication issues within the family can provide a great service by acting as an interpreter of the behavior. If the family situation and communication modes become more complex, the nurse can refer the patient and family to counseling services.

Grief

Cancer patients face many losses and have many reasons to grieve. It is now known that the stages of grief are less linear than first proposed by the classic grief research of Dr. Elisabeth Kübler-Ross. Kübler-Ross's proposed stages of grief—denial, anger, bargaining, depression, adjustment, and hope—have since been recategorized and defined by other researchers (CancerSource, 2006). Yet identifying stages of grief is still a helpful framework for the patient and family to understand their grief experience (Stephenson, 2004).

Grief reactions can be a response to tangible losses (e.g., health, death) or symbolic or psychological losses (e.g., roles in the family, attractiveness.) Appropriate grief-counseling interventions can validate the patient's grief experience, allowing a normal grief process to proceed (CancerSource, 2006; Goodell & Nail, 2005).

The process of grief—including mourning and bereavement—may include one or all of these characteristics (in no particular order or duration):

- somatic distress
- preoccupation with the image of the deceased
- guilt

FIGURE 20-1: COMPONENTS OF DISTRESS MANAGEMENT ASSESSMENT TOOL

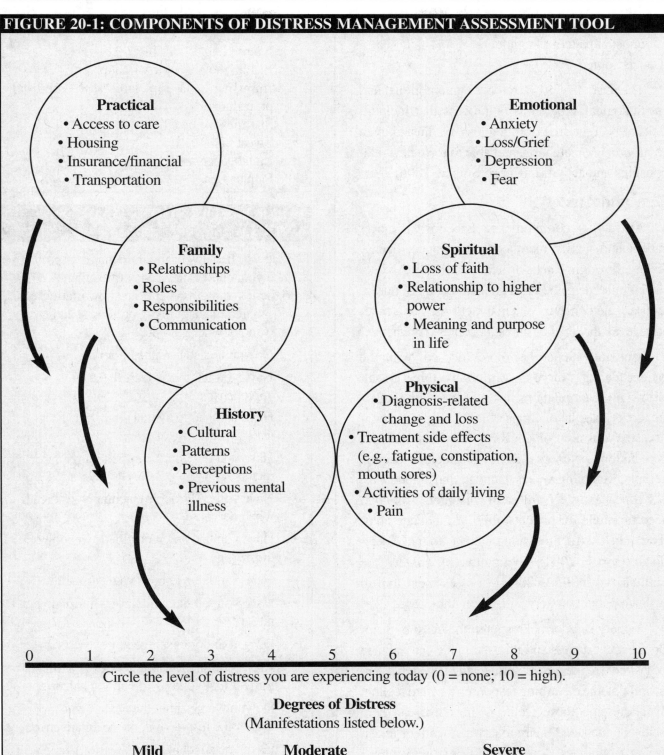

Practical
- Access to care
- Housing
- Insurance/financial
- Transportation

Emotional
- Anxiety
- Loss/Grief
- Depression
- Fear

Family
- Relationships
- Roles
- Responsibilities
- Communication

Spiritual
- Loss of faith
- Relationship to higher power
- Meaning and purpose in life

History
- Cultural
- Patterns
- Perceptions
- Previous mental illness

Physical
- Diagnosis-related change and loss
- Treatment side effects (e.g., fatigue, constipation, mouth sores)
- Activities of daily living
- Pain

```
0   1   2   3   4   5   6   7   8   9   10
```

Circle the level of distress you are experiencing today (0 = none; 10 = high).

Degrees of Distress
(Manifestations listed below.)

Mild	**Moderate**	**Severe**
Fatigue	Delirium	Depression
Sleep disturbance	Dementia	Anxiety
Cognitive dysfunction	Adjustment disorders	Posttraumatic stress disorder

(Cohen & Carlson, 2006; Grimm, 2005; National Comprehensive Cancer Network, 2005)

- hostile reactions
- unusual pattern of conduct.

(CancerSource, 2006)

The term *grief work* refers to an emotional and psychological experience or process that includes tasks to become free from the loss, readjusted to an environment or situation, and able to form new relationships and activities (CancerSource, 2006).

Fear and Anxiety

Anxiety—a common experience for the cancer patient and family members—is a vague, uneasy feeling. Its origin can be difficult to identify. Anxiety can be mild, described as a general feeling of unrest, arousal, and concern. When anxiety rises to a moderate level, the level of unrest becomes more acute.

Moderate anxiety is more focused, with the patient feeling a more uncomfortable threat to self or to significant relationships. Patients with moderate anxiety display feelings of unfocused apprehension, nervousness, or concern. They may express expectations of danger. Behaviors include pacing, tremors, trembling voices, tachycardia, diaphoresis, tachypnea, and sleep and eating disorders. Although uncomfortable for patients, mild to moderate anxiety can be useful, motivating patients to make decisions (Gobel, 2004). Symptoms of anxiety are summarized in Table 20-1. An assessment tool to evaluate patient anxiety is listed in Table 20-2.

Anxiety is a normal response to stress; by helping a patient understand this, the nurse can validate the patient's experience. Some patients benefit from prioritizing the disturbing responses they are feeling. By addressing those feelings, the nurse can help patients understand their anxiety and learn or revisit coping techniques. Among interventions to relieve anxiety are biofeedback and visualization. The administration of anxiety-reducing medications—such as benzodiazepines—can also help. Table 20-3 lists commonly prescribed benzodiazepines for cancer patients.

TABLE 20-1: SYMPTOMS OF ANXIETY

- Intense fear
- Inability to absorb information
- Inability to cooperate with medical procedures
- Shortness of breath
- Sweating
- Lightheadedness
- Palpitations

TABLE 20-2: QUESTIONS TO ASSESS ANXIETY

Have you had any of the following symptoms since your cancer diagnosis or treatment? When do these symptoms occur (i.e., how many days prior to treatment, at night, or at no specific time) and how long do they last?

- Do you feel shaky, jittery, or nervous?
- Have you felt tense, fearful, or apprehensive?
- Have you had to avoid certain places or activities because of fear?
- Have you felt your heart pounding or racing?
- Have you had trouble catching your breath when nervous?
- Have you had any unjustified sweating or trembling?
- Have you felt a knot in your stomach?
- Have you felt like you have a lump in your throat?
- Do you find yourself pacing?
- Are you afraid to close your eyes at night for fear that you may die in your sleep?
- Do you worry about the next diagnostic test, or the results of it, weeks in advance?
- Have you suddenly had a fear of losing control or going crazy?
- Have you suddenly had a fear of dying?
- Have you been confused or disoriented lately?

(CancerSource, 2005)

TABLE 20-3: COMMONLY PRESCRIBED BENZODIAZEPINES FOR CANCER PATIENTS

Short-acting
- Alprazolam
- Oxazepam
- Lorazepam
- Temazepam

Intermediate-acting
- Chlordiazepoxide

Long-acting
- Diazepam
- Clorazepate
- Clonazepam

Anxiety escalated beyond a mild to moderate level can become severe anxiety, manifesting as panic attacks. This state of anxiety can cause patients to be unfocused, stating feelings of dread, apprehension, concern, or nervousness. They may be inappropriately verbal or may not verbalize at all. These patients can be extremely agitated or immobile. They can have tachycardia, tachypnea, diaphoresis, increased muscle tension, dilated pupils, and pallor. They often have difficulty falling asleep. Sometimes these patients advance to a nonfunctional state; they become out of control and uncommunicative. Patients with severe anxiety usually require pharmacologic and psychiatric interventions (Gobel, 2004).

Depression

Depression is a common and normal reaction to a diagnosis of cancer or recurrent illness. Depression is usually an inevitable response to loss—anticipated or current. That loss can be the loss of a person (including oneself) or loss of many of life's substances and values, such as self-esteem, loss of control, or loss of a normal life. According to estimates, up to 25% of hospitalized cancer patients and 20% of adults with cancer have signs and symptoms of depression during the course of their disease (Grimm, 2005).

Table 20-4 lists cancer-related risk factors for depression.

TABLE 20-4: CANCER-RELATED RISK FACTORS FOR DEPRESSION

- Depression at time of cancer diagnosis
- Poorly controlled pain
- Advanced stage of cancer
- Additional concurrent life stressors
- Increased physical impairment or discomfort
- Pancreatic cancer
- Being unmarried
- Having head and neck cancer
- Treatment with certain medications
- Treatment with certain chemotherapeutic agents
- Metabolic changes
- Endocrine abnormalities

See Table 20-7 for more information.

(National Cancer Institute [NCI], 2007; Sharp, 2005)

Recognizing depression can be difficult. Depression is often intricately woven into a patient's disease process; determining the origin of depression can be complicated. Is it caused by the disease itself? The treatment? Both? Whatever the source or sources of depression, attempts to dissect the patient's depression can better lead to appropriate treatment or intervention. Table 20-5 lists common signs and symptoms of depression (Grimm, 2005). Table 20-6 summarizes indicators of depression.

Before their cancer experience, some patients have depression or are predisposed to depression. Thus, the new diagnosis of cancer may contribute to their underlying depression. Patients at high risk for depression include, but are not limited to, those with a history of depression, alcoholism, substance abuse, physical abuse, self-injury, or advanced stages of cancer; poorly controlled pain; concurrent illnesses; inadequate social support; impaired body image; or changed work and family roles (Barsevick & Much, 2004; Bennett & Badger, 2005; Grimm, 2005; Sharp, 2005).

TABLE 20-5: SIGNS AND SYMPTOMS OF DEPRESSION

(Patients may feel at least one of the following symptoms, lasting for a week or more.)

- Worthlessness
- Low spirits
- Inability to sleep, early awakening
- Decreased or increased appetite
- Irritability
- Loss of pleasure in life
- Withdrawal from others
- Feelings of sadness, tendency to cry easily
- Oversleeping
- Negative viewing of events
- Self-blame or self-criticism
- Death thoughts

TABLE 20-6: INDICATORS OF DEPRESSION THAT REQUIRE MORE FOCUSED OR INVOLVED INTERVENTIONS

- History of depression
- Weak social support system (not married, few friends, solitary work environment)
- Evidence of persistent irrational beliefs or negativistic thinking regarding the diagnosis
- More-serious prognosis
- Greater dysfunction related to cancer
- Depressed mood for most of the day on most days

In general, for more than 2 weeks:

- Diminished pleasure or interest in most activities
- Significant change in appetite and sleep patterns
- Psychomotor agitation or slowing
- Fatigue
- Feelings of worthlessness or excessive, inappropriate guilt
- Poor concentration
- Recurrent thoughts of death or suicide

(CancerSource, 2006)

Patients may avoid discussing depressive signs and symptoms unless asked, and some researchers believe that clinically significant depression is underdiagnosed and undertreated (Sharp, 2005). Moreover, a clear and definitive diagnosis of depression can be colored by patient behavior that may be seen as lazy, attention seeking, manipulative, or noncompliant. In addition, depression may cause the patient to be very fatigued, which may be initially attributed to the cancer itself or treatment side effects (Barsevick & Much, 2004; Sharp, 2005).

Depression can also be a side effect of some commonly used medications. These include analgesics, anti-inflammatory agents, antihistamines, antihypertensives, antimicrobials (e.g., amphotericin), antiparkinsonian agents, hormones, immunosuppressive agents, tranquilizers, stimulants, antineoplastics (e.g., vincristine, vinblastine, procarbazine, L-asparaginase, and interferon), anticonvulsants, and sedatives. Corticosteroids—commonly included in cancer treatment protocols—subject the patient to mood swings and periods of depression (Grimm, 2005; Sharp, 2005). Depression also is accentuated with alcohol consumption. Table 20-7 lists possible medical or medication-based causes of depression.

Severe Depression

If depression advances to a state of hopelessness, patients may report that they see limited or no available alternatives or personal choices and cannot mobilize energy on their own behalf. The hallmarks of hopelessness are extreme passivity, withdrawal, lack of initiative, and a more acute period of weight loss, decreased appetite, and sleep (Bennett & Badger, 2005).

Table 20-8 provides examples of questions to assess depression and suicide risk.

Antidepressants

Fortunately for many patients, antidepressants can be prescribed to address short-term or long-term periods of depression. Common antidepressants are listed in Table 20-9. Antidepressants should be one

TABLE 20-7: POSSIBLE MEDICAL CAUSES OF CANCER-RELATED DEPRESSION

Treatment with certain medications
- Corticosteroids
- Interferon-alfa and aldesleukin (interleukin-2 [IL-2])
- Methyldopa
- Reserpine
- Barbiturates
- Propranolol
- Some antibiotics (e.g., amphotericin B)

Treatment with certain chemotherapeutic agents
- Procarbazine
- L-asparaginase
- Interferon-alfa
- IL-2

Metabolic changes
- Hypercalcemia
- Sodium or potassium imbalance
- Anemia
- Vitamin B_{12} or folate deficiency
- Fever

Endocrine abnormalities
- Hyperthyroidism or hypothyroidism
- Adrenal insufficiency

(NCI, 2007)

TABLE 20-8: EXAMPLES OF ASSESSMENT QUESTIONS FOR DEPRESSION AND SUICIDE

Depression
- How well are you coping with your cancer?
- Do you cry sometimes? How often? Ever alone?
- What things do you still enjoy doing?
- Do you feel others would be better off without you?
- Is your pain under control?
- Do you feel you have any control over your care?
- Are you sleeping? Do you spend a lot of time in bed?
- What is your appetite like?
- Can you concentrate on things you want or need to do?

Suicide
- Have you ever had thoughts of not wanting to live or wishing you could hasten your death?
- Have you ever attempted suicide?
- Have you been treated for psychiatric problems before?
- Have you had a problem with alcohol or drugs?

(CancerSource, 2006)

component of a comprehensive approach to depression treatment, which should also include education, support, counseling, and additional pharmacologic and nonpharmacologic methods to help with sleeplessness, anxiety, and pain.

PSYCHOSOCIAL SUPPORT

All psychosocial issues for patients and families warrant the knowledgeable and caring touch of their health care team. Individual interventions vary by patient and family, but general approaches should include these measures:

1. Provide an honest, supportive environment for the patient to talk, cry, find solace, and share feelings. Listen. Encourage family and friends to be there for the patient. Be a conduit for support groups, information, clarification, and affirmation.

Studies continue to show that support of the patient is the foundation for dealing with psychosocial stressors. Studies show that patients seek support first from significant others, family, and friends. Then patients seek support from health care professionals. Frequently, talking through these feelings with a loved one, clergy, social worker, counselor, or support group can ease the grieving process (Sharp, 2005; Taylor, 2004).

TABLE 20-9: COMMON ANTIDEPRESSANTS

Tricyclic antidepressants
- amitriptyline (Elavil)
- clomipramine (Anafranil)
- desipramine (Norpramin)
- doxepin (Sinequan)
- imipramine (Tofranil)
- nortriptyline (Pamelor)

Selective Serotonin Reuptake Inhibitors
- citalopram (Celexa)
- fluoxetine (Prozac)
- fluvoxamine (Luvox)
- paroxetine (Paxil)
- sertraline (Zoloft)

Monoamine oxidase inhibitors
- tranylcypromine (Parnate)
- phenelzine (Nardil)

Atypical antidepressants
- bupropion (Wellbutrin)
- trazodone (Desyrel)
- nefazodone (Serzone)
- mirtazapine (Remeron)
- maprotiline (Ludiomil)
- venlafaxine (Effexor)

If a nurse cannot deal with these emotions, an immediate referral should be made to someone who can. Because patients in this situation are so vulnerable, it is imperative that their nurses have no agendas and seek help from resources that can help the patient.

2. Support the patient's sense of personal power and control. When possible, let the patient schedule some treatments or activities. Include the patient as much as possible in planning care and in setting goals and schedules.

3. Review coping strategies that the patient has used during other stressful times, and encourage the patient to apply those strategies to the current situation. Explore physical therapy, massage, biofeedback, relaxation techniques, self-hypnosis, and imagery to relieve pain, anxiety, and stress.

4. Teach with the goal of equipping the patient with the knowledge necessary to better understand the aspects of grief, mood swings, anxiety, and depression.

5. Foster an environment of hope. Review changes in health status. If treatment is going well, remind the patient of that reality.

   Help create a future perspective; talk about future goals.

   Support life-affirming activities, such as time with family (including grandchildren) and pets. Encourage the patient to tackle projects, enjoy hobbies, attend events, and arrange experiences that provide pleasure and joy (e.g., concerts, leisurely walks, a beautiful bouquet of flowers, or time to read a good book).

6. Clarify information. Confirm accurate perceptions and correct misconceptions and misinformation.

7. Support family members as they give support.

   Table 20-10 lists additional strategies to support coping behaviors.

Mental Health and Illness

Some patients have an underlying personality disorder or a history of psychiatric problems. When diagnosed with cancer and going through treatment, these patients may not have any successful coping skills and they may decompensate. For these patients, bringing a mental health team or specialist into the care team is the best intervention (Grimm, 2005).

Table 20-11 lists the American Psychiatric Association's (APA's) diagnostic criteria for adjustment disorders, which nurses may use to identify patients who need psychiatric treatment referral.

TABLE 20-10: COPING BEHAVIORS AND STRATEGIES TO SUPPORT PATIENTS AND FAMILY MEMBERS

- Provide information and teaching about the patient's disease.
- Provide information and teaching about coping behaviors and strategies.
- Facilitate and encourage helpful coping behaviors and strategies based on patient and family assessment.
- Provide an environment for therapeutic communication. Listen and accept.
- Provide ongoing and appropriate emotional support.
- Monitor and intervene to provide symptom control and comfort measures.
- Suggest or provide recreational and diversionary outlets.
- Support problem solving; optimize patient control.
- Initiate referrals to augment support (e.g., clergy, occupational, psychological).

(Ahles, & Henderson, 2004; Grimm, 2005; Manning-Walsh, 2005; NCCN, 2007; Skalla, Bakitas, Furstenberg, Taylor, 2004)

SEXUALITY AND BODY IMAGE

Cancer treatment can create issues with the patient's sexuality, which the nurse can address. The nurse's role is to convey accurate information and clarify concerns regarding these issues.

The following reviews some of these issues:

Sexual problems may stem from the patient's feelings about his or her medical condition or treatment as well as from the condition or treatment itself. These feelings are best explored, so that unrealistic expectations, self-consciousness, and anxiety are managed. Professionals can provide support and counseling. Other caregivers also may be able to offer guidance (Bakewell & Volker, 2005).

Treatment can leave patients with an altered body image (e.g., surgical removal of the breasts, alopecia, the tattoos necessary for radiation therapy [RT], or changes in pigmentation caused by treat-ment). Several resources are available to patients to answer questions and support positive feelings (see the Resources section at the end of the book).

Patients should be advised that cancer and its treatment can decrease their libido. Nurses can clarify the effects of cytotoxic agents or RT, which can affect sexual functioning.

Side effects of treatment can interfere with patients' sexual feelings, and treatments may leave them feeling nauseated and fatigued. Moreover, mucositis, stomatitis, and pain can make sexual activity uncomfortable. Patients can assure their partners that cancer is not contagious and that intimacy is possible (Bakewell & Volker, 2005).

Additional examples of tumor- or treatment-related effects include:

- Ovarian dysfunction may cause abnormally low estrogen levels and elevated follicle-stimulating hormone and leutinizing hormone levels. Symptoms include irregular menses, loss of libido, menopausal symptoms, and cessation of menses.

- Testicular dysfunction may cause decreased sperm production, decreased libido, impotence, and gynecomastia.

- Neurotoxicity may lead to decreased sensation, loss of deep tendon reflexes, ptosis, muscle pain, weakness, paralytic ileus, impotence, and constipation.

Chemotherapy, surgery, and RT can cause premature menopause or sterility. Chemotherapy affects the rapidly proliferating reproductive cells, just as it affects cells of the hematopoietic, gastrointestinal, and integumentary systems. The reproductive cells are prime targets of cytotoxic agents (Bakewell & Volker, 2005).

Temporary or permanent amenorrhea in women and oligospermia and azoospermia in men cause sterility. If patient protocols include agents known to cause permanent sterility, men can arrange for sperm banking. Although expensive, some women choose to harvest and store their eggs if treatment puts them at risk for sterility. These procedures

TABLE 20-11: DIAGNOSTIC CRITERIA FOR ADJUSTMENT DISORDERS

Criterion A

The development of emotional or behavioral symptoms in response to an identifiable stressor(s) occurring within 3 months of the onset of the stressor(s).

Criterion B

These symptoms or behaviors are clinically significant as evidenced by either of the following:
- Marked distress that is in excess of what would be expected from exposure to the stressor.
- Significant impairment in social or occupational (academic) functioning.

Criterion C

The stress-related disturbance does not meet the criteria for another specific Axis I disorder and is not merely an exacerbation of a preexisting Axis I or Axis II disorder.

Criterion D

The symptoms do not represent bereavement.

Criterion E

Once the stressor (or its consequences) has terminated, the symptoms do not persist for more than an additional 6 months. Specify:

Acute if the disturbance lasts less than 6 months.
Chronic if the disturbance lasts for 6 months or longer.
Specific subtypes represent the predominant symptoms and include:
- with depressed mood
- with anxiety
- with mixed anxiety and depressed mood
- with disturbance of conduct
- with mixed disturbance of emotions and conduct unspecified.

(APA, 2000)

require the nurse to provide patient teaching and credible resources (Bakewell & Volker, 2005).

The nurse can suggest methods to alleviate sources of discomfort (e.g., pain medication) or restore functioning (e.g., penile implants after prostate cancer surgery).

SUMMARY

Nurses are a vital and present source of psychosocial support for patients and families facing a cancer diagnosis and treatment. Interventions to help the patient and family members cope stem from appropriate assessments, which include grief, anxiety, and depression. Tailored supportive interventions can then follow, which help the patient and family members better cope.

EXAM QUESTIONS

CHAPTER 20
Questions 80-84

Note: Choose the option that BEST answers each question.

80. A psychological assessment of a cancer patient would include an assessment of

    a. depression.

    b. wound healing.

    c. emetic potential.

    d. mobility.

81. To best reduce a patient's anxiety, the nurse should

    a. revisit coping methods the patient has previously used.

    b. suggest that the patient take paroxetine.

    c. avoid confrontation with family members.

    d. enroll the patient in a cancer support group.

82. A sign of depression in a cancer patient includes

    a. oversleeping.

    b. agitation.

    c. watching the news on television.

    d. tingling in the extremities.

83. An intervention to help reduce a patient's depression is

    a. minimize visitors to reduce stress.

    b. encourage rest and sleep to promote coping.

    c. discuss use of an antidepressant with the patient's primary care provider.

    d. remind the patient not to be sad.

84. To support the patient's family members, which of the following responses from the nurse would be most helpful?

    a. "For the benefit of your mother, you've got to get a grip on yourself."

    b. "What is your annual income?"

    c. "What are some of the ways you've coped with past periods of stress in your life?"

    d. "Please refer all questions about the care of your mother to her doctor."

REFERENCES

American Psychiatric Association. (2000). *Diagnostic and statistical manual of mental disorders (DSM-IV-TR, 4th ed.)*. Washington, DC: American Psychiatric Association.

Bakewell, R., & Volker, D. (2005). Sexual dysfunction related to the treatment of young women with breast cancer. *Clinical Journal of Oncology Nursing, 9*(6), 697-702.

Barsevick, A., & Much, J. (2004). Depression. In C. Yarbro, M. Frogge, & M. Goodman (Eds.), *Cancer symptom management* (3rd ed., pp. 668-692). Sudbury, MA: Jones & Bartlett.

Bennett, G., & Badger, T. (2005). Depression in men with prostate cancer. *Oncology Nursing Forum, 32*(3), 545-556.

CancerSource. (2005). *Anxiety disorder.* Retrieved April 17, 2007, from http://www.cancersource.com/Search/37,CDR0000062818

CancerSource. (2006). *Loss, grief, and bereavement.* Retrieved April 17, 2007, from http://www.cancersource.com/Search/37,CDR0000062828

Cohen, M., & Carlson, E. (2006). Cancer-related distress. In C. Yarbro, M. Frogge & M. Goodman (Eds.), *Cancer nursing: Principles and practice* (6th ed., pp. 628-633). Sudbury: Jones & Bartlett.

Gobel, B. (2004). Anxiety. In C. Yarbro, M. Frogge, & M. Goodman (Eds.), *Cancer symptom management* (3rd ed., pp. 651-667). Sudbury, MA: Jones & Bartlett.

Goodell, T., & Nail, L. (2005). Operationalizing symptom distress in adults with cancer: A literature synthesis [Electronic version]. *Oncology Nursing Forum, 32*(2). Retrieved April 17, 2007, from http://www.ons.org/publications/journals/ONF/Volume32/Issue2/320242.asp

Grimm, P. (2005). Coping: Psychosocial issues. In J.K. Itano & K.N. Taoka (Eds.), *Core curriculum for oncology nursing* (4th ed., pp. 29-52). St. Louis: Elsevier.

Manning-Walsh, J. (2005). Psychospiritual well-being and symptom distress in women with breast cancer. *Oncology Nursing Forum, 32*(3), 543.

National Cancer Institute. (2007). *Depression (PDQ®).* Available from http://wwwicic.nci.nih.gov/cancertopics/pdq/supportivecare/depression

National Comprehensive Cancer Network. (2005). *Distress guidelines.* NCCN Clinical Practice Guidelines in Oncology. For latest guidelines, go to http://www.nccn.org/professionals/physician_gls/default.asp

National Comprehensive Cancer Network. (2007). Distress management [Electronic version]. In *NCCN clinical practice guidelines in oncology* (V.1.2007). Available from http://www.nccn.org/professionals/physician_gls/PDF/distress.pdf

Sharp, K. (2005). Depression: The essentials. *Clinical Journal of Oncology Nursing, 9*(5), 519-525.

Skalla, K., Bakitas, M., Furstenberg, C., Ahles, T., & Henderson, J. (2004). Patients' need for information about cancer therapy. *Oncology Nursing Forum, 31*(2), 313–319.

Stephenson, P. (2004). Understanding denial. *Oncology Nursing Forum, 31*(5), 985-988.

Taylor, E. (2004). Spiritual distress. In C. Yarbro, M. Frogge, & M. Goodman (Eds.), *Cancer symptom management* (3rd ed., pp. 693-705). Sudbury, MA: Jones & Bartlett.

CHAPTER 21

SPECIAL POPULATIONS

CHAPTER OBJECTIVE

After completing this chapter, the reader will be able to recognize concerns of special populations of cancer patients, including pediatrics, survivors, the elderly, multiracial populations, and patients with financial challenges.

LEARNING OBJECTIVES

After studying this chapter, the reader will be able to

1. recognize two late effects of childhood cancer treatment.

2. list two barriers for survivors of cancer.

3. name two strategies to assist patients with financial challenges related to their cancer care.

4. name two physiologic changes facing an elderly person with cancer.

INTRODUCTION

Several special populations of cancer patients—pediatrics, survivors, those faced with financial challenges, the elderly, and multiracial populations—have special needs. This chapter highlights some of those challenges, providing tools for assessment and resources to help better care for these patients (Jemal et al., 2004).

CHILDHOOD CANCERS

In the United States, cancer is second only to accidents as the leading cause of death in children between the ages of 1 and 14 years (American Cancer Society [ACS], 2006a). The most common cancers in this age-group are leukemia (especially acute lymphocytic leukemia—approximately one-third of cancer in children), cancer of the brain and nervous system, soft tissue sarcomas, Hodgkin's lymphoma, non-Hodgkin's lymphoma (NHL), and renal (Wilms) tumor. Still, cancer in children is relatively rare; on average, 1 to 2 children develop the disease each year for every 10,000 children in the United States (ACS, 2006a; National Cancer Institute [NCI], 2006b).

Over the past 30 years, the 5-year relative survival for many childhood cancers has improved, reflecting progress in early detection and treatment. Before the 1970s, the 5-year relative survival for all childhood cancers was less than 50%. In the late 1990s, 5-year relative survival improved to nearly 80% (ACS, 2006a).

Over the past 20 years, there has been some increase in the incidence of children diagnosed with all forms of invasive cancer, from 11.5 cases per 100,000 children in 1975 to 14.6 per 100,000 children in 2002. During this same time, however, death rates declined dramatically and survival rates increased for most childhood cancers (ACS, 2006a, 2006b).

Caring for Children with Cancer

Because of the uniqueness of childhood cancers, young patients are usually treated at major children's hospitals, university medical centers, and cancer centers. Table 21-1 lists possible causes of childhood cancer.

When treating children with cancer, nurses need to acknowledge developmental issues associated with their patients' age and maturity. Table 21-2 reviews some of the childhood developmental stages and corresponding behaviors that nurses should incorporate when providing care.

Secondary Malignancies

At 20 years, the cumulative incidence of secondary malignancies among survivors for 5+ years of childhood cancer was 5.2%. The highest risk of secondary malignancies is for those exposed to radiation therapy (RT) (Friedman et al., 2004). RT and a primary diagnosis of Hodgkin's lymphoma, neuroblastoma, or soft tissue sarcoma, were identified as independent risk factors for late secondary malignancies. Risk after 15 years is highest for second breast and thyroid cancers (Friedman et al., 2004).

One of the unfortunate by products of effective pediatric cancer care is the late effects from treatment for childhood cancer. Tables 21-3 and 21-4 on page 304 highlight some of those effects.

TABLE 21-1: CAUSES OF CHILDHOOD CANCER

- High levels of ionizing radiation from accidents or from RT have been linked with increased risk of some childhood cancers.
- Children treated with chemotherapy and RT for certain forms of childhood and adolescent cancers, such as Hodgkin's disease, brain tumors, sarcomas, and others, may develop a second primary malignancy (e.g., Hodgkin's lymphoma, breast cancer).
- Low levels of radiation exposure from radon are not significantly associated with childhood leukemias.
- Ultrasound use during pregnancy has not been linked with childhood cancer in numerous large studies.
- Residential magnetic field exposure from power lines has not been significantly associated with childhood leukemias.
- Certain types of chemotherapy, including alkylating agents or topoisomerase II inhibitors (e.g., epipodophyllotoxins), may cause increased risk of leukemia (in about 10% of cases).
- Pesticides have been suspected to be involved in the development of certain forms of childhood cancer based on interview data. However, interview results have been somewhat inconsistent and have not yet been validated by physical evidence of pesticides in the body or the environment .
- No consistent findings have been observed linking specific occupational exposures of parents to the development of childhood cancers.
- Several studies have found no link between maternal cigarette smoking before pregnancy and childhood cancers, but increased risks were related to the father's prenatal smoking habits in studies in the United Kingdom and China.
- Little evidence has been found to link specific viruses or other infectious agents to the development of most types of childhood cancers, though investigators worldwide are exploring the role of exposure of very young children to some common infectious agents that may protect children from, or put them at risk for, developing certain leukemias.
- Recent research has shown that children with acquired immunodeficiency syndrome (AIDS), like adults with AIDS, have an increased risk of developing certain cancers, predominantly NHL and Kaposi's sarcoma. These children also have an additional risk of developing leiomyosarcoma (a type of muscle cancer).
- Specific genetic syndromes, such as Li-Fraumeni syndrome and neurofibromatosis, have been linked to an increased risk of specific childhood cancers.

(NCI, 2005b, 2006b)

TABLE 21-2: DEVELOPMENTAL STAGES		
Age	**Issues and Behaviors**	**Examples of Care Strategies**
Infant < 1 year	Trust Separation Object permanence	Parents around as much as possible Nursing care given in tandem with parents
Toddler 1–3 years	Autonomy Independence Concrete thinking	Routine established Time for therapeutic play: drawing, games
Preschooler 4–6 years	New skills Increasing independence Differentiating	Routine continues Time for therapeutic play Simple explanations—use pictures and picture words
School Age 7–12 years	Concrete thinking	Routine continues Encourage opportunities to involve child in school events and be with classmates Competencies growing Honest explanations Allow control, when possible
Adolescent 13–18 years	Identity Abstract reasoning Body image Increased independence	Allow independence and control Encourage opportunities to involve child in school events and be with classmates Involve child in decisions Open communication; nurse is a listener

SURVIVORSHIP

Cancer survivors are living longer. As of 2006, the 5-year relative survival rate for all cancers was 66%, rising from 50% for the period 1974 to 1976. More than 10.5 million cancer survivors are alive in the United States, approximately 3.6% of the population. Approximately 14% of those survivors were diagnosed more than 20 years ago (NCI, 2006a). Figure 21-1 shows cancer survivors in the United States by site.

For a patient to be cured of his or her cancer, the standard measurement is no evidence of cancer 5 years after the patient's last treatment. With more successful outcomes from treatment, more and more patients can experience being survivors—with the emotional, spiritual, and financial issues that go along with it. Five-year survival rates are highest for prostate and female breast cancers and lowest for lung cancer (NCI, 2006a).

Some patients call themselves survivors from the day of diagnosis. Others see themselves as survivors when their medical team—based on statistical survival rates—declares them disease-free. That clinical declaration depends on the patient's disease and the number of years without evidence of disease.

Living as a Survivor

All survivors of cancer—no matter their individual profile—enter a new dimension of psychosocial coping. Their lives can take on elements of heartiness, advocacy, challenge, and euphoria. Due to advances in prevention, detection, treatment, and chronic care, patients who survive cancer join a

TABLE 21-3: RISK FACTORS FOR LATE EFFECTS

Tumor-related factors
- Direct tissue effects
- Tumor-induced organ dysfunction
- Mechanical effects

Treatment-related factors
- RT: Total dose and fraction size, organ or tissue volume, and machine energy are the most critical factors
- Chemotherapy: Agent type, single and cumulative dose, and schedule may modify risk
- Surgery: Technique and site are relevant

Host-related factors
- Developmental status
- Genetic predisposition
- Inherent tissue sensitivities and capacity for normal tissue repair
- Function of organs not affected by RT or chemotherapy
- Premorbid state

(NCI, 2006a, 2006b)

larger and larger group of cancer survivors. Stages of survivorship include acute, chronic, and permanent. Table 21-5 reviews the stages and the patient's needs during those stages.

However, the challenges of surviving cancer create a different set of barriers. Among them are:

- Fear of relapse and death. When new aches and pains occur, a preoccupation with minor physical problems begins.

- Guilt. Survivors sometimes feel guilty because they survived while others did not.

- Depression.

- Feelings of isolation. Survivors now have a history different—and sometimes alienating—from those who have not gone through a cancer diagnosis and treatment journey like themselves.

- Insurability. Patients with well-documented preexisting conditions may have difficulty finding health insurance.

TABLE 21-4: LATE EFFECTS ASSOCIATED WITH COMMON AGENTS

Agent/Agent Class/Modality	Affected Body System
Anthracyclines	Circulatory (cardiac) Respiratory (pulmonary)
Alkylating agents	Reproductive (gonadal) Second malignant neoplasms
Topoisomerase II inhibitors	Second malignant neoplasms
Platinums	Urinary (renal) Special senses (hearing) Second malignant neoplasms
Corticosteroids	Central nervous system Musculoskeletal (bone and body composition) Obesity
Intrathecal chemotherapy	Central nervous system
Bleomycin	Respiratory (pulmonary)
Methotrexate	Central nervous system
Vincristine	Digestive (dental)
Thioguanine	Digestive (hepatic)

(NCI, 2005, 2006b; NCCS, 2005)

FIGURE 21-1: ESTIMATED NUMBER OF PERSONS ALIVE IN THE UNITED STATES DIAGNOSED WITH CANCER, BY SITE (N = 10.1 M)

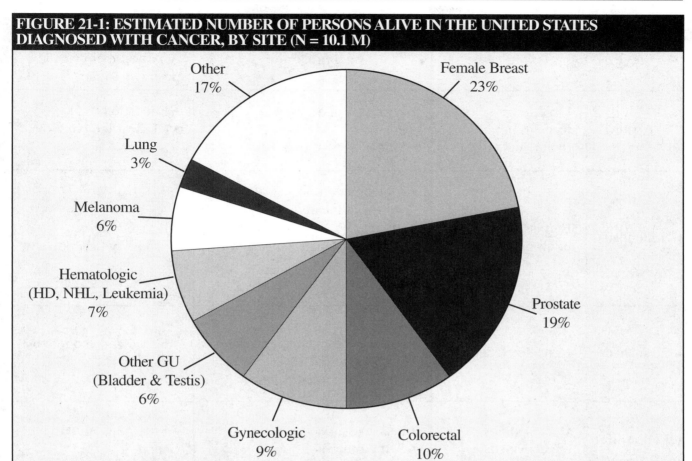

Other 17%

Female Breast 23%

Lung 3%

Melanoma 6%

Hematologic (HD, NHL, Leukemia) 7%

Other GU (Bladder & Testis) 6%

Prostate 19%

Gynecologic 9%

Colorectal 10%

Data Source: 2005 Submission. U.S. Estimated Prevalence counts were estimated by applying U.S. populations to SEER 9 and historical Connecticut Limited Duration Prevalence proportions and adjusted to represent complete prevalence. Populations from January 2003 were based on the average of the July 2002 and July 2003 population estimates from the U.S. Bureau of Census.

Note. From *Cancer Survivorship Research, Estimated US Cancer Prevalence, 2006,* by National Cancer Institute, Cancer Control and Population Sciences. National Cancer Institute, Cancer Control and Population Sciences.

- Employability, based on discrimination of employers who have an anachronistic view of the viability of employees treated for cancer. (One study estimated that 25% of cancer survivors have experienced some discrimination after returning to work [Fisher, 2006]).

- Fear to plan for the future; uncertainty.

- Persistent vulnerability. The sense of security in health and life have forever changed; survivors experience feelings of isolation and have to deal with chronic side effects.

(ACS, 2006b; CancerSource, 2006; Fisher, 2006; Hoffman, 2005).

The nurse's role with cancer survivors is to facilitate the transition from being sick to being able to function in society. This does not mean that the nurse is responsible for the transition but rather is a source of support, information, and perspective.

Referrals for cancer survivors may include occupational or physical therapy or referral to a social worker, the legal aid society, a mental health worker, or other supports in the community. A useful resource is the National Coalition for Cancer Survivorship (NCCS; www.cansearch.org). This nonprofit organization offers support groups, counseling, and advice about discrimination and financial concerns. It also lobbies Washington on behalf of cancer survivors (NCCS, 2005).

A 2006 report from the National Cancer Policy Board, the Institute of Medicine, and the National Research Council called on health professionals, insurers, advocates, and the government to work together to improve follow-up care for the 10 mil-

TABLE 21-5: STAGES OF CANCER SURVIVORSHIP

Stage	Time Frame	Facing/Coping	Focus of Needs (any need below can be prominent in any stage)
Acute	First diagnosis through initial treatment	• Fear and anxiety • Pain • Side effects of treatment	• Education • Clinical interventions • Support
Extended	Remission through point of "cure"	• Adjustment to less contact with health care team • Anxiety • Some continued physical limitations • Long-term side effects	• Rehabilitation • Emotional support
Permanent	Considered "cured"	• Adaptation • Social and economic challenges • Fear of recurrence • Chronic effects of treatment	• Social and economic support
End of life	Occurs at any of the above stages	• Fear and anxiety • Symptom relief	• Symptom relief • Social and emotional support • Spiritual support

(Centers for Disease Control and Prevention, 2004)

lion cancer survivors in the United States. Recommendations from the report, *From Cancer Patient to Cancer Survivor: Lost in Transition*, attempt to address the long-term consequences of cancer and its treatments. Among the recommendations are:

• Improving ongoing care for cancer survivors and allow them to maintain comprehensive summaries of their cancer care and detailed plans for follow-up care.

• Developing more evidence-based guidelines to standardize what that follow-up care should be

• Creating a system to monitor the quality of that care

• Providing more continuing education programs for health care providers about survivorship care

• Supporting demonstration programs to test new ways to deliver survivorship care (an example of a promising model has nurses with the primary responsibility for cancer follow up; another model is to set up specialized cancer survivorship clinics)

• Improving insurance coverage for cancer survivors to fill gaps in standard coverage from Medicare or other policies (Hewitt, Greenfield, & Stovall, 2006).

ECONOMIC FACTORS

Of all the challenges to providing quality nursing care, public access to that care is one of the most difficult. This challenge continues to stretch an already overwhelmed health care system.

Cancer care brings with it daunting financial burdens, which not only include hospital bills but also the costs to cover treatments and drugs, transportation, and home care costs. Increasingly, clinical nurses have had to absorb knowledge and skills related to insurance and reimbursement strategies to provide care to patients.

Here are a few statistics related to the costs of health care:

- In 2005, the official poverty rate in the United States was 12.6%, or 37 million people.

- In 2005, an estimated 15.9% of the population (46.6 million) was without health insurance. This is an increase from 15.6% in 2004 (DeNavas-Walt, Proctor, & Lee, 2006).

- Government-covered health insurance programs (Medicaid and Medicare) cover 27.3% of health care bills in the United States (DeNavas-Walt et al., 2006). Medicare does not cover certain cancer care expenses, such as oral medicines commonly used to treat cancers of the breast and prostate.

- Minorities make up 34% of the nonelderly population but account for more than half (52%) of the uninsured (Ward et al., 2004).

- In 2013, national health care spending is expected to reach $3.4 trillion, or 18.4% of the gross domestic product. This rise is at an annual growth rate of 7.3% during the period 2002 to 2013.

- In 2026, the Medicare program alone is expected to consume 20% of all government revenue. The majority of baby boomers will be retiring in the next 5 years. In the next 25 years, the number of people in retirement programs will increase from 48 million to 84 million (Miller-Murphy et al., 2005).

Paying for Cancer Care

Health care, and cancer care especially, is expensive. The cost to treat, which can include multimodality, sophisticated, and investigational therapies,

can determine whether a patient receives appropriate therapy. Patients with health care through health maintenance organizations (HMOs) often are deterred from appropriate treatments because their HMO policies do not cover all the costs of cancer treatment (Cohen & Martinez, 2005).

Between 1995 and 2004, the overall costs of treating cancer increased by 75%. In 2004, cancer treatment accounted for an estimated $72.1 billion. In 2004, the total economic burden of cancer-related illness was estimated at $190 billion (NCI, 2005a).

Table 21-6 shows the estimated costs for the 15 most common cancer diagnoses. Out-of-pocket costs may add as much as 10% to these estimates. Among the four most common cancers, the first-year costs for lung and colorectal cancer are higher because screening is not commonly used in the detection of these cancers (CancerSource, 2005, 2006; Loney, 2005).

Cancer costs are expected to increase at a faster rate than overall medical expenditures. As the population ages, the absolute number of people treated for cancer will increase faster than the overall population. Moreover, costs are expected to climb due to the cost of manufacturers' recouping costs for development of new therapies. For example, new cancer therapies for advanced colorectal cancer have almost doubled the life expectancy for patients. In a disease that has had very few changes in disease reduction and overall survival, new drugs added to the armamentarium of chemotherapy agents effective in the treatment of advanced colorectal cancer are exciting but expensive (CancerSource, 2005; Loney, 2005; Maltzman, 2004; NCI, 2005a; Wagner & Lacey, 2004).

Assistance Programs

Medical reimbursement programs are sometimes available through cancer organizations, such as the ACS, the Leukemia and Lymphoma Society, CancerCare; the United Way; area offices on aging; and local community organizations (NCI, 2007).

TABLE 21-6: COSTS OF CANCER CARE

Estimates of national expenditures for medical treatment for the 15 most common cancers (based on cancer prevalence in 1998 and cancer-specific costs for 1997-1999, projected to 2004 using the medical care component of the Consumer Price Index)

Cancer	Percent of all new cancers (1998)	Expenditures (billions; in 2004 dollars)	Percent of all cancer treatment expenditures	Average Medicare payments* per individual in first year following diagnosis (2004 dollars)
Lung	12.7%	$9.6	13.3%	$24,700
Breast	15.9%	$8.1	11.2%	$11,000
Colorectal	10.7%	$8.4	11.7%	$24,200
Prostate	16.8%	$8.0	11.1%	$11,000
Lymphoma	4.6%	$4.6	6.3%	$21,500
Head/Neck	2.8%	$3.2	4.4%	$18,000
Bladder	4.4%	$2.9	4.0%	$12,300
Leukemia	2.4%	$2.6	3.7%	$18,000
Ovary	1.9%	$2.2	3.1%	$36,800
Kidney	2.6%	$1.9	2.7%	$25,300
Endometrial	2.9%	$1.8	2.5%	$16,200
Cervix	0.8%	$1.7	2.4%	$20,100
Pancreas	2.3%	$1.5	2.1%	$26,600
Melanoma	4.0%	$1.5	2.0%	$4,800
Esophagus	1.0%	$0.8	1.1%	$30,500
All other	14.0%	$13.4	18.5%	$20,400
Total	**100%**	**$72.1**	**100%**	

Note. Based on methods described in: Brown ML, Riley GF, Schussler N, Etzioni RD. Estimating health care costs related to cancer treatment from SEER-Medicare data. *Medical Care;* 2002 Aug 40(8 Suppl):IV-104-17. Phase-specific prevalence and cost estimates are for SEER-Medicare cases diagnosed between 1996-1999, with costs expressed in 2001 dollars using CMS cost adjusters. Estimates are updated to 2004 using the medical care services component of the Consumer Price Index: U.S. Department of Labor, Bureau of Labor Statistics: *CPI Detailed Report and Producer Price Indexes.* Washington. U.S. Government Printing Office. Monthly reports for January 1999-March 2004.
*Medicare payments include copayments and deductibles paid by patient.
Note. From *Cancer trends progress report: 2005 update: Costs of cancer* by National Cancer Institute (2005). Retrieved April 17, 2007, from http://progressreport.cancer.gov/doc_detail.asp?pid=1&did=2005&chid=25&coid=226&mid

Other support is possible from private agencies and foundations. Federal, state, and local governments offer entitlement programs and other services. Table 21-7 highlights some of the community-supported programs that can pay for pharmaceuticals or out-of-pocket costs of treatment.

Many pharmaceutical manufacturers have established programs to provide medications for patients who cannot pay for their drugs. Table 21-8 lists some of the manufacturers with patient assistance programs.

An important element of cancer nursing competency continues to be how to pursue care reimbursement. Those skills begin with the ability to read and interpret insurance policies as well as tap into a network of people, contacts, resources, and services that allow that care to happen.

To help nurses navigate patients through insurance issues, Table 21-9 (on page 314) provides a list of questions that patients can use as a guide to better understand their insurance coverage.

TABLE 21-7: ORGANIZATIONS OFFERING FINANCIAL ASSISTANCE PROGRAMS (1 OF 3)

American Cancer Society (ACS)
Telephone: 1-800-227-2345 (1-800-ACS-2345)
Web site: http://www.cancer.org

Cancer Care
Telephone: 1-800-813-4673 (1-800-813-HOPE)
Web site: http://www.cancercare.org

Candlelighters Childhood Cancer Foundation (CCCF)
Telephone: 1-800-366-2223 (1-800-366-CCCF)
Web site: http://www.candlelighters.org

Community voluntary agencies and service organizations, such as the Salvation Army, Lutheran Social Services, Jewish Social Services, Catholic Charities, and the Lions Club, may offer help. These organizations are listed in a local phone directory. Some churches and synagogues may provide financial help or services to their members.

Fund-raising is another mechanism to consider. Some patients find that friends, family, and community members are willing to contribute financially if they are aware of a difficult situation. Contact your local library for information about how to organize fund-raising efforts.

General Assistance programs provide food, housing, prescription drugs, and other medical expenses for those who are not eligible for other programs. Funds are often limited. Information can be obtained by contacting your state or local department of social services; this number can be found in a local telephone directory.

Hill-Burton is a program through which hospitals receive construction funds from the federal government. Hospitals that receive Hill-Burton funds are required by law to provide some services to people who cannot afford to pay for their hospitalization. Information about which facilities are part of this program is available by calling the toll-free number or visiting the Web site shown below. A brochure about the program is available in Spanish.

Telephone: 1-800-638-0742
Web site: http://www.hrsa.gov/osp/dfcr/obtain/consfaq.htm

Income tax deductions: Medical costs that are not covered by insurance policies sometimes can be deducted from annual income before taxes. Examples of tax-deductible expenses might include mileage for trips to and from medical appointments; out-of-pocket costs for treatment, prescription drugs, or equipment; and the cost of meals during lengthy medical visits. The local Internal Revenue Service office, tax consultants, or certified public accountants can determine medical costs that are tax deductible. These telephone numbers are available in a local telephone directory.

Web site: http://www.irs.ustreas.gov

The **Leukemia and Lymphoma Society** (LLS) offers information and financial aid to patients who have leukemia, NHL, Hodgkin's lymphoma, or multiple myeloma. Callers may request a booklet describing LLS's Patient Aid Program or the telephone number for their local LLS office. Some publications are available in Spanish.

Telephone: 1-800-955-4572
Web site: http://www.leukemia-lymphoma.org

TABLE 21-7: ORGANIZATIONS OFFERING FINANCIAL ASSISTANCE PROGRAMS (2 OF 3)

Medicaid, a jointly funded, federal-state health insurance program for people who need financial assistance for medical expenses, is coordinated by the Centers for Medicare & Medicaid Services (CMS), formerly the Health Care Financing Administration. At a minimum, states must provide home care services to people who receive federal income assistance, such as Social Security income and aid to families with dependent children. Medicaid coverage includes part-time nursing care, home care aide services, and medical supplies and equipment. Information about coverage is available from local state welfare offices, state health departments, state social services agencies, or the state Medicaid office. Check the local telephone directory for the number to call. Information about specific state contacts is also available on the Web site listed below. Spanish-speaking staff are available in some offices.

Web site: http://www.cms.gov/medicaid/consumer.asp

Medicare is a federal health insurance program also administered by the CMS. Eligible individuals include those who are 65 or older, people of any age with permanent kidney failure, and disabled people under age 65. Medicare may offer reimbursement for some home care services. Cancer patients who qualify for Medicare may also be eligible for coverage of hospice services if they are accepted into a Medicare-certified hospice program. To receive information on eligibility, explanations of coverage, and related publications, call Medicare at the number listed below or visit their Web site. Some publications are available in Spanish. Spanish-speaking staff are available.

Telephone: 1-800-633-4227 (1-800-MEDICARE)
TTY: 1-877-486-2048
Web site: http://www.medicare.gov

The **Patient Advocate Foundation** (PAF) provides education, legal counseling, and referrals to cancer patients and survivors concerning managed care, insurance, financial issues, job discrimination, and debt crisis matters. The **Patient Assistance Program** is a subsidiary of PAF. It provides financial assistance to patients who meet certain qualifications. The toll-free number is 1-866-512-3861.

Telephone: 1-800-532-5274
Web site: http://www.patientadvocate.org

Patient assistance programs are offered by some pharmaceutical manufacturers to help pay for medications. To learn whether a specific drug might be available at reduced cost through such a program, talk with a physician or a medical social worker.

The **Social Security Administration** (SSA) is the government agency that oversees Social Security and Supplemental Security Income. A description of each of these programs follows. More information about these and other SSA programs is available by calling the toll-free number listed below. Spanish-speaking staff are available.

Telephone: 1-800-772-1213
TTY: 1-800-325-0778

Social Security provides a monthly income for eligible elderly and disabled individuals. Information on eligibility, coverage, and application for benefits is available from the SSA.

Web site: http://www.ssa.gov

TABLE 21-7: ORGANIZATIONS OFFERING FINANCIAL ASSISTANCE PROGRAMS (3 OF 3)

Supplemental Security Income (SSI) supplements Social Security payments for individuals who have certain income and resource levels. SSI is administered by the SSA. Information on eligibility, coverage, and claim procedures is available from the SSA.

Web site: http://www.socialsecurity.gov/ssi/index.htm

The **State Children's Health Insurance Program** (SCHIP) is a federal-state partnership that offers low-cost or free health insurance coverage to uninsured children of low-wage, working parents. Callers will be referred to the SCHIP program in their state for further information about what the program covers, who is eligible, and the minimum qualifications.

Telephone: 1-877-543-7669 (1-877-KIDS-NOW)
Web site: http://www.insurekidsnow.gov

Transportation: Certain nonprofit organizations arrange free or reduced-cost air transportation for cancer patients going to or from cancer treatment centers. Financial need is not always a requirement. To find out about these programs, talk with a medical social worker. Ground transportation services may be offered or mileage reimbursed through the local ACS or the state or local department of social services.

Veterans Benefits: Eligible veterans and their dependents may receive cancer treatment at a Veterans Administration medical center. Treatment for service-connected conditions is provided, and treatment for other conditions may be available based on the veteran's financial need. Some publications are available in Spanish. Spanish-speaking staff are available in some offices.

Telephone: 1-877-222-8387 (1-877-222-VETS)
Web site: http://www1.va.gov/health

CANCER AND THE ELDERLY

For most cancers, the rate of incidence increases with age. Therefore, with a steadily growing population that is living longer, the elderly will continue to be a prominent subcategory of patients needing cancer care (Given & Sherwood, 2006; Greco, 2006).

To put the growing elderly population in perspective, here are some statistics:

- **40.2 million**—By 2010, the number of people age 65 and older projected to live in the United States. By 2010, this age-group will account for 13% of the total population (Federal Interagency Forum on Aging-Related Statistics [FIFARS], 2006).

- **86.7 million**—By 2050, projected population of people age 65 and older. People in this age-group will comprise 20.6% of the population (FIFARS, 2006).

- **147%**—Projected percentage increase in the 65-and-older population between 2000 and 2050. By comparison, the population as a whole will increase by only 49% over the same period (DeNavas-Walt et al., 2006).

- **483 million**—Current world population age 65 and older. By 2030, projections indicate the number will increase to 974 million (DeNavas-Walt et al., 2006; FIFARS, 2006).

When a cancer diagnosis and accompanying treatment are added to the challenge of geriatric care, cancer nurses are faced with an additional area of competencies.

Elderly Care

Among major issues affecting the elderly with cancer is their access to care. In the past, physicians

TABLE 21-8: DIRECTORY OF PhRMA MEMBER COMPANY PATIENT ASSISTANCE PROGRAMS (1 OF 3)

PhRMA companies have long been worldwide leaders not only in pharmaceutical innovation, but also in philanthropic initiatives—and their long-standing patient assistance programs are especially helpful. This Directory, www.PPARx.org and 1-888-4PPA-NOW (1-888-477-2669), further their goal of helping to make medicines available to those who need them.

3M Pharmaceuticals
3M Pharmaceuticals Patient Assistance Program
P 1-800-328-0255 | F 1-651-733-6068

■ Abbott Laboratories
Abbott Patient Assistance Program
P 1-800-222-6885 | F 1-866-898-1473

Abbott Virology Patient Assistance Program
P 1-800-222-6885 | F 1-866-483-1305

HUMIRA Patient Assistance Program
P 1-800-448-6472 | F 1-866-323-0661

Ross Medical Nutritionals Patient Assistance Program
P 1-800-222-6885 | F 1-866-483-1305

Ross Metabolic Formula and Elecare Patient Assistance Program
P 1-800-222-6885 | F 1-866-483-1305

Zemplar Patient Assistance Program
P 1-877-936-7527 | F 1-877-936-7528

■ Amgen
Encourage Foundation® (Enbrel)
P 1-888-436-2735 | F 1-888-508-8083

Safety Net Foundation for Kineret
P 1-866-546-3738 | F 1-866-203-4926

Safety Net Foundation for Sensipar
P 1-800-272-9376 | F 1-800-508-8090

Safety Net Program
P 1-800-272-9376 | F 1-888-508-8090

■ Amylin Pharmaceuticals, Inc.
Amylin Patient Assistance Program
P 1-800-330-7647

■ Astellas Pharma US Inc.
Prograf and Protopic Patient Assistance Programs
P 1-800-477-6472

■ AstraZeneca Pharmaceuticals, LP
AstraZeneca Foundation Patient Assistance Program
P 1-800-424-3727

Aventis Pharmaceuticals Inc.
Lovenox Reimbursement Services and Patient Assistance Program
P 1-888-632-8607 | F 1-888-875-9951

Sanofi-Aventis Patient Assistance Program
P 1-800-221-4025

■ Bayer Pharmaceuticals Corporation
Bayer Patient Assistance Program
P 1-800-998-9180

Nexavar REACH Program
P 1-866-639-2827

■ Berlex Laboratories, Inc.
Arch Foundation
P 1-877-393-9071

Berlex Inc. Patient Assistance Program
P 1-888-237-5394, option 6
F 1-973-305-3545

Berlex Oncology Reimbursement Support Line P 1-800-321-4669

The Betaseron Foundation
P 1-800-948-5777 | F 1-877-744-5615

■ Boehringer Ingelheim Pharmaceuticals, Inc.
Boehringer Ingelheim CARES Foundation, Inc.
P 1-800-556-8317 | F 1-866-851-2827

■ Bristol-Myers Squibb Company
Bristol-Myers Squibb Patient Assistance Foundation, Inc.
P 1-800-736-0003 | F 1-800-736-1611

Bristol-Myers Squibb Patient Assistance Foundation, Inc. (Abilify)
P 1-800-736-0003 | F 1-800-598-5561

Bristol-Myers Squibb Patient Assistance Foundation, Inc. (Oncology/Virology)
P 1-800-736-0003 | F 1-866-694-2545

■ Celgene Corporation
Patient Support Solutions
P 1-888-423-5436, option 3
F 1-800-822-2496

■ Centocor, Inc.
Patient Assistance Program for Remicade
P 1-866-489-5957 | F 1-866-489-5958

■ Cephalon, Inc.
Actiq PAP
P 1-888-337-2579 | F 1-240-632-3092

Gabitril PAP
P 1-866-209-7589 | F 1-866-209-7596

Provigil PAP
P 1-800-675-8415

■ Eisai Inc.
Aciphex Patient Assistance Program
P 1-800-523-5870 | F 1-800-526-6651

Aricept Patient Assistance Program
P 1-800-226-2072 | F 1-800-226-2059

Fragmin Patient Assistance Program
P 1-866-272-8804 | F 1-866-272-8805

Patients in Need (Zonegran)
P 1-866-694-2550 | F 1-866-801-5631

■ Eli Lilly and Company
Lilly Cares
P 1-800-545-6962

■ Enzon Pharmaceuticals, Inc.
Enzon Hotline for Abelcet, Depocyt, and Oncaspar
P 1-800-345-2252

■ Genzyme Corporation
The Charitable Access Program (CAP)
P 1-800-745-4447, ext. 16634

■ GlaxoSmithKline
Bridges to Access
P 1-866-728-4368

Commitment to Access
P 1-866-265-6491

■ Janssen L.P.
Johnson & Johnson Health Care Systems Patient Assistance Program
P 1-800-652-6227 | F 1-888-526-5168

■ Johnson & Johnson WoundManagement, A Division of Ethicon, Inc.
Johnson & Johnson Health Care Systems Patient Assistance Program
P 1-800-652-6227 | F 1-888-526-5168

■ McNeil Consumer and Specialty Pharmaceuticals
Johnson & Johnson Health Care Systems Patient Assistance Program
P 1-800-652-6227 | F 1-888-526-5168

■ Merck and Co., Inc.
ACT (Accessing Coverage Today) for EMEND
P 1-866-363-6379 | F 1-866-363-6389

The Merck Patient Assistance Program
P 1-800-727-5400

Merck Prescription Discount Card
P 1-800-506-3725

The SUPPORT Program for Crixivan Reimbursement Support and Patient Assistance Services for Crixivan
P 1-800-850-3430

■ Merck/Schering-Plough Pharmaceuticals
Merck/Schering-Plough Patient Assistance Program
P 1-800-347-7503

■ Millennium Pharmaceuticals, Inc.
VELCADE Reimbursement Assistance Program
P 1-866-835-2233

■ Novartis Pharmaceuticals Corporation
Clozaril Patient Assistance Program
P 1-800-277-2254

Gleevec Patient Assistance Program
P 1-800-277-2254

Novartis Oncology Patient Assistance Program
P 1-800-277-2254

TABLE 21-8: DIRECTORY OF PhRMA MEMBER COMPANY PATIENT ASSISTANCE PROGRAMS (2 OF 3)

Novartis Patient Assistance Program for Transplant Patients
P 1-800-277-2254

Novartis Pharmaceuticals Corporation Patient Assistance Program
P 1-800-277-2254

Sandostatin/Sandostatin LAR Patient Assistance Program
P 1-800-277-2254

Visudyne Patient Assistance Program
P 1-877-736-2778

■ **Novo Nordisk, Inc.**
Novo Nordisk Diabetes Patient Assistance Program
P 1-866-310-7549 | **F** 1-908-429-8764

Novo Nordisk Hormone Therapy Patient Assistance Program
P 1-866-668-6336

■ **Ortho Biotech Products, L.P.**
DOXILine
P 1-800-609-1083 | **F** 1-800-987-5572
ORTHOVISCline
P 1-866-633-8472 | **F** 1-800-987-5572
PROCRITline
P 1-800-553-3851 | **F** 1-800-987-5572

■ **Ortho-McNeil Neurologics, Inc.**
Johnson & Johnson Health Care Systems Patient Assistance Program
P 1-800-652-6227 | **F** 1-888-526-5168

■ **Ortho Women's Health & Urology, A Unit of Ortho-McNeil Pharmaceutical, Inc.**
Johnson & Johnson Health Care Systems Patient Assistance Program
P 1-800-652-6227 | **F** 1-888-526-5168
OrthoNeutrogena, A Division of Ortho-McNeil

■ **Pharmaceutical, Inc.**
Johnson & Johnson Health Care Systems Patient Assistance Program
P 1-800-652-6227 | **F** 1-888-526-5168

■ **Pfizer, Inc.**
Pfizer Helpful Answers
P 1-800-706-2400

Single point of access to all Pfizer programs
Aricept Patient Assistance Program
P 1-800-226-2072 | **F** 1-800-226-2059
Connection to Care
P 1-800-707-8990 | **F** 1-866-470-1748
FirstRESOURCE (Oncology)
P 1-877-744-5675 | **F** 1-800-708-3430
Fragmin Patient Assistance Program
P 1-866-272-8804 | **F** 1-866-272-8805
Macugen Access Program
P 1-866-272-8838
Pfizer Bridge Program (Endocrine care)
P 1-800-645-1280 | **F** 1-800-479-2562

Pfizer Pfriends Savings Program
P 1-800-706-2400
Revatio Patient Assistance Program
P 1-888-327-7787
Tikosyn Patient Assistance Program
P 1-877-845-6796, option 6
Zyvox/Vfend RSVP Hotline
P 1-888-327-7787

■ **PriCara, Unit of Ortho-McNeil, Inc.**
Johnson & Johnson Health Care Systems Patient Assistance Program
P 1-800-652-6227 | **F** 1-888-526-5168

■ **Procter & Gamble Pharmaceuticals**
Procter & Gamble Pharmaceuticals Patient Assistance Program
P 1-800-830-9049 | **F** 1-866-277-9329

■ **Roche Laboratories Inc.**
Boniva Patient Assistance Program
P 1-888-587-9438
Fuzeon Patient Assistance Program
P 1-866-487-8591
ONCOLINE Patient Assistance Program
P 1-800-443-6676, option 2
Pegassist Patient Assistance Program
P 1-877-734-2797
Roche HIV Therapy Assistance Program
P 1-800-282-7780
Roche Laboratories Patient Assistance Program
P 1-877-757-6243 or 1-800-285-4484
Roche Transplant Patient Assistance Program
P 1-800-772-5790

■ **Sankyo Pharma, Inc.**
Sankyo Pharma Open Care Program
P 1-866-268-7327
Sanofi Pasteur
Sanofi Pasteur Indigent Patient Program
P 1-877-798-8716
Sanofi-Aventis
Eligard Reimbursement Hotline and Patient Assistance Program
P 1-877-354-4273 | **F** 1-866-354-4273
PACT+ Program
P 1-800-996-6626 | **F** 1-800-996-6627
Hyalgan Reimbursement Hotline and Patient Assistance Program
P 1-800-992-9022 | **F** 1-877-366-0584
Sanofi-Aventis Patient Assistance Program
P 1-800-446-6267

■ **Sanofi-Aventis Oncology**
PACT+ Program
P 1-800-996-6626 | **F** 1-800-996-6627
Schering-Plough Corporation Commitment to Care
P 1-800-521-7157

SP-Cares Patient Assistance Program
P 1-800-656-9485

■ **Schwarz Pharma, Inc.**
Schwarz Pharma, Inc. Patient Assistance Program
P 1-800-558-5114 | **F** 1-262-238-5317

■ **Scios, Inc.**
NATRECOR Patient Assistance Program
P 1-888-667-3212 | **F** 1-877-576-3346

■ **Serono, Inc.**
MS LifeLines Patient Assistance Program
P 1-877-447-3243
Serostim PAP (McKesson)
P 1-888-628-6673 | **F** 1-203-798-2289
Saizen PAP (McKesson)
P 1-800-582-7989 | **F** 1-877-408-4288
Serono Compassionate Care (Medical Information)
P 1-888-275-7376 | **F** 1-781-681-2940

■ **Sigma-Tau Pharmaceuticals, Inc.**
Carnitor Drug Assistance Program (NORD)
P 1-800-999-6673 | **F** 1-203-798-2291
Matulane Patient Assistance Program (NORD)
P 1-800-999-6673 | **F** 1-203-798-2291

■ **Solvay Pharmaceuticals Incorporated**
Solvay Pharmaceuticals Incorporated Patient Assistance Program
P 1-800-256-8918 | **F** 1-800-276-9901

■ **Takeda Pharmaceuticals North America, Inc.**
Takeda Patient Assistance Program
P 1-800-830-9159 or 1-877-582-5332
F 1-800-497-0928

■ **Together Rx Access™**
A free savings program sponsored by Abbott, AstraZeneca, Bristol-Myers Squibb, GlaxoSmithKline, members of the Johnson & Johnson Family of Companies, Novartis, Pfizer, Sanofi-Aventis Group, Takeda and TAP Pharmaceutical Products Inc.
P 1-800-444-4106

■ **Valeant Pharmaceuticals International**
Valeant Pharmaceuticals International Patient Assistance Program
P 1-800-548-5100

■ **Vistakon Pharmaceuticals, LLC**
Johnson & Johnson Health Care Systems Patient Assistance Program
P 1-800-652-6227 or 1-866-815-6874
F 1-800-544-2987

TABLE 21-8: DIRECTORY OF PhRMA MEMBER COMPANY PATIENT ASSISTANCE PROGRAMS (3 OF 3)

■ **Wyeth** RapAssist (Rapamune Patient Assistance Program) **P** 1-877-472-7268 | **F** 1-800-378-7645	Wyeth Hemophilia Patient Assistance Program **P** 1-888-999-2349 | **F** 1-703-310-2524	Wyeth Oncology Patient Assistance Program **P** 1-888-638-6342 | **F** 1-866-836-0819 Wyeth Patient Assistance Program **P** 1-800-568-9938

Note. From *Directory of PhRMA Member Company Patient Assistance Programs,* by PhRMA, 2006. Washington, DC: Author.

TABLE 21-9: WHAT QUESTIONS SHOULD I BE ABLE TO ANSWER ABOUT MY INSURANCE?

- What are the benefits of my insurance plan?
    - What cancer treatments and care does it cover?
    - Do I have a primary care provider? Can I use only certain "preferred providers" under my plan?
    - Am I entitled to a yearly checkup or does my plan cover office visits only when I am sick?
    - What are the benefits if I go outside of my health plan to obtain care?
- What are the rules of my insurance plan?
    - Do I need a referral from a primary care provider?
    - Do I need a written referral form?
    - Do I need to get approval from my health plan (precertification) before seeing a specialist; obtaining treatment, tests, medical equipment, or physical therapy services; or going to the emergency room or a hospital?
    - Does my lab work, including blood work or Pap smear need to go to a special lab?
- Do I have to pay a certain amount (co-pay) at the time of my visit?
- Do I have an amount that I must pay for medical expenses (annual deductible) before the insurance pays for services?
- Do I have a lifetime or annual limit on how much is covered for medical expenses?
- Is there a special pharmacy where I need to get my medications?
- Are all tests and procedures covered both as an inpatient and outpatient?

(NCI, 2007)

presenting treatment options to older patients might limit the choices, especially those considered aggressive treatment protocols. Moreover, symptom treatment of the elderly—whether it is because of their disease or treatment—may not be as standard or comprehensive because of advanced age. (And often, the perceptions of the limitations of age are the beliefs of younger caregivers.)

Among issues of particular importance to the elderly are:

- treatment protocols, acknowledging age factors
- altered symptom responses
- concurrent illnesses that impact treatment
- quality-of-life issues
- spiritual care
- insurance coverage, including cost of medications
- legal issues.

(Cope, 2006; Overcash, 2006; Reb, 2006; Sinding, Wiernikowski, & Aronson, 2005; Xakellis et al., 2004)

Physiologic changes and other health challenges also play a large part in the ongoing care of older patients with cancer (Cope, 2006; Green & Hacker, 2004; Overcash, 2006; Reiner & Lacasse, 2006). Table 21-10 highlights some of the challenges facing older patients with cancer.

TABLE 21-10: CHALLENGES OF ELDERLY CANCER PATIENTS
• Comorbidities (more than 80% of people older than age 65 have at least one chronic condition, such as hypertension, heart disease, hearing impairment, cataracts, sinusitis, diabetes)
• Polypharmacy (older adults take at least four medications per day; the elderly are twice as likely to experience drug interactions)

• Age-related physiologic changes
    - Gastrointestinal system—decreased motility, saliva production, and secretion of gastric acid and prolonged gastric emptying
    - Renal system—decreased glomerular filtration rate, decreased urinary concentrating ability, and limited ability to excrete water and certain electrolytes
    - Hepatic system—increased susceptibility to toxicities from chemotherapy (myelotoxicity, cardiotoxicity, mucosal toxicity, neurotoxicity)
    - Body composition—decreased plasma volume, total body water, and lead body weight to fat ratio
    - Hematopoiesis—diminished ability to mobilize stem cells from the bone marrow
    - Hematopoietic defenses—at greater risk for myelosuppression

• Falls due to dizziness, orthostatic hypotension, impaired mobility, muscle weakness, and cognitive impairment
(Cope, 2006; Green & Hacker, 2004; Lewis & McBride, 2004; Overcash, 2006; Sinding et al., 2005)

MULTICULTURAL CARE

Providing quality health care to patients in this day and age requires a knowledge of and respect for cultural beliefs and practices of different ethnic and cultural groups (Freeman, 2004; Phillips & Williams-Brown, 2005; Robinson, Sandoval, Baldwin, & Sanderson, 2005; Schultz, Stava, Beck, & Vassilopoulou-Sellin, 2004).

The concepts of health, the perceptions of treatment, and a wide range of quality-of-life issues now present a cultural component in the practice of cancer care (Ashing-Giwa & Kagawa-Singer, 2006; Kemp, 2005). For example, because African Americans men are at high risk for prostate cancer, African American concepts and perceptions of health are of great concern. One issue in particular is the patient's fear of diagnosis and treatment side effects. Other issues are underlying factors that contribute to the high incidence rate of prostate cancer (e.g., tobacco exposure, diet, socioeconomic conditions) (Adams-Campbell et al., 2004; Hamilton & Sandelowski, 2004).

Examples of multicultural influences on cancer care include the settings for effective preventive care and screening (Burhansstipanov & Olsen, 2004; Gill & Yankaskas, 2004; Kim & Sarna, 2004; Lee-Lin & Menon, 2005) and caregiver training for families caring for patients in the home (Morgan et al., 2005; Ward et al., 2004).

Minority Groups and Cancer

In the United States, African Americans are more likely to develop and die from cancer than any other ethnic group (ACS, 2006a). The death rate from cancer for African American males is 40% higher than the death rate for Caucasian males; for African American females, the death rate is 18% higher than that for Caucasian females (ACS, 2006a). African Americans have higher mortality and incidence rates than Caucasians for the major cancers (colorectal, lung, and prostate) (ACS, 2006a).

For other ethnic groups (Asian Americans, American Indians, Hispanics), the incidence rates are higher for these cancer sites: stomach, liver, uterine cervix. The incidence rate for liver cancer in Asian American and Pacific Islander men is twice the rate of African American men and three times the rate of Caucasian men. The incidence rate of cervical cancer is highest in Hispanic women.

Access to prevention and early detection strategies and consistent quality health care remains an obstacle for many ethnic minorities due to the challenges of low income, inner city environments, language barriers, racial bias, and stereotyping (ACS, 2006a). Of African Americans, 20% live below the poverty line and 20% do not have health insurance. Of Hispanics and Latinos, 22% live below the poverty line and 32% are uninsured. Of Caucasians, 11% do not have health insurance.

Social inequalities and cultural barriers can contribute many factors that limit the care a patient receives. Limited access means that patient treatment can also be delayed (Freeman, 2004).

Culturally Sensitive Health Care Delivery

The disparities in health status among racial and ethnic minority populations are well known. Culturally sensitive education of nurses, which leads to culturally appropriate communication and behavioral strategies, is clearly needed in any health care setting.

So where does one start in providing culturally sensitive care? Figure 21-2 provides a transcultural nursing assessment model that focuses on different categories as points of reference: communication, space, time, social orientation, environmental control, and biological variation. Table 21-11 provides examples of how cultural differences can affect nursing care.

SUMMARY

This chapter reviewed several special populations of cancer patients—pediatric patients, survivors of cancer, those faced with financial challenges, the elderly, and patients from diverse cultural backgrounds. Due to the special challenges that these patient groups face, nurses providing care need to be prepared to offer more customized interventions and comprehensive resources.

FIGURE 21-2: GIGER AND DAVIDHIZAR'S TRANSCULTURAL ASSESSMENT MODEL

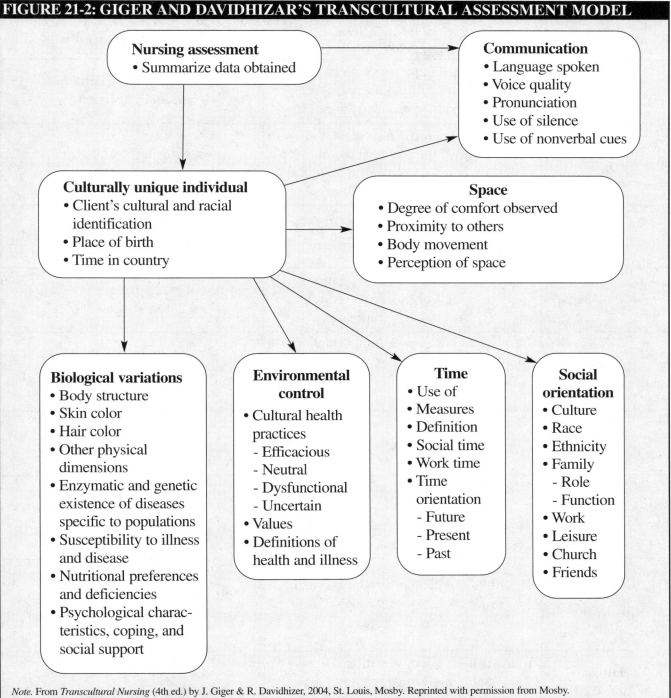

Nursing assessment
- Summarize data obtained

Communication
- Language spoken
- Voice quality
- Pronunciation
- Use of silence
- Use of nonverbal cues

Culturally unique individual
- Client's cultural and racial identification
- Place of birth
- Time in country

Space
- Degree of comfort observed
- Proximity to others
- Body movement
- Perception of space

Biological variations
- Body structure
- Skin color
- Hair color
- Other physical dimensions
- Enzymatic and genetic existence of diseases specific to populations
- Susceptibility to illness and disease
- Nutritional preferences and deficiencies
- Psychological characteristics, coping, and social support

Environmental control
- Cultural health practices
  - Efficacious
  - Neutral
  - Dysfunctional
  - Uncertain
- Values
- Definitions of health and illness

Time
- Use of
- Measures
- Definition
- Social time
- Work time
- Time orientation
  - Future
  - Present
  - Past

Social orientation
- Culture
- Race
- Ethnicity
- Family
  - Role
  - Function
- Work
- Leisure
- Church
- Friends

Note. From *Transcultural Nursing* (4th ed.) by J. Giger & R. Davidhizer, 2004, St. Louis, Mosby. Reprinted with permission from Mosby.

TABLE 21-11: CULTURAL BEHAVIORS RELATED TO HEALTH ASSESSMENT

Cultural Group	Cultural Variations (*common belief/practice*)	Nursing Implications
African Americans	Dialect and slang terms require careful communication to prevent error (e.g., "bad" may mean "good").	Question the client's meaning or intent.
Mexican Americans	Eye behavior is important. An individual who looks at and admires a child without touching the child has given the child the "evil eye."	Always touch the child you are examining.
American Indians	Eye contact is considered a sign of disrespect and is thus avoided.	Recognize that the client may be attentive and interested even though eye contact is avoided.
Appalachians	Eye contact is considered impolite or a sign of hostility. Verbal patter may be confusing.	Avoid excessive eye contact. Clarify statements.
American Eskimos	Body language is very important. The individual seldom disagrees publically with others. Client may nod yes to be polite, even if not in agreement.	Closely monitor own body language as well as client's to detect meaning.
Jewish Americans	Orthodox Jews may consider excessive touching, particularly from members of the opposite sex, offensive.	Establish whether client is Orthodox Jew and, if so, avoid excessive touching.
Chinese Americans	Individual may nod head to indicate yes or shake head to confirm no. Excessive eye contact indicates rudeness. Excessive touch is offensive.	Ask questions carefully and clarify responses. Avoid eye contact and touch.
Filipino Americans	Offending people is to be avoided at all cost. Nonverbal behavior is very important.	Monitor nonverbal behaviors of self and client, being sensitive to physical and emotional discomfort or concerns of the client.
Haitian Americans	Touch is used in conversation. Direct eye contact is used to gain attention and respect during communication.	Use direct eye contact when communicating.
East Indian-Hindu Americans	Women avoid eye contact as a sign of respect.	Be aware that men may view eye contact by women as offensive. Avoid eye contact.
Vietnamese Americans	Avoidance of eye contact is a sign of respect. The head is considered sacred; it is not polite to pat the head. An upturned palm is offensive in communication.	Touch the head only when mandated and explain clearly before proceeding to do so. Avoid hand gesturing.

Note. From *Transcultural Nursing* (4th ed.) by J. Giger & R. Davidhizer, 2004, St. Louis, Mosby. Reprinted with permission from Mosby.

EXAM QUESTIONS

CHAPTER 21
Questions 85-88

Note: Choose the option that BEST answers each question.

85. A late effect of childhood cancer treatment using an alkylating agent may involve the

    a. digestive system.

    b. central nervous system.

    c. reproductive system.

    d. respiratory system.

86. A survivor of cancer may face

    a. easy insurability.

    b. overly enthusiastic confidence.

    c. job discrimination.

    d. extended periods of euphoria.

87. To help a patient facing financial challenges, the nurse could

    a. provide a bank loan.

    b. provide the patient with cancer patient resources.

    c. call the patient's family members.

    d. start a fund, based on contributions from staff.

88. A physiological change that elderly cancer patients experience related to aging is

    a. a slow gastrointestinal tract.

    b. increased muscle tone in the lower extremities.

    c. increased renal function.

    d. increased plasma volume.

REFERENCES

Adams-Campbell, L. L., Ahaghotu, C., Gaskins, M., Dawkins, F. W., Smoot, D., Polk, O. D., et al. (2004). Enrollment of African Americans into clinical treatment trials: Study design barriers. *Journal of Clinical Oncology, 22*(4), 730-734.

American Cancer Society. (2006a). *Cancer facts & figures 2006*. Atlanta: Author.

American Cancer Society. (2006b). Cancer survivors need better long-term follow-up. *CA: Cancer Journal for Clinicians, 56,* 65-67.

Ashing-Giwa, K., & Kagawa-Singer, M. (2006). Infusing culture into oncology research on quality of life. *Oncology Nursing Forum, 33*(1 Suppl.), 31-36.

Burhansstipanov, L., & Olsen, S. (2004). Cancer prevention and early detection in American Indian and Alaska native populations. *Clinical Journal of Oncology Nursing, 8*(2), 182-186.

CancerSource. (2005). Paying for chemotherapy. Retrieved October 31, 2006, from http://www.cancersource.com/Search/45,25469-11

CancerSource. (2006). Work and money concerns. Available from http://www.cancersource.com/CopeWithCancer/WorkAndMoneyIssues/

Centers for Disease Control and Prevention. (2004). *A national action plan for cancer survivorship: Advancing public health strategies.* Retrieved October 31, 2006, from http://www.cdc.gov/cancer/survivorship/pdf/plan.pdf

Cohen, R., & Martinez, M. (2005). *Health insurance coverage: Estimates from the National Health Interview Survey, January–June 2005.* Retrieved October 31, 2006, from http://www.cdc.gov/nchs/data/nhis/earlyrelease/insur200512.pdf

Cope, D. (2006). Cancer and the aging population. In D. Cope & A. Reb (Eds.), *An evidence-based approach to the treatment and care of the older adult with cancer* (pp. 1-10). St. Louis: Elsevier.

DeNavas-Walt, C., Proctor, B., & Lee, C. H. (2006). *Income, poverty, and health insurance coverage in the United States: 2005.* Retrieved October 31, 2006, from http://www.census.gov/prod/2006pubs/p60-231.pdf

Federal Interagency Forum on Aging-Related Statistics. (2006). *Older amercians update 2006.* Available from http://www.agingstats.gov/agingstatsdotnet/Main_Site/Data/Data_2006.aspx

Fisher, P. (2006). Survivorship. In L. Clarke & M. Dropkin (Eds.), *Site-specific cancer series: Head and neck cancer,* reprinted in *Clinical Journal of Oncology Nursing, 10*(1), 93-98.

Freeman, H.P. (2004). Poverty, culture, and social injustice: Determinants of cancer disparities. *CA: Cancer Journal for Clinicians, 54*(2), 72-77.

Friedman, D. L., Whitton, J., Yasui, Y., Mertens, A. C., Hammond, S., Stovall, M., et al. (2004). Risk of second malignant neoplasms (SMN) 20 years after childhood cancer: The updated experience of the Childhood Cancer Survivor Study (CCSS) [Abstract 8509]. Proceedings of the *American Society of Clinical Oncology, 22,* 801s.

Giger, J., & Davidhizar, R. (2004). Introduction to transcultural nursing. In J. Giger & R. Davidhizar (Eds.), *Transcultural nursing: Assessment & intervention* (4th ed., pp. 1-15). St. Louis: Mosby.

Gill, K., & Yankaskas, B. (2004). Screening mammography performance and cancer detection among black women and white women in community practice. *Cancer, 100*(1), 139-148.

Given, B., & Sherwood, P. (2006). Family care for the older person with cancer. *Seminars in Oncology Nursing, 22*(1), 43-50.

Greco, K. (2006). Cancer screening in older adults in an era of genomics and longevity. *Seminars in Oncology Nursing, 22*(1), 10-19.

Green, J., & Hacker, E. (2004). Chemotherapy in the geriatric population. *Clinical Journal of Oncology Nursing, 8*(6), 591-597.

Hamilton, J., & Sandelowski, M. (2004). Types of social support in African Americans with cancer. *Oncology Nursing Forum, 31*(4), 792-800.

Hewitt, M., Greenfield, S., & Stovall, E. (2006). *Executive summary: From cancer patient to cancer survivor: Lost in transition.* Available from http://books.nap.edu/openbook.php?record_id=11468&page=1

Hoffman, B. (2005). Cancer survivors at work: A generation of progress. *CA: Cancer Journal for Clinicians, 55*(5), 271-280

Jemal, A., Tiwari, R. C., Murray, T., Ghafoor, A., Samuels, A., Ward, E., et al. (2004). Cancer statistics, 2004. *CA: Cancer Journal for Clinicians, 54*(1), 8-29.

Kemp, C. (2005). Cultural issues in palliative care. *Seminars in Oncology Nursing, 21*(1), 44-52.

Kim, Y. H., & Sarna, L. (2004). An intervention to increase mammography use by Korean American women. *Oncology Nursing Forum, 31*(1), 105-110.

Lee-Lin, F., & Menon, U. (2005). Breast and cervical cancer screening practices and interventions among Chinese, Japanese, and Vietnamese Americans. *Oncology Nursing Forum, 32*(5), 995-1003.

Lewis, I. D., & McBride, M. (2004). Anticipatory grief and chronicity: Elders and families in racial/ethnic minority groups. *Geriatric Nursing, 25*(1), 44-47.

Loney, M. (2005). Cancer economics and health care reform. In J. K. Itano & K. N. Taoka (Eds.), *Core curriculum for oncology nursing* (4th ed., pp. 921-932). St. Louis: Elsevier.

Maltzman, J. (2004). *Drug reimbursement.* Available from http://www.oncolink.upenn.edu

Miller-Murphy, C., Ballon, L., Culhane, B., Mafrica, L., McCorkle, M., & Worrall, L. (2005). Oncology Nursing Society environmental scan 2004. *Oncology Nursing Forum, 32*(4), 742.

Morgan, P., Fogel, J., Rose, L., Barnett, K., Mock, V., Davis, B., et al. (2005). African American couples merging strengths to successfully cope with breast cancer. *Oncology Nursing Forum, 32*(5), 979-987.

National Cancer Institute. (2005a). *Cancer trends progress report—2005 update: Costs of cancer care.* Retrieved April 17, 2007, from http://progressreport.cancer.gov/doc_detail.asp?pid=1&did=2005&chid=25&coid=226&mid=

National Cancer Institute. (2005b). *National Cancer Institute research on childhood cancers.* Retrieved October 31, 2006, from http://www.cancer.gov/cancertopics/factsheet/Sites-Types/childhood

National Cancer Institute. (2006a). *Cancer trends progress report—2005 update: Life after cancer.* Retrieved October 31, 2006, from http://progressreport.cancer.gov/doc.asp?pid=1&did=2005&mid=vcol&chid=25

National Cancer Institute. (2006b). Childhood cancers. Retrieved October 31, 2006, from http://www.cancer.gov/cancertopics/types/childhoodcancers

National Cancer Institute. (2007). Financial assistance and other resources for people with cancer. Retrieved October 31, 2006, from http://www.cancer.gov/cancertopics/factsheet/support/financial-assistance

National Cancer Institute, Cancer Control and Population Sciences. (2006). *Cancer survivorship research, Estimated U.S. cancer prevalence.* National Cancer Institute, Cancer Control and Population Sciences. Available from http://cancercontrol.cancer.gov/ocs/index.html

National Coalition for Cancer Survivorship. (2005). *Cancer facts & stats.* Retrieved October 31, 2006, from http://www.canceradvocacy.org/news/pdf/IOM/Facts%20Stats.pdf

Overcash, J. (2006). Comprehensive geriatric assessment. In D. Cope & A. Reb (Eds.), *An evidence-based approach to the treatment and care of the older adult with cancer* (pp. 57-72). St. Louis: Elsevier.

Phillips, J., & Williams-Brown, S. (2005). Cultural issues in palliative care. *Seminars in Oncology Nursing, 21*(4), 278-285.

PhRMA. (2006). *Directory of PhRMA member company patient assistance programs.* Washington, DC: Author. Retrieved April 17, 2007, from https://www.pparx.org/ViewCompanies.php

Reb, A. (2006). Cancer screening in the older adult. In D. Cope & A. Reb (Eds.), *An evidence-based approach to the treatment and care of the older adult with cancer* (pp. 75-84). St. Louis: Elsevier.

Reiner, A., & Lacasse, C. (2006). Symptom correlates in the gero-oncology populations. *Seminars in Oncology Nursing, 22*(1), 20-30.

Robinson, F., Sandoval, N., Baldwin, J., & Sanderson, P. (2005). Breast cancer education for Native American women: Creating culturally relevant communications. *Clinical Journal of Oncology Nursing, 9*(6), 689-692.

Schultz, P. N., Stava, C., Beck, M. L., & Vassilopoulou-Sellin, R. (2004). Ethnic/racial influences on the physiologic health of cancer survivors. *Cancer, 100*(1), 156-164.

Sinding, C., Wiernikowski, J., & Aronson, J. (2005). Cancer care from the perspectives of older women. *Oncology Nursing Forum, 32*(6), 1169-1175.

Wagner, L., & Lacey, M. (2004). The hidden costs of cancer care: An overview with implications and referral resources for oncology nurses. *Clinical Journal of Oncology Nursing, 8*(3), 279-287.

Ward, E., Jemal, A., Cokkinides, V., Singh, G. K., Cardinez, C., Ghafoor, A., et al. (2004). Cancer disparities by race/ethnicity and socioeconomic status. *CA: Cancer Journal for Clinicians, 54*(2), 78-93.

Xakellis, G., Brangman, S. A., Hinton, W. L., Jones, V. Y., Masterman, D., Pan, C. X., et al. (2004). Curricular framework: Core competencies in multicultural geriatric care. *Journal of the American Geriatrics Society, 52*(1), 137-142.

CHAPTER 22

PALLIATIVE CARE

CHAPTER OBJECTIVE

After completing this chapter, the reader will be able to discuss important aspects of palliative care, including end-of-life care, the hospice model, pain management, and quality-of-life issues.

LEARNING OBJECTIVES

After studying this chapter, the reader will be able to

1. list two elements of quality palliative care.

2. recognize two strategies to help patients and families transition to palliative care.

3. identify three principles of appropriate cancer pain management.

4. recognize two side effects of pain medications.

INTRODUCTION

Palliative care is based on a broad foundation of knowledge that includes providing physical, emotional, psychological, and spiritual comfort to the patient and family members. To honor the final days of a patient and best take care of his or her needs, the nurse should be equipped with knowledge about the keystone principles of palliative care, including communication skills, family dynamics of decision making, physical care of the patient, and

pain management. This chapter provides a review of the important elements of palliative care.

OVERVIEW

Palliative care focuses on the prevention and relief of pain and suffering. It encompasses the physical, emotional, spiritual, and practical needs of terminal patients. Palliative care regards dying as a normal process and neither hastens nor postpones death.

One of the first goals of palliative care involves a struggle of patient and family to accept a pure focus of palliative care for the patient. There can be a constant feeling of crossover—curative intent juxtaposed to pure palliative care—before comprehensive palliative care becomes the reality.

In 2002, the World Health Organization (WHO) broadened its definition of palliative care, expanding it beyond a focus on disease. It now is based on a cancer model of care, which includes a priority of effective cancer pain management (Kuebler, 2005; WHO, n.d.).

This broadened palliative care definition integrates a focus on pain and symptom management earlier in the course of various diseases. Among symptoms that palliative care can address are dyspnea, nausea and vomiting, sleepiness, congestion, confusion, restlessness, anorexia, fatigue, and urinary incontinence. Palliative care also acknowledges the multidimensional needs of patients, families, and communities. Table 22-1 lists domains of quality palliative care.

TABLE 22-1: CLINICAL PRACTICE GUIDELINES DOMAINS OF QUALITY PALLIATIVE CARE

Structure and Processes of Care

Aspects of Care:
- Physical
- Psychological and psychiatric
- Social
- Spiritual, religious, existential
- Cultural
- Ethical and legal

Care of the Imminently Dying Patient

(National Concensus Project for Quality Palliative Care [NCPQPC], 2004)

Palliative Care Guidelines

Education in palliative care is meaningless without a supportive context in clinical practice to promote application of that knowledge. The National Consensus Project for Quality Palliative Care (NCPQPC) guidelines provide a clinical practice framework for palliative care in the clinical community (Ferrell, 2005a). These guidelines were developed to apply palliative care principles in intensive care units, cardiac care settings, home care, long-term care, and the many and varied settings where patients are cared for at end of life (Ferrell, 2005a).

Based on those guidelines, Table 22-2 provides a list of best practices when providing an integrated approach to care at end of life.

TABLE 22-2: PALLIATIVE CARE BEST PRACTICES

- Cure when possible
- Disease modification and management
- Informed decision making
- Coordinated care
- Symptom control (a priority)
- Optimization of quality of life
- End-of-life care

(Cooney, 2005)

Palliative care relies on communication, clarity, compassion, and a clear focus on care versus cure. Among many areas of concern are fear, abandonment, meaning and value, family relationships, unfinished business, and legacies.

The public, by and large, still has fear and misinformation about death. There may be an assumption that pain and misery at death are inevitable. Many methods exist to reduce suffering at the end of life, but many patients and families still do not know what they are. Therefore, the nurse can serve as a pivotal resource for that information as well as a provider of caring interventions (Rutledge & Kuebler, 2005).

HOSPICE AS A MODEL OF CARE

The approach of hospice care is now a familiar concept, transferred from England and nurtured toward acceptance over the last 30 years in the United States. The goals of hospice care—the operational venue of palliative care—are to keep the dying individual free from pain and other symptoms and to provide emotional support for the family and patient. In concert with hospice staff, family members are the fulcrum of caregiving.

Hospice stresses quality of life—peace, comfort, and dignity—that also keeps the patient in as much control of the process as possible (Volker, Kahn, & Penticuff, 2004). This means that, at its best, hospice care has provided the patient control of pain and other symptoms so that she or he is as alert and comfortable as possible. Hospice services are available to persons who can no longer benefit from curative treatment. The typical hospice patient has a life expectancy of 6 months or less.

A study of 28,777 Medicare patients (age 65 or older), who died of cancer between 1993 and 1996 reported that patients receiving active treatment within 2 weeks of death increased from 13.8% in 1993 to 18.5% in 1996. The study also showed that use of the hospice model of care for Medicare patients increased from 28.3% (in 1993) to 38.8% (in 1996) (p < 0.001). The study reported that hospice referrals within the last 3 days of life increased from 14.3% to 17.0% from 1993 to 1996 (Cooney, 2005). The report concluded that the treatment of cancer patients near death is becoming increasingly aggressive over time. This appears to contribute to later hospice referrals (Cooney, 2005). Also, because of advances in treatment technologies and supportive care, the boundaries between control of disease and palliation remain blurred. Patients with advanced cancer can decide to continue treatment with palliative chemotherapy, which may prolong survival while maintaining their quality of life (Cooney, 2005).

Supporting Transitions to Palliation

Since the transition from care to palliation can be so difficult for patients and families, knowing the underlying reasons for reluctance can assist the nurse in helping the family make the shift with minimal anguish.

Hospice care continues to be considered by many as preceding imminent death, rather than optimizing quality of life. Therefore, a transition to palliation requires acknowledgement of the pace and timing of the decision. The nurse, with the hospice team, can address the fears and misunderstandings of the patient and family members and the vision of palliative care allowing for "a good death," with peace, limited suffering, and life lived to the fullest (Duggleby & Berry, 2005).

Research indicates that as much as 50% of people cannot make their own decisions when they near death, and significant others often do not know their loved ones' views about decisions regarding death (Duggleby & Berry, 2005). In addition, health care professionals traditionally continue to treat when uncertain about a person's wishes. Therefore, a discussion about advance directives is a major element of providing quality palliative care. Table 22-3 pro-

vides a list of questions that can guide a discussion about advance directives.

A suggested framework of care used by the palliative nurse to ease transition and discussion includes:

- respectful listening and gentle exploration, with honest explanation of the options (including hospice and palliative care)

- discussing what illness means to the patient and his or her family

- validating the patient's thoughts, fears, and feelings

- discussing issues related to advance care planning (i.e., what "living well" means to the patient).

- gaining a clear understanding of the patient and family's goals, hopes, and needs

- understanding that adjustment to death is a process and cannot be rushed; it is different for everyone

- listening and honoring the wishes of the patient and family members with an open mind

- preserving the patient's control over decisions, with the hospice and palliative care team acting as guides and facilitators.

(Duggleby & Berry, 2005)

Table 22-4 lists questions and concerns of patients and families when the patient has transitioned to end-of-life care. Table 22-5 provides a grief assessment focused on strengths and stressors. Elements of this assessment can be incorporated in the patient's plan of care, especially during discussions about next steps.

Hospice Care in Different Settings

The Medicare Hospice Benefit was created in the early 1980s. The concept of hospice care is not limited to a building, although many free-standing hospices exist. Hospice care can be provided in a home or within a hospital or nursing home. In the United States, more than 3000 hospices and more than 1500 palliative care programs currently serve those facing end of life (Ferrell, 2005b).

TABLE 22-3: ADVANCE DIRECTIVES: GUIDELINES FOR DISCUSSION

1. **What rights do patients have regarding their medical treatment?**

   Patients are entitled to complete information about their illness and how it may affect their lives, and they have the right to share or withhold that information from others. Patients have the right to make decisions about their own treatment. These decisions may change over time.

   Sometimes a patient is unable to make decisions due to severe illness or a change in mental condition. That is why it is important for people with cancer to make their wishes known in advance.

2. **What is end-of-life care? What are advance directives?**

   End-of-life care is a general term that refers to the medical and psychosocial care given in the advanced or terminal stages of illness. Advance directives are legal documents, such as a living will, durable power of attorney, and health care proxy, that allow people to convey their decisions about end-of-life care ahead of time.

   Ideally, the process of discussing and writing advance directives should be ongoing, rather than a single event. Advance directives can be modified as a patient's situation changes. Even after advance directives have been signed, patients can change their minds at any time.

3. **Why are advance directives important?**

   Complex choices about end-of-life care are difficult even when people are well. If a person is seriously ill, these decisions can seem overwhelming. Communicating wishes about end-of-life care ensures that people with cancer face the end of their lives with dignity and with the same values by which they have lived.

4. **What is a living will?**

   A living will is a set of instructions documenting a person's wishes about medical care intended to sustain life. A living will protects the patient's rights and removes the burden of making decisions from family, friends, and physicians.

   There are many types of life-sustaining care that should be taken into consideration when drafting a living will. These include:
   - the use of life-sustaining equipment (dialysis machines, ventilators, and respirators)
   - "do not resuscitate" orders; that is, instructions not to use cardiopulmonary resusitation if breathing or heartbeat stops
   - artificial hydration and nutrition (tube feeding)
   - withholding of food and fluids
   - palliative and comfort care
   - organ and tissue donation.

   It is also important to understand that a decision not to receive "aggressive medical treatment" is not the same as withholding all medical care. A patient can still receive antibiotics, nutrition, pain medication, radiation therapy, and other interventions when the goal of treatment becomes comfort rather than cure. This is called *palliative care*, and its primary focus is helping the patient remain as comfortable as possible.

   Once a living will has been drawn up, patients may want to talk about their decisions with the people who matter most to them, explaining the values underlying their decisions.

5. **What is a health care proxy and durable power of attorney for health care?**

   A health care proxy is an agent (a person) appointed to make a patient's medical decisions if the patient is unable to do so.

   The durable power of attorney for health care is the legal document that names a patient's health care proxy. Once written, it should be signed, dated, witnessed, notarized, copied, distributed, and incorporated into the patient's medical record.

6. **Where can people with cancer get assistance with their advance directives?**

   Although a lawyer is not needed to complete an advance directive, it is important to be aware that each state has its own laws for creating advance directives. Because these laws can vary in important details, special care should be taken to adhere to the laws of the state a patient lives in or is treated in. It is possible that a living will or durable power of attorney signed in one state may not be recognized in another. Appropriate forms can be obtained from health care providers, legal offices, offices on aging, and state health departments.

(National Cancer Institute [NCI], 2005)

TABLE 22-4: END-OF-LIFE DECISION MAKING: ANTICIPATING QUESTIONS AND CONCERNS OF PATIENTS AND THEIR FAMILIES

1. **What do the patient and family understand?**
   A. How well do they understand the severity of the illness and prognosis?
   B. How well are they coping?
   C. What are the overall goals of care?

2. **What information do they need about artificial nutrition and hydration?**
   A. Explain the difference in response that is expected in a healthy versus a terminally ill patient.
   B. Explain the risks and benefits for this specific patient in this situation.
   C. Discuss whether artificial nutrition and hydration will help the patient achieve desired goals of care.

3. **What guidelines should be followed in negotiating a solution?**
   A. Learn who the "stakeholders" are and try to determine what each person wants.
   B. Consider all perspectives where possible: patient, family, and clinicians.
   C. Acknowledge the emotional aspects of these decisions.
   D. Negotiate agreement; try to satisfy all parties: "Let's see how we can best care for _____ in a way that moves toward his or her goals."
   E. Reframe and summarize to ensure all understand: "Let's sum this up. This is what I understand…"

4. **Pitfalls to avoid during negotiations:**
   A. Do not try to avoid conflict; rather, learn how to manage it.
   B. Do not assume that you know or understand "the whole story"; remember the adage: "Seek first to understand."
   C. Do not repeatedly try to convince; rather use "Help me understand your concerns…."
   D. Do not "label" family members; instead, try to learn about their positions and behaviors.
   E. Remember that the family may not view artificial nutrition and hydration as "futile care;" the health care team has a responsibility to meet them "where they are."
   F. If all else fails:
      1. Consult your ethics team.
      2. Bring in a consultant to assist.
      3. Transfer care to another provider.

(Bouton, 2005a)

Palliative care in acute care settings is becoming more common. But the approach can be a difficult transition for acute care staff when the focus has traditionally been on curative goals. Because this transition or paradigm shift can be uncomfortable, referrals to palliative care teams and a coordinated plan of care can be delayed. Unfortunately, referrals to palliative care teams may be initiated by acute care staff only when the patient's death is imminent (Cooney, 2005).

Increasing awareness about care options, both by professionals and the public, is a first step in changing the perspective that considers all palliative care as hospice or end-of-life care (Beach, 2004).

Still, the average time from referral to palliative care services and the patient's death is, on average, 2 weeks (CancerSource, 2005; Duggleby & Berry, 2005; NCPQPC, 2004).

To qualify for Medicare reimbursement, hospices must offer 16 core and noncore services. Core services include bereavement counseling, dietary and nutritional services, and physician and skilled nursing services. Noncore services include continuous home care, physical therapy, medications, personal care, and homemaker and household services (Carlson, Gallo, & Bradley, 2004).

TABLE 22-5: GRIEF ASSESSMENT: STRENGTHS AND STRESSORS

Physical	Psychological	Spiritual	Strengths and Stressors
Preexisting health concerns	Emotional concerns	Involvement in faith community	Access to support
Increased visits to physicians	Obvious mental health problems	Importance of beliefs and faith	Satisfaction with social interaction
Health insurance coverage	History of mental health concerns	Sense of spirituality or meaning	Experience of disenfranchised grief
Change in health status	Suicide ideation or plans	Satisfaction with funeral, memorial ritual	Adequate financial resources
Change in energy level	Extreme dependency	Signs of spiritual strength	Change in activity level
Exhaustion	Extreme anger	Signs of spiritual distress	Legal concerns
Sleep changes	Extreme fearfulness		Employment status
Appetite changes	Extreme guilt		Day-to-day living concerns
Weight gain or loss	Attitude (optimism versus pessimism)		Advance preparation for death
Neglect of appearance			
Recent accidents	Current therapeutic interventions		Circumstances of death
Alcohol or substance abuse			

(Bouton, 2005b)

END-OF-LIFE CARE

End-of-life care that is compassionate and knowledgeable has emerged as an important phase in the continuum of cancer care. In an environment of pervasive technology and science-driven care, patients and families are beginning to question how they want to spend their final days together and how to die with dignity. The process of empowerment and control over one's fate also brings a series of complex and stressful decisions. The amount of decisions—colored by nuance and emotion—can tax patients and families at their most vulnerable time.

Support and education—covering physical, emotional, spiritual, ethical, and cultural concerns—are the foundation of quality end-of-life care. Communication skills and the ability to compassionately deal with difficult issues are the main competencies the nurse brings to the patient and family (Chochinov, 2006; Kinlaw, 2005).

In addition to using an advance directive to ensure a palliative approach to care, patients and their families are beginning to use a relatively new tool to clarify end-of-life wishes—a values history. The values history is a method of discovery and documentation that more fully informs decisions made in an advance directive. Table 22-6 highlights questions that would be included in a values history.

Several assessment tools can help the nurse monitor a patient's performance status, thereby ensuring the provision of appropriate and timely interventions as patients approach end of life. Table 22-7 provides a review of common performance status scales.

As a guide to family members and caregivers, Table 22-8 lists situations that would prompt a hospice team member to be called in to help, especially when a patient's symptoms become frightening to family members. Table 22-9 lists the symptoms prevalent during a patient's last week of life.

Some of the ongoing research being pursued about end-of-life care includes a discussion of the focus of nursing education. Nurses face many challenges in providing quality, ethical end-of-life care. For example, a patient or family member may ask a nurse to assist with acceleration of the dying process (NCPQPC, 2004; Northouse, 2005). With well-grounded education and research-based information, those ethical and legal issues can be clarified for the nurse as he or she faces these requests.

Artificial Nutrition and Hydration

One of the ethical questions that face hospice caregivers is the scope of providing artificial nutrition and hydration during the final days of a patient's life. A framework to discuss this issue from an ethical perspective includes these considerations:

- Decisions about artificial nutrition and hydration should be made based on a pros-and-cons evaluation, similar to any other treatment decision.

- The withholding and withdrawing of artificial nutrition and hydration are morally and ethically equivalent.

- Decisions to stop artificial nutrition and hydration can be made with reasonable evidence of a patient's preference.

- Decisions to stop artificial nutrition and hydration can ethically be made without evidence of preferences.

- Whatever the decision about withholding artificial nutrition and hydration, all patients deserve high-quality hospice and palliative care.

(Bouton, 2005a)

In our society, food is equated with nourishment (both physical and emotional), tradition, and history, and it connotes images and memories of family and social gatherings and celebrations. The concepts of "withholding" nutrition and hydration may be difficult for families to embrace. When the decision and timing of the decision conflict the patient and family, the hospice nurse can provide a forum for clarity, emotional support, and resolution. Sometimes a family conference can be a reasonable and productive way to accomplish consensus about withholding nutrition or hydration.

Providing Contact after Death

Some health care providers who care for patients during their final days make contact with the families after the death. Studies show that contact can have a very positive effect on a family's experience and may help prevent some of the problems that are associated with poor coping (decline in health; inappropriate use of the health care system; increased risk of depression; sleep disruption; increased consumption of tobacco, alcohol, and sedatives; increased suicide risk; and death).

Such contact facilitates the healthy adaptation process of families, provides appropriate and definitive closure to the relationship between the family and health care providers, and creates an opportunity for clinicians to encourage the family to contact appropriate community resources for bereavement follow-up (Bouton, 2005a).

TABLE 22-6: VALUES HISTORY QUESTIONS (1 OF 2)

Overall Attitude Toward Life and Health

- What would you like to say to someone reading this document about your overall attitude toward life?
- What goals do you have for the future?
- How satisfied are you with what you have achieved in your life?
- What, for you, makes life worth living?
- What do you fear most? What frightens or upsets you?
- What activities do you enjoy (e.g., hobbies, watching television)?
- How would you describe your current state of health?
- If you currently have any health problems or disabilities, how do they affect: you? your family? your work? your ability to function?
- If you have health problems or disabilities, how do you feel about them? What would you like others (family, friends, doctors) to know about this?
- Do you have difficulties in getting through the day with activities such as: eating? preparing food? sleeping? dressing and bathing?
- What would you like to say to someone reading this document about your general health?

Personal Relationships

- What role do family and friends play in your life?
- How do you expect friends, family, and others to support your decisions regarding medical treatment you may need now or in the future?
- Have you made any arrangements for family or friends to make medical treatment decisions on your behalf? If so, who has agreed to make decisions for you and in what circumstances?
- What general comments would you like to make about the personal relationships in your life?

Thoughts About Independence and Self-Sufficiency

- How does independence or dependence affect your life?
- If you were to experience decreased physical and mental abilities, how would that affect your attitude toward independence and self-sufficiency?
- If your current physical or mental health gets worse, how would you feel?

Living Environment

- Have you lived alone or with others over the last 10 years?
- How comfortable have you been in your surroundings? How might illness, disability, or age affect this?
- What general comments would you like to make about your surroundings?

Religious Background and Beliefs

- What is your spiritual and religious background?
- How do your beliefs affect your feelings toward serious, chronic or terminal illness?
- How does your faith community, church, or synagogue support you?
- What general comments would you like to make about your beliefs?

Relationships with Doctors and Other Health Caregivers

- How do you relate to your doctors? Please comment on trust, decision making, time for satisfactory communication, and respectful treatment.
- How do you feel about other caregivers, including nurses, therapists, chaplains, and social workers?
- What else would you like to say about doctors and other caregivers?

Thoughts About Illness, Dying, and Death

- What general comments would you like to make about illness, dying, and death?
- What will be important to you when you are dying (e.g., physical comfort, no pain, family members present)?
- Where would you prefer to die?
- How do you feel about the use of life-sustaining measures if you were suffering from an irreversible chronic illness (e.g., Alzheimer's disease), terminally ill, or in a permanent coma?
- What general comments would you like to make about medical treatment?

TABLE 22-6: VALUES HISTORY QUESTIONS (2 OF 2)

Finances
- What general comments would you like to make about your finances and the cost of health care?
- What are your feelings about having enough money to provide for your care?

Funeral Plans
- What general comments would you like to make about your funeral and burial or cremation?
- Have you made your funeral arrangements? If so, with whom?

Optional Questions
- How would you like your obituary (announcement of your death) to read?
- Write yourself a brief eulogy (a statement about yourself to be read at your funeral).
- What would you like to say to someone reading this values history form?

Note. From *Values history,* by University of New Mexico Institute for Ethics, 2001. Retrieved April 17, 2007, from http://hsc.unm.edu/ethics/pdf/Values_History.doc

Spiritual Care

Spirituality encompasses a broad scope involving the patient's and family's self-awareness, faith, and expression. Quality end-of-life care incorporates open-mindedness to a patient's spiritual beliefs and a readiness by all team members to support and sustain those beliefs. To accomplish that, providers of end-of-life care are best equipped when they practice the art of self-awareness (Quiles, 2005). Therefore, providers should ask themselves: "What is spirituality to me?" This question prompts a personal response from each of us that includes the definition of our families, our upbringing, our moral and emotional development, and our religious background (NCPQPC, 2004; Quiles, 2005). The process of self-reflection or self-inquiry can lead to a better understanding of how we function with and around our patients and families.

Those who have self-understanding about their spiritual issues—values, meaning of life and death, relationships—can better gain an understanding of how they function with patients and families. This process of inquiry can be constant for each individual, ever moving and changing (Duggleby & Berry, 2005).

Access to Hospice Care

Access to Hospice Care: Expanding Boundaries, Overcoming Barriers is a seminal report drawn from a 3-year study that identifies both the values that drive and hinder access to hospice care (Carlson et al., 2004; National Home and Hospice Care Data, 2004). According to the survey, specific areas where the most significant barriers exist are:

- laws, policies, and regulations that affect the organization, financing, and delivery of care

- attitudes and practices of health care providers, including referring physicians and hospice professionals themselves, who are considered "gatekeepers" of the health care system

- consumer misunderstandings, misinformation, and stigmas about hospice care.

The survey results indicate that deliberate barriers are not the principal problem. For the most part, the impediments to hospice access are not deliberate but indirect and subtle (Carlson et al., 2004). Occasionally, access is blocked by the patient's and family's ability to pay (Bouton, 2005a).

Families as Caregivers

One of the underpinnings of end-of-life care is that more and more family caregivers have the responsibilities of end-of-life treatment coordination, symptom management, and comfort. With patients increasingly treated in outpatient facilities or quickly discharged from hospitals, the place of care switches to home, coordinated by lay caregivers. As the end-of-life process progresses, the

TABLE 22-7: PERFORMANCE STATUS SCALES

WHO§	ECOG*	SWOGª	Karnofsky	Activity	Restrictions	Care	Disease
0	0		100%	Fully active	Able to carry on all predisease performance without restrictions	No special care or complaints	Asymptomatic
1	1		90%	Active			Minor signs and symptoms of disease
			80%	Normal activity with effort	Restricted in physically strenuous activity	No special care	
2	2		70%	Ambulatory	Unable to work	Able to live at home, but some assistance needed	
			60%		Up and about more than 50% of waking hours	Able to care for most needs but requires occasional assistance	
3			50%		Requires frequent medical care and considerable assistance		
			40%	Disabled	Confined to bed or chair more than 50% of waking hours	Requires specialized medical care and assistance	Disease may be progressing
	3		30%	Severely disabled		Limited self-care; hospitalization is indicated	
			20%	Completely disabled	Hospitalization necessary	No self-care; totally confined to bed	Very sick; active supportive treatment necessary
4	4		10%	Moribund			Fatal processes progressing rapidly
	5		0%	Dead			

§ World Health Organization
* Eastern Cooperative Oncology Group
ª Southwest Oncology Group

(Razilla & Anderson, 2001)

tasks can become overwhelming and unsettling (Northouse, 2005).

To better profile caregiving, here are a few statistics:

- Family caregivers provide the overwhelming majority (approximately 80%) of home care services in the United States.

- More than 50 million people provide care for a chronically ill, disabled, or aged family member or friend during any given year

- Caregiving is no longer predominantly a women's issue. Men now make up 44% of the caregiving population.

TABLE 22-8: WHEN TO CALL FOR HELP

- The patient is in pain that is not relieved by the prescribed dose of pain medication
- The patient shows discomfort, such as grimacing or moaning
- The patient is having trouble breathing and seems upset
- The patient is unable to urinate or empty the bowels
- The patient has fallen
- The patient is very depressed or talking about committing suicide
- The caregiver has difficulty giving medication to the patient
- The caregiver is overwhelmed by caring for the patient or is too grief-stricken or afraid to be with the patient
- At any time, the caregiver does not know how to handle a situation

- The value of the services family caregivers provide for "free" is estimated to be $257 billion a year. This is twice as much as is actually spent on home care and nursing home services.
- Caregiving families tend to have lower incomes than noncaregiving families. In the United States, 35% of households have incomes less than $30,000. Among caregiving families, the percentage is 43%.
- Elderly spousal caregivers with a history of chronic illness who are experiencing caregiving-related stress have a 63% higher mortality rate than their noncaregiving peers.
- Family caregivers who provide care 36 or more hours weekly are more likely than noncaregivers to experience symptoms of depression or anxiety. For spouses, the rate is six times higher; for those caring for a parent, the rate is twice as high.

TABLE 22-9: SYMPTOM PREVALENCE IN THE LAST WEEK OF LIFE

(Note: The presence of one or more of these symptoms does not necessarily indicate that the patient is close to death.)

- **Drowsiness**, increased sleep, or unresponsiveness (caused by changes in the patient's metabolism)
- **Confusion** about time, place, or identity of loved ones; restlessness; visions of people and places that are not present; pulling at bed linens or clothing (caused in part by changes in the patient's metabolism)
- **Decreased socialization and withdrawal** (caused by decreased oxygen to the brain, decreased blood flow, and mental preparation for dying)
- **Decreased need for food and fluids** and loss of appetite (caused by the body's need to conserve energy and its decreasing ability to use food and fluids properly)
- **Loss of bladder or bowel control** (caused by the relaxing of muscles in the pelvic area)
- **Darkened urine or decreased amount of urine** (caused by slowing of kidney function or decreased fluid intake)
- **Skin becomes cool to the touch,** particularly the hands and feet; skin may become bluish in color, especially on the underside of the body (caused by decreased circulation to the extremities)
- **Rattling or gurgling sounds while breathing,** which may be loud; breathing that is irregular and shallow; decreased number of breaths per minute; breathing that alternates between rapid and slow (caused by congestion from decreased fluid consumption, a buildup of waste products in the body, or a decrease in circulation to the organs)
- **Turning the head toward a light source** (caused by decreasing vision)
- **Increased difficulty controlling pain** (caused by progression of the disease)
- **Involuntary movements** (called *myoclonus*), changes in heart rate, and loss of reflexes in the legs and arms

(NCI, 2002)

- By the year 2030, nearly 150 million American caregivers will have developed some type of chronic illness, a 50% increase since 1995.

- More than 40% of family caregivers provide some type of "nursing care" for their loved ones, such as giving medications, changing bandages, managing machinery, and monitoring vital signs.

- One-third of family caregivers who change dressings and manage machines receive no instructions

(National Family Caregivers Association [NFCA], 2006).

Family members of patients with cancer experience extreme distress as a result of caregiving roles. This distress has been shown to continue over time and can worsen with changes in the patient's condition (CancerSource, 2006; Given et al., 2004). Caregiver stress can become anxiety, depression, helplessness, feelings of being burdened, and fear.

Adult children caregivers of cancer patients who are employed out of the home have been shown to develop depression. These caregivers, according to studies, feel abandoned (a portion of caregiver burden)—especially when the caregiver is female and a nonspouse. Studies have also shown that caregivers who care for patients with a rapid course from diagnosis to death report the highest depressive symptoms, burden, and impact on schedule. Thus, these caregivers are at greater risk for burnout and should be targeted for additional support by the hospice team (Given et al., 2004; Northouse, 2005).

PAIN MANAGEMENT

As mentioned earlier, WHO has broadened its definition of palliative care to encompass improving quality of life and reducing suffering. Still, a major focus of palliative care is the priority of effective cancer pain management "through the effective early identification and impeccable assessment and treatment of pain" (WHO, 2004).

Although pain management for cancer patients is one of the most important goals of compassionate care, it is surprisingly lacking for many cancer patients. Studies indicate that many barriers prevent patients from the pain management they deserve. Among those barriers are:

- lack of an ideal analgesic or set of analgesics

- intolerable side effects of pain agents

- lack of an institutional commitment to pain management

- complex attitudes and fears of patients and their families and caregivers

- complex attitudes and fears of health care providers toward pain management.

(Dawson et al., 2005; McMillan, Tittle, Hagan, & Small, 2005; Vallerand, Riley-Doucet, Hasenau, & Templin, 2004)

In addition to the list of patient-centered barriers to effective pain management, the health care system—including physicians and nurses—can contribute to ineffective pain management, despite having appropriate orders and education.

Too frequently, the patient, family members and health care providers believe that a cancer patient on pain medication will become addicted (develop a psychological dependence) or develop an inappropriate analgesic tolerance (physical dependence) (Dawson et al., 2005; McMillan et al., 2005; Vallerand et al., 2004). For proper pain management of cancer patients, educating the patient and family about addiction and tolerance to medication is important. Myths about pain medication and its effects should be reviewed. Some of these myths and barriers are:

- inaccurate knowledge (patient, family members, health care team) about appropriate choice and dosing of analgesics

- pain relief as an inappropriate goal of treatment

- fear of addition, sedation, and respiratory depression

- disconnect of pain perceptions—patient versus health care team

- fear of regulatory scrutiny when prescribing narcotics.

(Coyne, Smith, Laird, Hansen, & Drake, 2005)

Research on cancer pain management has demonstrated that provider and patient education interventions can significantly affect patients' knowledge or concerns about pain management as well as their compliance with pain management regimens (Dawson et al., 2005). Continual assessment of a patient's pain, coupled with knowing the patient's beliefs about pain medication and management, can establish why pain management may be ineffective (Dawson et al., 2005).

Studies have also reported that pain management of cancer patients is frequently under the direction of the primary care provider, with one study reporting that 42% of cancer patients received narcotic prescriptions from their primary physician (Dawson et al., 2005). Another study reported that home care nurses are on the front line of cancer pain management, having control over translating to patients and their families the implications of medications, anticipated side effects, and benefits and challenges of the medication regimen (Vallerand et al., 2004).

Inadequate communication is associated with poor symptom control and patient dissatisfaction. Thus, collaboration and effective written and oral communication are vital when pain treatment plans are established (Dawson et al., 2005).

Types of Pain

Pain can be acute or chronic. Acute pain is a response to an initial stimuli that excites or stimulates sensory nerve endings. The substances released from an acute pain stimulus include prostaglandins, serotonin, histamine, bradykinin, substance P, and other substances. By definition,

acute pain resolves, although it can sometimes last as long as 6 months (Brant, 2005).

Pain medication for acute pain is administered to interfere with the release of the substances released when nerve endings are stimulated. These stimulated nerve endings can send messages—via neurons—from the periphery to the spinal cord. Further administration of pain medication for acute pain targets the neurotransmitters in the spinal column.

Chronic pain persists beyond an acute pain stimulus. Its source can be nonmalignant or from tumor growth. Usually, chronic pain lasts longer than 3 months (Brant, 2005). Mechanisms that contribute to chronic pain are thought to include direct damage or prolonged stimulation of sensory neurons. Fatigue and depression contribute to the patient's perception of the severity of chronic pain.

Cancer pain is sometimes defined separately from acute or chronic pain, although it can be acute, chronic, or both.

Cancer Pain

Pain associated with a cancer diagnosis or tumor growth can be caused by a variety of factors. Pain from the cancer itself can be divided into two categories:

1. **Nociceptive pain or damage to tissue.** This pain is usually described as sharp, aching, or throbbing pain. Nociceptive pain may be caused by tumor cells growing and expanding, a blocked organ, or swelling that originates from the blockage.

2. **Neuropathic pain.** This pain is caused by nerve damage. It can burn or be a heavy sensation or numbness. The pain can emanate from a tumor pressing or infiltrating a nerve or a group of nerves.

Treatment-Related Pain

Surgery for cancer treatment can cause pain. As with any postoperative pain, this type of pain can pass with healing and can be managed with pain medication and nonpharmacologic pain management methods.

Chemotherapy may cause pain if some selected vesicant agents infiltrate tissue during improper administration. This infiltration—called *extravasation*—can lead to necrosis. (Chapter 8, Figure 8-2 reviews response to extravasation.)

Some patients report highly discomforting pain from routine needlesticks associated with blood draws or the intravenous (IV) administration of chemotherapy. To avoid multiple needlesticks, patients may be candidates for central venous access devices.

Some chemotherapies can cause painful sores in the mouth (stomatitis) and in the lining of the intestines (mucositis). This pain can be managed with medication and prevention strategies. (See Chapter 11, Table 11-10.)

Other selected chemotherapies, such as vincristine (Oncovin), cisplatin (Platinol), paclitaxel (Taxol), vinblastine (Velban), and ifosfamide (IFEX), can cause peripheral neuropathy—a tingling, numbness, or pain in the extremities (hands, fingers, toes, and feet). Neuropathic pain can also occur, especially when chemotherapy is given long-term or in high doses. To manage neuropathic pain, therapy dosing and schedules can be adjusted or substituted.

Radiation therapy (RT) affects normal cells while damaging cancer cells. Sometimes this effect on normal cells and tissues can cause pain and discomfort. Skin desquamation, difficulty swallowing, and mucositis of membranes may occur. (See Chapter 11 for ways to manage these side effects.)

Assessment

Pain management begins and continues with thorough, confident, frequent pain assessments. In 1999, The Joint Commission (formerly the Joint Commission on Accreditation of Healthcare Organizations, or JCAHO) added pain as the fifth vital sign to its provision of care standards. Since then, pain assessment has been much more integrated into nursing practice (JCAHO, 2006). Table 22-10 highlights pain standards from The Joint Commission.

TABLE 22-10: HIGHLIGHTS FROM THE JOINT COMMISSION PAIN STANDARDS
• Patients should be involved with all aspects of their care.
• Patients have the right to appropriate assessment and management of pain.
• Pain should be assessed in all patients.
• Policies and procedures should support safe medication prescription and ordering.
• The patient should be monitored during the post procedure period.
• Patients should be educated about pain and pain management as part of treatment, as appropriate.
• The follow-up process should provide for continuing care based on the patient's assessed needs.
• The organization should collect data to monitor its performance.
(JCAHO, 2006)

In addition to asking appropriate questions about a patient's pain, the nurse should use pain assessment tools that patients can clearly understand. (Figure 22-1 shows the main elements of a pain assessment.)

In addition to the level of pain, other areas of pain assessment are:

- duration
- location
- quality
- timing
- methods to control
- anxiety
- sleep
- depression
- alleviating and aggravating symptoms.

FIGURE 22-1: PAIN ASSESSMENT

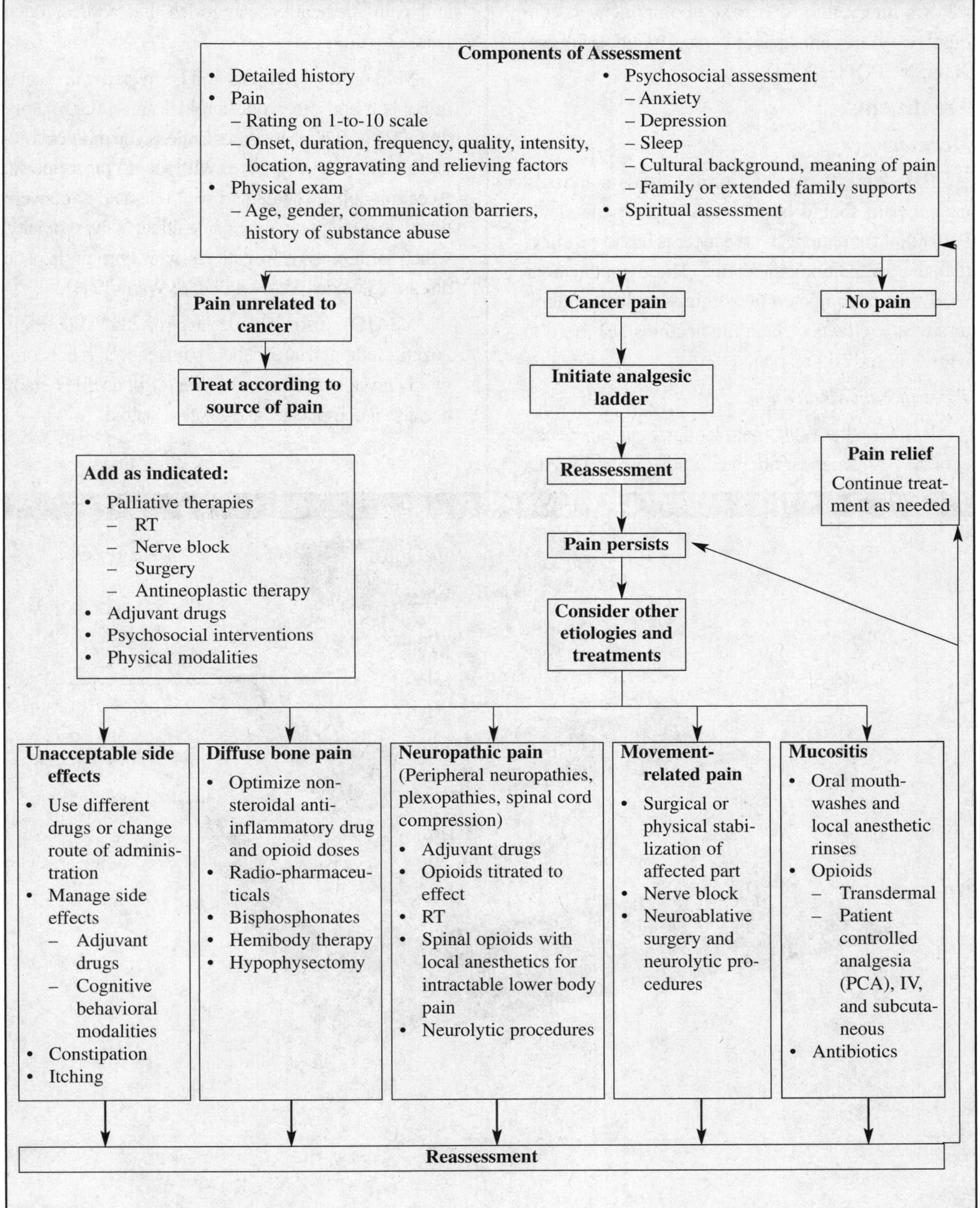

Components of Assessment

- Detailed history
- Pain
  - Rating on 1-to-10 scale
  - Onset, duration, frequency, quality, intensity, location, aggravating and relieving factors
- Physical exam
  - Age, gender, communication barriers, history of substance abuse

- Psychosocial assessment
  - Anxiety
  - Depression
  - Sleep
  - Cultural background, meaning of pain
  - Family or extended family supports
- Spiritual assessment

↓

Pain unrelated to cancer

↓

Treat according to source of pain

Add as indicated:

- Palliative therapies
  - RT
  - Nerve block
  - Surgery
  - Antineoplastic therapy
- Adjuvant drugs
- Psychosocial interventions
- Physical modalities

Cancer pain

↓

Initiate analgesic ladder

↓

Reassessment

↓

Pain persists

↓

Consider other etiologies and treatments

No pain

Pain relief

Continue treatment as needed

Unacceptable side effects

- Use different drugs or change route of administration
- Manage side effects
  - Adjuvant drugs
  - Cognitive behavioral modalities
- Constipation
- Itching

Diffuse bone pain

- Optimize non-steroidal anti-inflammatory drug and opioid doses
- Radio-pharmaceuticals
- Bisphosphonates
- Hemibody therapy
- Hypophysectomy

Neuropathic pain
(Peripheral neuropathies, plexopathies, spinal cord compression)

- Adjuvant drugs
- Opioids titrated to effect
- RT
- Spinal opioids with local anesthetics for intractable lower body pain
- Neurolytic procedures

Movement-related pain

- Surgical or physical stabilization of affected part
- Nerve block
- Neuroablative surgery and neurolytic procedures

Mucositis

- Oral mouthwashes and local anesthetic rinses
- Opioids
  - Transdermal
  - Patient controlled analgesia (PCA), IV, and subcutaneous
- Antibiotics

↓

Reassessment

(Brant, 2005; CancerSource 2005; Dawson et al., 2005.)

Ongoing documentation, which precedes and follows interventions, is a key component in adequately addressing patient pain (CancerSource, 2005; NCPQPC, 2004).

Treatments

Medication

Based on The Joint Commission's standards, patient pain should be assessed at each encounter. Pain relief for patients with cancer is based on effective use of pain medications. These medications work when competently administered and monitored. Side effects of pain medications also need to be monitored and managed.

Types of Pain Medication

Based on the WHO pain ladder, pain can be categorized as mild, moderate, and severe (WHO, n.d.). Figure 22-2 illustrates the WHO pain ladder and pain medication categories that address each level of pain.

Mild or low-level pain can be treated with acetaminophen and other nonsteroidal anti-inflammatory drugs (NSAIDs). Most medications for mild or low-level pain are available without a prescription. Acetaminophen is safe and well tolerated at conventional doses; its only major side effect is liver toxicity, which is rare, even in patients with chronic hepatic disease (Stockler, Vardy, Pillai, & Warr, 2004).

NSAIDs also include aspirin and ibuprofen. Aspirin, although an excellent pain reliever, is not commonly given to patients receiving RT or chemotherapy because it complicates coagulation status.

FIGURE 22-2: WHO'S PAIN RELIEF LADDER

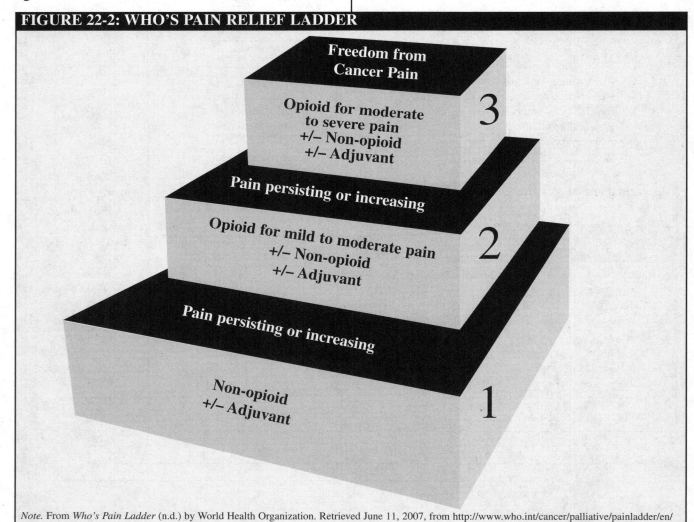

Note. From *Who's Pain Ladder* (n.d.) by World Health Organization. Retrieved June 11, 2007, from http://www.who.int/cancer/palliative/painladder/en/index.html

For moderate to severe pain, patients are given opioids. Opioids are type-2 narcotics, which require a physician's written prescription. Examples of opioids are morphine, fentanyl, hydromorphone, oxycodone, and codeine. They can be taken by mouth (pill or liquid), by a patch on the body (e.g., fentanyl), or as a suppository. Some can also be given IV.

Pain can be controlled by increasing the dose or frequency of the medication, based on the patient's disease process. If a medication is not providing adequate pain control, a different but equivalent medication can be used (Portenoy, 2005).

Cancer patients with histories of substance abuse who are on long-term opioid therapy for cancer pain rarely become addicted to their pain medication (less than 1% of patients) (Lussier & Pappagallo, 2004). Although addiction is not an issue in cancer pain management, patients can become tolerant of medications or doses, so that higher doses (or a change of medication) may be warranted.

Antidepressants may be used to address nerve pain (burning and tingling). They can serve as adjunct treatments to an overall pain management strategy. Examples of antidepressants are amitriptyline, imipramine, and the antiseizure medications carbamazepine (Tegretol) and gabapentin (Neurontin).

Additional pain management strategies are based on the synergy of combining pain medications, effective dosing, and scheduling (Portenoy, 2005). Table 22-11 reviews pain medications used to treat cancer pain.

Pain Management Strategies

Around-the-Clock Dosing

To avoid the ups and downs of maintaining a steady state of pain medication in the bloodstream, good pain management for cancer patients is based on around-the-clock (ATC) dosing, or round-the-clock dosing. For example, a patient's dose may be one Percocet (oxycodone and acetaminophen) every 6 hours. For best effect of the drug and dosing, the Percocet needs to be taken every 6 hours ATC rather than as needed.

Adjuvant Pain Methods

In many cases, opioid doses are not adequate to completely control pain. A strategy to address ineffective pain control is to add a coanalgesic or mild pain medication—such as acetaminophen or an NSAID—to the opioid regimen. This creates a synergy between the two medications that adequately controls the pain. By adding a mild pain medication, rather than increasing the opioid dose, the side effects of a higher opioid dose (e.g., drowsiness, somnolence, constipation) can be avoided or lessened (Stockler et al., 2004).

To alleviate swelling, patients can be given steroids, such as prednisone and dexamethasone. When patients are on steroids, the dose needs to be titrated.

Breakthrough Pain

When ATC dosing is not effective, an additional medication may be added for breakthrough pain. The breakthrough medication addresses episodes of short, intermittent pain, also known as *breakthrough pain*. Breakthrough pain can be prompted by various activities (incident pain), be entirely unpredictable (idiopathic pain), or occur toward the end of ATC medication (end-of-dose failure) (Rhiner, Palos, & Termini, 2004).

Breakthrough pain occurs in as much as 86% of patients with cancer, even when persistent pain is well controlled (Rhiner et al., 2004). An example of breakthrough pain medication is the elixir form of Vicodin. It can be added for breakthrough pain and is prescribed to be taken between Percocet dosing, timed during the breakthrough pain periods (Rhiner et al., 2004).

Keep in mind, the need for breakthrough medication can suggest that the main pain medication, dosed ATC, may need to be higher or—for some medications—administered more frequently. In this

TABLE 22-11: PAIN MANAGEMENT AGENTS (1 OF 4)

FIRST STEP: NON-OPIOID ANALGESICS FOR MILD TO MODERATE PAIN

Class	Generic Name	Half-Life (hours) (approx.)	Dosing Schedule	Recommended Starting Dose (mg/d)	Maximum Recommended Dose (mg/d)
p-Aminophenol	Acetaminophen (paracetamol)	2-4	q4-6h	2,600	4,000
COX-2 selective inhibitors	Celecoxib	11	q12h	200	600
Salicylates	Aspirin	3-12	q4-6h	2,600	6,000
	Choline magnesium trisalicylate	9-17	q12h	1,500 x 1, then 1,000 q12h	4,000
	Diflunisal	8-12	q12h	1,000 x 1, then 500 q12h	1,500
	Salsalate	8-12	q12h	1,500 x 1, then 1,000 q12h	4,000
Propionic acids	Fenoprofen	2-3	q4-6h	800	200
	Flurbiprofen	5-6	q8-12h	100	1,200
	Ibuprofen	1.8-2	q4-8h	1,200	200
	Ketoprofen	2-3	q6-8h	150	300
	Naproxen	13	q12h	500	1,000
	Naproxen sodium	13	q12h	550	1,100
	Oxaprozin	42-50	q24h	600	1,800
Acetic acids	Diclofenac	2	q6h	150	200
	Etodolac	7	q6-8h	600	1,200
	Indomethacin	4-5	q8-12h	75	200
	Ketorolac	4-7	q6h	15-30 q6h IV, IM 10 q6h PO	120 IV, IM 40 PO
	Sulindac	7.8	q12h	300	400
	Tolmetin	2	q6-8h	600	1,800
Naphthyl-alkanone	Nabumetone	20-35	q24h	1,000	2,000
Oxycams	Meloxicam	15-20	q24h	7.5	15
	Piroxicam	50	q24h	20	40
Fenamates	Meclofenamic acid	1.3	q6-8h	150	400
	Mefenamic acid	2	q6h	500 x 1, then 250 q6h	1,000
Pyrazole	Phenylbutazone	50-100	q6-8h	300	400

TABLE 22-11: PAIN MANAGEMENT AGENTS (2 OF 4)					
SECOND STEP: SHORT-ACTING OPIOIDS FOR MODERATE PAIN					
Class	**Generic Name**	**Dose (mg)** Equianalgesic to aspirin 650 mg	**Half-Life (hours)**	**Peak Effect (hours)**	**Duration (hours)**
Morphine-like agonists	Codeine	32-65	2-3	1.5-2	3-6
	Dihydrocodeine	15-20	–	–	4-5
	Hydrocodone	–	4	0.5-1	4-6
	Meperidine (pethidine)	50	3-4	1-2	3-5
	Oxycodone	2.5	–	1	3-6
	Propoxyphene hydrochloride	65-130	12	2-2.5	3-6
	Propoxyphene napsylate	100-200	12	2-2.5	3-6
Agonist-antagonist	Pentazocine	30	2-3	1.5-2	2-4
Other	Tramadol	–	6-7	2-3	4-6

Table continues on next page.

situation, reevaluate the pain management regimen based on assessments.

Pain Medication Administration

Pain medication is available in many forms and can be administered in many different ways. If one route does not work well, another route can be used. According to experts in cancer pain, 85% to 95% of cancer pain can be effectively relieved using oral medications. (Oral medications are generally more convenient and less expensive than other routes.) The other 5% to 15% of patients may need to have a different route of administration or have more sophisticated pain management requirements (Portenoy, 2005). Table 22-12 lists medication routes for patients who cannot swallow pills.

Other routes to administer pain medication are

- rectal
- transdermal (for fentanyl)
- parenteral route such as
  - intramuscular (IM) injections
  - subcutaneously under the skin
  - IV
- intraspinal (through the spinal fluid)
- intraventricular (through brain ventricles).

Changing the route of administration from oral to IV should be considered for patients who do not achieve satisfactory pain relief and for those who require rapid onset of analgesia. Many patients already have a central line device (for example, Port-a-Cath) that can be used rather than using a subcutaneous route. Ideally, administration of pain medication through a central line should be started in a monitored inpatient setting.

Patient-controlled analgesia (PCA) is an optional delivery strategy. With PCA, infusion systems or pumps allow the patient to control medication delivery within limits set by the physician. PCA routes of administration can be IV, subcutaneous, and intraspinal. PCA infusion systems can be programmed to allow the patient to access extra doses (boluses) of pain medication when breakthrough pain occurs.

TABLE 22-11: PAIN MANAGEMENT AGENTS (3 OF 4)

THIRD STEP: SHORT- AND LONG-ACTING OPIOIDS FOR MODERATE TO SEVERE PAIN

Class	Generic Name	Dose (mg) Equianalgesic to morphine 10 mg IM	Half-Life (hours)	Peak Effect (hours)	Duration (hours)
Morphine-like agonists	Fentanyl transdermal system	25 mcg/h	17	24-72	72
	Hydromorphone	1.5 IM 7.5 PO	2-3 –	0.5-1 1-2	4-5 4-5
	Extended-release hydromorphone	7.5 PO	2-3	3-4	24
	Levorphanol	2 IM 4 PO	11-16	0.5-1	6-8
	Meperidine (pethidine)	75 IM 300 PO	3-4	0.5-1 1-2	2-4 3-6
	Methadone	10 IM 20 PO	15-150+	0.5-1.5	4-8
	Morphine	10 IM 20-60 PO	3 2-4	0.5-1 1.5-2	6 4-7
	Modified-release morphine	20-60 PO	2-3	3-4	8-24
	Oxycodone	20-30 PO	2-4	1	3-6
	Modified-release oxycodone	20-30 PO	2-4	3-4	8-12
	Oxymorphone	1 IM 10 PR		0.5-1 1.5-3	3-6 4-6
Partial agonist	Buprenorphine	0.4 IM	2-5	0.5-1	6-8
Mixed agonists-antagonists	Butorphanol	2 IM	2-3	0.5-1	3-4
	Nalbuphine	10 IM	4-6	0.5-1	3-6
	Pentazocine	60 IM 180 PO	2-3 –	0.5-1	3-6

Table continues on next page.

The two intraspinal routes—epidural and intrathecal—deliver low-dose opioids to the spaces around the spinal cord. For short-term analgesia, the epidural route is more common, although it is rarely used in outpatient settings. For longer-term therapy, the intrathecal route is preferred because it is more efficient and less expensive over time. *Note:* Intraspinal doses are approximately 1/10 (epidural) to 1/100 (intrathecal) of the IV dose. (Bourdeanu, Loseth, & Funk, 2005).

Side Effects of Pain Medication

For pain medication to be effective, the side effects from these agents must be managed. Among side effects of pain medications, especially opioids, are:

• Constipation

TABLE 22-11: PAIN MANAGEMENT AGENTS (4 OF 4)

ADJUVANT ANALGESICS: Adjuvant analgesics comprise diverse classes of drugs that have other indications. They should be used when specific indications exist.

Class	Rationale for Use	Application	Examples	Dosing Schedule	Starting Dose (mg/d)	Usual Daily Dose (mg/d)
Anticonvulsants	Extensive survey data and controlled trials support efficacy in neuropathic pain	Neuropathic pain	Carbamazepine, clonazepam, gabepentin, lamotrigine, levetiracetam, oxcarbazepine, phenytoin, tiagabine, topiramate, valproate, zonisamide	Variable	Variable	Variable
Oral local anesthetics	Controlled studies in painful diabetic neuropathy	Neuropathic pain	Mexiletine	q8h	450	600-900
Antidepressants	Proven analgesics in a variety of nonmalignant pain states	Neuropathic pain, pain complicated by depression or insomnia	tricyclic antidepressants, selective serotonin reuptake inhibitors, and serotonin-norepinephrine reuptake inhibitors, others	Variable	Variable	Variable
Corticosteroids	Extensive anecdotal experience in the treatment of pain and other symptoms confirmed by a single controlled study of methylprednisolone	Pain from infiltration of neural structures, bone pain, pain in patients with far advanced diseases	Dexamethasone	q6-12h	Variable (e.g., 10-20 mg x 1, then 4 mg q6h or less)	2-24
Miscellaneous	Controlled study in trigeminal neuralgia	Neuropathic pain	Baclofen	q8h	15	30-120
	Controlled study and anecdotal reports	Refractory bone pain and neuropathic pain	Calcitonin	q12h	200 IU	200-400 IU
	Controlled studies and anecdotal reports	Refractory bone pain	Bisphosphonates (pamidronate)	Repeat monthly	60	–
	Controlled study	Refractory bone pain	Strontium 89, samarium 153	–	–	–
	Anecdotal reports	Pain due to bowel obstruction	Anticholinergic drugs (e.g., scopolamine and glycopyrrolate), octreotide	Variable	Variable	Variable
Psychostimulants	Clinical experience and controlled trials of dextroamphetamine in postoperative pain and methyl-phenidate in cancer pain	Reversal of opioid-induced sedation	Methylphenidate, dextroamphetamine, pemoline, modafinil	bid bid bid qd	5 5 18.75 100	10-40 10-40 37.5-70 200

(Portenoy, 2006)

TABLE 22-12: MEDICATION ROUTES FOR PATIENTS WHO CANNOT SWALLOW PILLS

- Liquids or crushable medications (opioids and lorazepam are available as concentrated liquids)
- Rectal medications
- Transdermal patches (e.g., fentanyl)
- Subcutaneous route to administer:
  - Opioids: hydromorphone, morphine, fentanyl, oxymorphone, methadone
  - Benzodiazepines: midazolam, lorazepam
  - Antiemetics: metoclopramide, haloperidol, hydroxyzine, chlorpromazine
  - Anticholinergics: glycopyrrolate, scopolamine

Constipation is not difficult to control but proactive methods best manage it. Among strategies to decreased or eliminate constipation

- eating lots of fruits and vegetables and drinking lots of water and fruit juices
- eating foods high in fiber, such as prunes and grains
- if possible, staying physically active
- administering or taking maintenance laxatives or stool softener regimens, as appropriate.

Chapter 11 reviews other interventions for constipation.

- Pruritus (itching)
  If possible, prevent pruritus by keeping skin moist and lubricated with creams, lotions, and moisturizing agents. Administration of over-the-counter diphenhydramine (Benadryl) and hydrocortisone cream can help. If pruritus is unmanageable, consider changing pain medications to an agent that provokes less itching for the patient.

- Nausea and vomiting
  If nausea and vomiting occur, they usually accompany the initial administration of pain medications and resolve later. To manage:

  - administer antiemetic medication (encourage the patient to lie down after taking the medicine and to take the medicine with food, unless otherwise indicated)
  - avoid spicy or fatty foods
  - eat several small meals a day
  - eat foods such as dry toast, crackers, pretzels, and sherbet
  - drink plenty of clear liquids
  - use relaxation or visualization techniques to minimize the feeling of nausea.

- Drowsiness
  Drowsiness can pass after the initial period of medication administration. Doses can be adjusted.

  Opioid-induced sedation occurs in 20% to 60% of patients receiving opioids. In patients with cancer, pronounced opioid-induced sedation is usually an unacceptable and undesirable side effect that affects quality of life. Sedation is a dose-dependent effect of opioids. Patients can develop tolerance to the sedative effects of opioids within a few days (Bourdeanu et al., 2005). Therefore, assessment can provide strategies to limit drowsiness:

  - Carefully reduce the dose by as much as 50% when pain is controlled. For example, gradually reduce morphine 10 mg/hr to 8 mg/hr, while constantly assessing pain control and any side effects. During assessment, attention to withdrawal symptoms is important. (Withdrawal symptoms can include sweating, runny nose, cramping, tearing, and tachycardia.)
  - Combine opioid administration with other agents. For example, adding amphetamines in some well-selected situations is an accepted therapy for opioid-induced sedation. (*Note:* Amphetamines are contraindicated in patients with a history of psychiatric disorders, a history of substance abuse, and paroxysmal tachyarrhythmia). Potential side effects of amphetamines include weight loss, anxiety, and exacerbation of delirium.

Tolerance to the effects of psychostimulants is also a potential problem.

Another example of combining agents is adding an adjuvant agent—such as acetaminophen—to opioids, such as hydrocodone or oxycodone. These adjuvant-with-opioid combinations can allow good pain management with a lower opioid dose, thus reducing opioid-induced sedation (Brant, 2005).

– Opioid rotation, or changing an opioid-induced sedation agent to another in its class, allows for equianalgesia while reducing drowsiness (Bourdeanu et al., 2005). For example, a 24-hour equivalent dose of morphine changed to an alternative opioid, such as a 24-hour equivalent dose of hydromorphone—can reduce the opioid dosing by approximately 20% to 25%. Then, after the switch, titrate hydromorphone to the effective dose, as needed.

Other Pain Management Methods

Surgery, RT, chemotherapy, and biotherapy can lessen and control pain caused by tumors. These modalities can remove or reduce the size of the tumor. For example, Table 22-13 lists types of pain that can be treated with RT.

Nonpharmacologic pain management strategies can be helpful alone or as complements to the administration of pain medication:

- Heat relaxes the muscles and gives a sense of comfort. Warm showers, baths, hot water bottles, and warm washcloths can be soothing.

- Using cool cloths and ice to cool the skin and muscles can soothe pain, especially any pain that comes from inflammation or swelling.

- Relaxation and meditation can help reduce tension and stress. Techniques include simple breathing exercises, progressive muscle relaxation, and visualization.

- Distraction allows the patient a brief time away from pain. Popular methods are listening to

---

TABLE 22-13: COMMON INDICATIONS FOR PALLIATIVE RADIOTHERAPY

- Pain relief
  - Bone metastases
  - Painful lung cancer
  - Soft-tissue infiltration
- Control of bleeding
  - Hemoptysis
  - Vaginal or rectal bleeding
- Control of fungal wound and ulceration
- Relief of impending or actual obstruction
  - Esophagus
  - Bronchus
  - Rectum
- Shrinkage of tumor mass causing distressing symptoms
  - Brain metastases
  - Skin lesions
- Prevention of significant functional morbidity and pain
  - Impending bone fracture (long bones, vertebral bodies, ribs)
  - Spinal cord compression
  - Superior mediastinal obstruction

---

music, watching television, reading, cooking, and talking to family and friends.

- The use of guided imagery helps to gain pain control. This method allows the mind and powers of concentration to focus on soothing images. It is a way of further extending the benefits of relaxation and distraction.

- Skin stimulation can include massage, heating pads, or ice packs. It can be used alone or in combination with other methods for relieving pain, such as transcutaneous electrical nerve stimulation.

- Exercise can help relieve tension, depression, and fatigue.

- Support groups, facilitated either by a trained professional or peers, can offer pain relief or ideas on pain control.

EDUCATING HEALTH CARE PROVIDERS

Continuing the education of health care providers is essential to improving palliative care (McMillan et al., 2005). Much is known about pain management, but study results indicate that nurses still lack knowledge and harbor unsuitable attitudes about appropriate pain management practices. Studies that have looked at changes in pain management behavior as a result of nursing education are limited. Those that have been conducted involved short-term programs, and results were not encouraging. What is known is that more education is needed, not only in basic nursing curricula but also in continuing education programs for practicing nurses (McMillan et al., 2005).

An example of a model program is **H**ome care **O**utreach for **P**alliative care **E**ducation (HOPE), which was funded by the NCI and coordinated by the City of Hope National Medical Center in Duarte, California. This five-part curriculum teaches key modules of end-of-life care, including an overview of palliative care and home care, pain management, symptom management, communication, and preparation for death at home. In addition to nurses, the program materials target nursing assistants and unlicensed personnel.

Other model programs include the PERT curriculum (**P**alliative care **E**ducational **R**esource **T**eam)—emphasizing goals of care, pain and symptom management, communication, culture, spiritual care, and grief—and a case-study-based project at the Institute for Palliative and Hospice Training in Alexandria, Virginia. This program emphasizes assessing and reporting pain and symptoms, understanding psychosocial needs, and identifying signs of approaching death (Ferrell, 2005b).

Yet another training strategy was developed by the End of Life Nursing Education Consortium (ELNEC). The project consists of nine modules covering such topics as palliative nursing, pain management, symptom management, culture, communication, ethical issues, care at the time of death, and quality improvement. The ELNEC project is a "train-the-trainer" design in which those who participate in the ELNEC training are taught not only the content but also teaching strategies. The participants of the ELNEC training then return to their own settings with established goals to implement the material they learned from the modules. As of 2005, more than 2000 nurses had been trained through the core ELNEC project, with thousands of others trained through efforts by these participants after their training (Ferrell, 2005a).

SUMMARY

Cancer care at its very best adheres to the principles and guidelines of palliative care, providing physical, emotional, psychological, and spiritual comfort to the patient and family members. This chapter reviewed the main components of providing quality palliative care, including strategies for communication, a review of family dynamics and decision making, components of end-of-life care, and principles of pain management for cancer pain.

CHAPTER 22
Questions 89-92

Note: Choose the option that BEST answers each question.

89. Quality palliative care includes

    a. family distanced from the patient.

    b. administration of new treatments.

    c. adequate symptom management.

    d. weight gain.

90. To help patients and families transition to palliative care, the nurse can

    a. discuss the issues.

    b. provide distraction.

    c. provide pain medication.

    d. have the physician order psychotherapy.

91. Appropriate cancer pain management includes

    a. administering medications on an as-needed basis.

    b. restricting the use of opioids.

    c. avoiding heat and cold therapies.

    d. ATC dosing.

92. A side effect of pain medications is

    a. insomnia.

    b. alopecia.

    c. constipation.

    d. diarrhea.

REFERENCES

Beach, P. (2004). Palliative care in an acute care setting. *Clinical Journal of Oncology Nursing, 8(2)*, 202-203.

Bourdeanu, L., Loseth, D., & Funk, M. (2005). Management of opioid-induced sedation in patients with cancer. *Clinical Journal of Oncology Nursing, 9(6)*, 705-711.

Bouton, B. (2005a). *Ethical "hot buttons in hospice care."* Session in *Highlights of the Sixth Annual Clinical Team Conference of the National Hospice and Palliative Care Organization (NHPCO).* Retrieved April 17, 2007, from http://www.medscape.com/viewprogram/4128

Bouton, B. (2005b). *Understanding grief.* Session in *Highlights of the Sixth Annual Clinical Team Conference of the National Hospice and Palliative Care Organization (NHPCO).* Retrieved April 17, 2007, from http://www.medscape.com/viewprogram/4128

Brant, J. (2005). Comfort. In J.K. Itano & K.N. Taoka (Eds.), *Core curriculum for oncology nursing* (4th ed., pp. 3-28). St. Louis: Elsevier.

CancerSource. (2005). *End of life issues.* Available from http://www.cancersource.com

CancerSource. (2006). *Loss, grief, and bereavement.* Available from http://www.cancersource.com/Search/37,CDR0000062828

Carlson, M.D., Gallo, W.T., & Bradley, E.H. (2004). Ownership status and patterns of care in hospice: Results from the National Home and Hospice Care Survey. *Medical Care, 42(5)*, 432-438.

Chochinov, H. (2006). Dying, dignity, and new horizons in palliative end-of-life care. *CA: Cancer Journal for Clinicians, 56(2)*, 84-103.

Cooney, G. (2005). *Integrating curative and palliative care: It can be done.* Session in *Highlights of the Sixth Annual Clinical Team Conference of the National Hospice and Palliative Care Organization (NHPCO).* Retrieved April 17, 2007, from http://www.medscape.com/viewprogram/4128

Coyne, P., Smith, T., Laird, J., Hansen, L., & Drake, D. (2005). Effectively starting and titrating intrathecal analgesic therapy in patients with refractory cancer pain. *Clinical Journal of Oncology Nursing, 9(5)*, 581-583.

Dawson, R., Sellers, D., Spross, J., Jablonski, E., Hoyer, D., & Solomon, M. (2005). Do patients' beliefs act as barriers to effective pain management behaviors and outcomes in patients with cancer-related or noncancer-related pain? *Oncology Nursing Forum, 32(2)*, 363-374.

Duggleby, W., & Berry, P. (2005). Transitions and shifting goals of care for palliative patients and their families. *Clinical Journal of Oncology Nursing, 9(4)*, 425-428.

Ferrell, B. (2005a). *National guidelines for quality palliative care.* From session at *Annual Assembly of the American Academy of Hospice and Palliative Medicine and the Hospice and Palliative Nurses Association.* Available from http://www.medscape.com/viewprogram/3782

Ferrell, B. (2005b). *Nursing education in palliative care*. From session at *Annual Assembly of the American Academy of Hospice and Palliative Medicine and the Hospice and Palliative Nurses Association*. Available from http://www.medscape.com/viewprogram/3782

Given, B., Wyatt, G., Given, C., Sherwood, P, Gift, A., DeVoss, D., & Rahbar, M. (2004). Burden and depression among caregivers of patients with cancer at the end of life. *Oncology Nursing Forum, 31*(6), 1105-1117.

Kinlaw, K. (2005). Ethical issues in palliative care. *Seminars in Oncology Nursing, 21*(1), 63-68.

Kuebler, K. (2005). Palliative care. *Clinical Journal of Oncology Nursing, 9*(5), 617–620.

Lussier, D., & Pappagallo, M. (2004). 10 most commonly asked questions about the use of opioids for chronic pain. *Neurologist, 10*(4), 221-224.

McMillan, S., Tittle, M., Hagan, S., & Small, B. (2005). Training pain resource nurses: Changes in their knowledge and attitudes. *Oncology Nursing Forum, 32*(4), 835-842.

National Cancer Institute. (2002). *End of life care: Questions and answers*. Retrieved June 11, 2007, from http://www.cancer.gov/cancer-topics/factsheet/support/end-of-life-care

National Cancer Institute. (2005). *Advance directives*. Retrieved October 31, 2006, from http://www.cancer.gov/cancertopics/factsheet/support/advance-directives

National Consensus Project for Quality Palliative Care. (2004). *Clinical practice guidelines for quality palliative care*. Retrieved October 31, 2006, from http://www.nationalconsensusproject.org/Guideline.pdf

National Family Caregivers Association. (2006). *Caregiver statistics*. Retrieved October 31, 2006, from http://www.thefamilycaregiver.org/who/stats.cfm#1

National Home and Hospice Care Data. (2004). National Center for Health Statistics. *Access to hospice care: Expanding bounderies, overcoming barriers*. Available from http://www.cdc.gov/nchs/about/major/nhhcsd/nhhcsdes.htm

Northouse, L. (2005). Helping families of patients with cancer. *Oncology Nursing Forum, 32*(4), 743-750.

Portenoy, R. (2005). Three-step analgesic ladder for management of cancer pain. *Oncology Special Edition, 8*, 1-4.

Quiles, K. (2005). *Spiritual awareness and the interdisciplinary team*. Session in *Highlights of the Sixth Annual Clinical Team Conference of the National Hospice and Palliative Care Organization (NHPCO)*. Retrieved April 17, 2007, from http://www.medscape.com/viewprogram/4128

Razilla, R., Anderson, J. (2001) An overview of oncology clinical trials. From *Oncology special edition* (4th ed., pp 115-120). New York: McMahon.

Rhiner, M., Palos, G., & Termini, M. (2004). Managing breakthrough pain: A clinical review with three case studies using oral transmucosal fentanyl citrate. *Clinical Journal of Oncology Nursing, 8*(5), 507-512.

Rutledge, D., & Kuebler, K. (2005). Applying evidence to palliative care. *Seminars in Oncology Nursing, 21*(1), 36-43.

Stockler, M., Vardy, J., Pillai, A., & Warr, D. (2004). Acetaminophen (paracetamol) improves pain and well-being in people with advanced cancer already receiving a strong opioid regimen: A randomized, double-blind, placebo-controlled cross-over trial. *Journal of Clinical Oncology, 22*(16), 3389-3394.

The Joint Commission on Accreditation of Healthcare Organizations. (2006). *Comprehensive accreditation manual for hospitals: The official handbook (CAMH).* Available from http://www.jcrinc.com

University of New Mexico. (2001). Values history. Retrieved April 17, 2007, from http://hsc.unm.edu/ethics/pdf/Values_History.doc

Vallerand, A., Riley-Doucet, C., Hasenau, S., & Templin, T. (2004). Improving cancer pain management by homecare nurses. *Oncology Nursing Forum, 31*(4), 809–816.

Volker, D., Kahn, D., & Penticuff, J. (2004). Patient control and end-of-life care, Part II: The advanced practice nurse perspective. *Oncology Nursing Forum, 31*(5), 954–960.

World Health Organization. (n.d.). *WHO's pain ladder.* Retrieved June 11, 2007, from http://www.who.int/cancer/palliative/painladder/en/index.html

CHAPTER 23

INTERNET USE AND CANCER CARE

CHAPTER OBJECTIVE

After completing this chapter, the reader will be able to recall ways to evaluate content disseminated on the Internet and relate ways to access accurate, timely, and understandable cancer content.

LEARNING OBJECTIVES

After studying this chapter, the reader will be able

1. identify subpopulations that most frequently seek health-related information online.

2. specify sites on the Internet that provide accurate and timely cancer-related information.

3. identify guidelines for patients who seek cancer-related information on the Internet.

4. list criteria to evaluate Internet web sites.

INTRODUCTION

The Internet is now a part of clinical practice. Patients, family members, and colleagues keep up with the explosion of information now readily available via the World Wide Web. To make sure that patients best use the Web, nurses should share with them guidelines for assessing Web-based information. Using the web for communication and support is also integral to providing comprehensive care.

EXPLOSION OF INTERNET USE

The World Wide Web offers an unprecedented tool of convenience and personal control to access abundant cancer-related information. Yet not all information on the Internet is timely and accurate. With the bounty of possibilities that go with being online, patients and professionals need to know how to search for quality information and where to find it (CancerSource, 2005; National Cancer Institute [NCI], 2005; Oncology Nursing Society [ONS], 2006).

Health care professionals search the Web for research findings, new treatments, and information to better understand their patients' diseases. Health care professionals have learned to rely on Web sites that provide clear and accurate information for their practices and their patients.

Patients and Family Members Seeking Information

Accessing medical information from the Internet has been shown to be more common among those with higher incomes, with higher education and from a nonminority race (Nguyen, Hara, & Chlebowski, 2005). Nevertheless, more people representing multiethnic, multilingual, and lower socioeconomic groups are using the Internet to access health care information (Nguyen et al., 2005). An estimated 73% of adults in the United

States are online, with 65% of them having access at home. Of those, 7% are 65 years or older (Murphy et al., 2005).

Those who research the experience of consumers who use the Web for information estimate that 6% to 43% of cancer patients seek information about their disease and treatment using the Internet (Nguyen et al., 2005).

Results from 2003 surveys estimate that 80% of Internet users (about 93 million Americans, or half of American adults) have searched the Internet for health information. The majority of those seeking health-related information said that information found on the Internet was useful; 47% of health seekers reported that the information influenced their health care decisions and provider interactions (Dickerson, Boehmke, Ogle, & Brown, 2005).

The majority of those who use the Internet for information bring that information to their physicians and nurses. In another study, nurses reported increased frequency of patient encounters involving discussions of Internet information (Dickerson et al., 2005; Dickerson, Boehmke, Ogle, & Brown, 2006).

EVALUATING INFORMATION

Internet-based and disseminated information continues to flourish with limited regulation. No one, accepted oversight body guarantees the veracity of Internet-based information. Therefore, those using the Internet need to establish criteria to identify reliable information and health care advice.

Several organizations offer criteria lists to guide Internet searches. Table 23-1 provides one of the published criteria. The Internet Health care Coalition offers a set of tips to guide Internet information searches (see Table 23-2).

Oncology nurses can coach patients and family members to look for key pieces of information on a Web site's home page, including the date the site

---

TABLE 23-1: SUGGESTED CRITERIA TO EVALUATE HEALTH CARE WEB SITES

Principles of the Health on the Net Foundation Code of Conduct

- Authority
- Complementarity
- Confidentiality
- Attribution
- Justifiability
- Transparency of authorship
- Transparency of sponsorship
- Honesty in advertising and editorial policy

Note. From "HON code of conduct for medical and health web sites," by Health on the Net Foundation, 2006. Retrieved October 31, 2006, from http://www.hon.ch/HONcode/conduct.html

---

TABLE 23-2: TIPS TO ACCESS RELIABLE INTERNET CONTENT

1. Choose an online health information source like you would choose your doctor.

2. Make sure you can validate the source of information.

3. Question sites that claim they are the only source of information.

4. Do not be fooled by comprehensive lists of links.

5. Find out if a site is professionally managed and guided by an editorial board of experts.

6. For clinical content, make sure the site includes the date of publication and when it was last modified.

7. Any sponsorship, advertising, underwriting, or potential conflicts of interest should be stated and separated from the editorial content.

8. Avoid online physicians who claim to be able to treat you.

9. Review the Web's privacy statement. Make sure any information you provide is kept absolutely confidential.

10. Use your common sense. Get more than one opinion. Shop around.

(Internet Healthcare Coalition, 2006)

was last updated, links to a disclosure of funding, privacy statement, and descriptions of the qualifications of the information provider.

Cancer-Related Web Sites

Credible, reliable web sites for cancer-related information have emerged, augmenting reliable information available from textbooks and peer-reviewed journals. Table 23-3 provides a list of selected sites known for their reliability and ongoing attention to providing timely, updated information. Many sites have categorized information, geared to specific cancers and treatments as well as target readerships (professionals, patients, the general public).

In addition to cancer information provided online by the NCI or the American Cancer Society (ACS), other reliable sites are those sponsored by nonprofit organizations (e.g., ONS Online, CancerCare, Oncolink) or hospital or health care facility web sites (University of Texas M.D. Anderson Cancer Center, Fox Chase Cancer Center, Dana-Farber Harvard Cancer Center).

Keeping the criteria for evaluating web sites in mind, sources of cancer information can be categorized into these areas:

- **Familiar resources:** Example: NCI
- **Activist organizations:** Examples: ACS, Leukemia and Lymphoma Society
- **Health portals:** Example: CancerSource
- **Pharmaceutical and biotechnology companies:** Examples: Amgen, Bristol-Myers Squibb, Novartis
- **Professional organizations:** Examples: ONS, American Society of Clinical Oncology (http://www.asco.org), Oncolink (published by the University of Pennsylvania; www.oncolink.upenn.edu)
- **Individual information provider:** Individual health care professionals and patients

E-MAIL AS A FORM OF COMMUNICATION

E-mail is a way for patients to exchange information with their health care team and one another. Thus, e-mail provides a built-in form of documentation for exchanges with patients. That said, when using e-mail, nurses must remember to protect confidentiality of information and communication. Here are some technical aspects of using e-mail for patient communication:

- **Turn-around time:** Both parties should agree on an acceptable turn-around time for e-mail and conditions when a telephone call or a page should be used instead of e-mail.

TABLE 23-3: SELECTED WEB SITES: GENERAL INFORMATION

American Cancer Society (ACS)	http://www.cancer.org
Cancer Care	http://www.cancercare.org
CancerSource	http://cancersource.com
Cancer Patient Education Network (CPEN)	http://cpen.nci.nih.gov
National Cancer Institute at National Institutes of Health	http://www.cancernet.nci.nih.gov
National Cancer Institute (NCI)	http://www.cancer.gov
National Cancer Institute (NCI), CancerNet™	
National Cancer Institute (NCI), CancerTrials	
National Cancer Institute (NCI), Cancer Information Service	
OncoLink	http://www.oncolink.upenn.edu
Oncology Nursing Society	http://www.ons.org
People living with Cancer	http://www.plwc.org

- **Privacy:** Patients should be notified if office staff triages e-mail and should be given the opportunity to "opt-out" of e-mail communication for this reason.

- **Content:** Human immunodeficiency virus testing, workers' compensation, mental illness, and other sensitive issues are best discussed in person, or at least over the telephone.

- **Archiving messages:** Patients should know what happens to their e-mail messages after they are received, whether they are placed in the medical record or archived in some other way.

(Dickerson et al., 2006)

INTERNET SUPPORT GROUPS

Patient use of the Internet to make connections and feel supported continues to expand, crossing previously distinct ethnic, geographic, cultural, and socioeconomic boundaries. For example, men have been shown to gravitate to the advantages of online support opportunities; women have long sought support and are expanding that need by participating in online forums (Im, Chee, Tsai, Lin, & Cheng, 2005).

Patients report that Internet-based support groups, blogs, and online connections offer many advantages. Among them:

- retrieving and filtering Internet information according to personal situation by Internet-savvy people in patient support networks

- seeking hope from the newest treatment options while coping with fear in manageable "bytes," self-care for personal illness situations with meaningful information regarding symptom management

- empowering patients as partners when Internet information serves as a second opinion in decision making and validating treatment decisions

- providing peer support—for example, patients using the Internet to find support and information have discovered ways to live with cancer as a chronic illness instead of a death sentence.

(CancerSource, 2005; Dickerson et al., 2006)

Table 23-4 provides a list of Internet-based support groups for cancer patients. This list represents only a fraction of online support groups that exist and continue to flourish using the Web.

To put patients' use of Internet support groups in context, a 2005 survey reported these insights from nurses in practice:

- Patient support networks are important in processing information.

- Internet use encourages patients' desire for involvement in care decisions.

- The necessity for nurses' Internet use is patient driven.

- Nurses should be aware of the social influence of technology in affecting trust and confidence in health care providers, as well as encouraging or discouraging partner relationships.

(Dickerson et al., 2006)

A clearinghouse found on the Web, the Association of Cancer Online Resources, Inc., maintains a large collection of cancer-related resources. OncoChat (www.oncochat.org) is a peer support resource site for cancer patients to share experiences.

Worth repeating, the burgeoning use of the Internet provides a wealth of forums and cancer information. But the accuracy of the information in circulation—exchanged in these chat rooms and support groups—can be suspect. Health care professionals need to be vigilant in monitoring their patients' understanding of their diseases and treatments, providing the accuracy check for any information they hear from other venues (Murphy et al., 2005). These forums have no quality control on accuracy or perspective (Cancerindex, 2004).

TABLE 23-4: SELECTED ONLINE SUPPORT GROUPS

Cancer Pain

http://cancer-pain.org/
This site was created to help cancer patients receive the pain treatment they deserve. It contains information about cancer pain, its causes and available treatments as well as links to online groups.

General

http://www.oncochat.org/
OncoChat is a real-time global support community for people whose lives have been touched by cancer. Oncochat does not offer medical advice or professional counseling. Oncochat does offer lots of hugs and understanding from people who share similar experiences and emotions.

Disease-Specific Sites

http://www.leiomyosarcoma.info/
A patient-oriented site devoted to esophageal cancer, the EC Cafe contains information gathered by esophageal cancer patients and nonmedical caregivers. The purpose is to help others that are coping with esophageal cancer, possibly for the first time, to gain insight into this disease.

http://www.liferaftgroup.org/
A patient-oriented site devoted to gastrointestinal stromal tumor (GIST). The Life Raft Group (LRG) provides support, through information, education, and innovative research to patients with GIST.

http://www.acor.org/leukemia/
Leukemia Links is a guide to Internet accessible information about all types of leukemia. The site is maintained by two cancer patients.

http://www.acor.org/mm/
Stories of multiple myeloma survivors. This site is dedicated to the memory of June Brazil, one of the original list owners of the MYELOMA list.

http://blcwebcafe.org/
Bladder Cancer WebCafe is an online community for bladder cancer patients and those who care for them. It covers treatment options, chemoprevention guidelines, survivor stories, a support group, and more.

http://www.pancreatica.org/
This site provides a wealth of information about pancreatic cancer, as well as access to the world's largest listing of clinical trials against pancreatic cancer.

http://www.lungcanceronline.org/
Lung Cancer Online is a gateway to lung cancer resources for the benefit of people with lung cancer and their families. It is intended to facilitate the time-consuming and often frustrating process of learning about lung cancer, treatment options, and support services.

http://www.acor.org/tcrc/
The Testicular Cancer Resource Center is a charitable organization devoted to helping people understand testicular and extragonadal germ cell tumors. Specifically, it provides accurate and timely information about these tumors and their treatment to anyone and everyone interested. The site has information for patients, caregivers, family, friends, and physicians. The site maintainers rely on the support of some of the finest doctors in the field.

http://www.ccalliance.org/
The Colon Cancer Alliance is an organization of colon and rectal cancer survivors, caregivers, people with a genetic predisposition to the disease, and other individuals touched by colorectal cancer. Colorectal cancer is the second leading cancer killer in the United States. The Colon Cancer Alliance is committed to ending the suffering caused by cancers of the colon, rectum, appendix, and anus.

http://www.myeloma.org/
The International Myeloma Foundation helps everyone battling multiple myeloma (patients, families, friends, caregivers, and the medical community).

Note. From *Special Online Resources for Support and Information*, by Association of Cancer Online Resources, 2007. Retrieved June 11, 2007, from http://www.acor.org/support.html

Patients, especially those familiar with navigating the Internet and open-forum sites, can present nurses with all sorts of information. Nurses cannot dissuade patients from visiting those forums but can coach patients on how to evaluate what they are reading. To better guide patients as they visit these sites, nurses need to share the criteria approaches that Internet experts have developed (Dickerson et al., 2006). Nurses can enhance the trust of a nurse-patient relationship by continuing to be an advocate and primary information source for quality Web-based information (ACS, 2006; Dickerson et al., 2006).

SUMMARY

Because the Internet is the tool of our time—and for generations to come—it is important for nurses to coach patients on how to best use it. This includes recommending reliable Web sites for information and support and teaching patients how best to assess the accuracy of Web-based information. E-mail, blogs, and support groups speed up and broaden the network of information available. Providing education to patients about astute use of the Internet should be part of any nurse's state-of-the-art practice.

EXAM QUESTIONS

CHAPTER 23
Questions 93-96

Note: Choose the option that BEST answers each question.

93. Surveys indicate that those who seek health care information on the Internet have

    a. higher incomes than the rest of the population.

    b. many children.

    c. a minority race heritage.

    d. a fear of information.

94. A site that presents reliable oncology information is

    a. www.cancer.org.

    b. www.Ihavecancer.com.

    c. www.cancercures.com.

    d. www.yourmd.com.

95. To evaluate the reliability and credibility of content on the Internet, nurses should consider

    a. the Web site's source of funding.

    b. the volume of data on the site.

    c. the graphics on the site.

    d. the ease of the Web site navigation.

96. One indication that a Web site has reliable information is it provides

    a. many links to other sites.

    b. content with dates posted 1995 and earlier.

    c. no posted sponsorship or stated conflict of interest.

    d. reputable, validated information.

REFERENCES

American Cancer Society. (2006). *Cancer information on the internet.* Available from http://www.cancer.org

Association of Cancer Online Resources. (2007). *Special online resources for support and information.* Retrieved June 11, 2007, from http://www.acor.org/support.html

Cancerindex. (2004). *Guide to Internet resources for cancer.* Retrieved October 31, 2006, from http://www.cancerindex.org/clinks1.htm

CancerSource. (2005). *How to evaluate health information on the Internet: Questions and answers.* Retrieved April 17, 2007, from http://www.cancersource.com/Search/45,NCIWeb

Dickerson, S., Boehmke, M., Ogle, C., & Brown, J., (2005). Out of necessity: Oncology nurses' experiences integrating the Internet into practice. *Oncology Nursing Forum, 32*(2), 355-362.

Dickerson, S., Boehmke, M., Ogle, C., & Brown, J. (2006). Seeking and managing hope: Patients' experiences using the Internet for cancer care [Electronic version]. *Oncology Nursing Forum, 33*(1), E8-17. Retrieved October 31, 2006, from http://www.ons.org/publications/journals/ONF/volume33/issue1/330138.asp

Health on the Net Foundation. (2006). *HON code of conduct for medical and health web sites.* Retrieved October 31, 2006, from http://www.hon.ch/HONcode/conduct.html

Im, E., Chee, W., Tsai, H., Lin, L., & Cheng, C. (2005). Internet cancer support groups: A feminist analysis. *Cancer Nursing, 28*(1), 1-7.

Internet Healthcare Coalition. (2006). *Tips to access reliable Internet content.* Available from http://www.ihealthcoalition.org/content/tips.html

Murphy, C., Ballon, L., Culhane, B., Mafrica, L., McCorkle, M., & Worrall, L. (2005). Oncology Nursing Society Environmental Scan 2004 [Electronic version]. *Oncology Nursing Forum, 32*(4), 742. Retrieved October 31, 2006, from http://www.ons.org/publications/journals/ONF/Volume32/Issue4/3204742.asp

National Cancer Institute. (2005). *Cancer information sources.* Retrieved October 31, 2006, from http://www.cancer.gov/cancertopics/factsheet/Information/sources

Nguyen, K., Hara, B., & Chlebowski, R. (2005). Utility of two cancer organization websites for a multiethnic, public hospital oncology population: Comparative cross-sectional survey. *Journal of Medical Internet Research, 7*(3), e28.

Oncology Nursing Society. (2006). *Website reviews and awards.* Retrieved October 31, 2006, from http://www.ons.org/about/sitereviews.shtml

CHAPTER 24

PROFESSIONAL ISSUES IN ONCOLOGY NURSING

CHAPTER OBJECTIVE

After completing this chapter, the reader will be able to identify selected professional issues important to oncology nursing.

LEARNING OBJECTIVES

After studying this chapter, the reader will be able to

1. recognize one component of an ethical assessment.

2. identify two factors that affect the workplace of oncology nurses.

3. identify three categories in the OCN blueprint.

4. list two components of the Oncology Nursing Society's strategic plan for 2006.

INTRODUCTION

Oncology nurses face many challenges in their career that fall under the umbrella of professional practice. Among these challenges are workplace issues of retention, ethical behavior, and job burnout as well as educational and practice issues that are based on standards and guidelines of practice. This chapter highlights some of the issues facing the professional oncology nurse and reviews a few of the foundations for continued quality in professional practice.

ETHICAL ISSUES

Among the challenges of cancer nursing are the ethical issues that arise in providing care. Those that affect oncology nurses are:

*   open communication, including shared decision making among patients, family members ,and health care providers

*   informed consent, which includes providing information about benefits, risks, and alternatives of treatments; protecting the patient; ensuring autonomy of choice; and ensuring responsibility of actions by health care providers

*   communicating bad news

*   obligation to minimize pain and suffering

*   privacy and confidentiality.

(Nelson-Marten & Glover, 2005)

A key role in the nurse-patient relationship in cancer care is the role of the nurse as advocate. Advocacy is the active support of an important cause or assertion of a patient's choices or desires. To advocate for a patient, the nurse must know the patient's values. Moreover, to advocate successfully, the nurse should recognize his or her own set of values and identify any areas of conflict. Components of an ethical assessment are listed in Table 24-1.

TABLE 24-1: ETHICAL PRINCIPLES AND PRACTICAL EXAMPLES

Ethical Principle	Definition	Clinical Practice
Autonomy	Individual has the right to choose	Patient chooses to have advance directive
Beneficence	The act of doing good	Patient provided optimal mouth care
Fidelity	Being faithful in providing professional care	Patient given enough pain medication
Justice	Ensuring individuals receive their due	All patients treated with dignity and respect
Nonmalfeasance	Above all else, do no harm	Provide and ensure safe practice of delivering intravenous chemotherapy
Veracity	Truth telling	Inform patient about risks of clinical trials

Note. From "Ethical Dimensions in Cancer Care," by C. Sheridan, 2000. In B. Nevidjon & K. Sowers (Eds.), *A nurse's guide to cancer care* (p. 469-478). Philadelphia: Lippincott (http://lww.com). Reprinted with permission.

PROFESSIONALISM OF THE ONCOLOGY NURSE

Workplace Issues

Those who choose oncology nursing as the focus of their practice do so within an environment of significant workplace issues. Among them:

- More than 1 million new and replacement nurses will be needed to take care of our nation's population by 2012. From 2002 to 2012, the projected increase of nurses needed is 27% (Gullatte & Jirasakhiran, 2005).

- According to the U.S. Department of Labor, nursing is the top occupation in terms of job growth through 2012. By 2020, the nursing shortage is expected to affect at least 44 states as well as the District of Columbia.

- The number of first-time, U.S.-educated nursing school graduates who sat for their licensing exam declined by 10% from 1995 to 2004.

- In 2005, the average turnover rate of nurses leaving their positions was 13.9%. The vacancy rate was 16.1%. The registered nurse (RN) cost-per-hire was $2,821. Three-fourths of vacancies in hospitals are for nursing positions. In 2002, an estimated one in seven hospitals reported a severe nursing vacancy rate of more than 20% (Miller-Murphy et al., 2005). Job satisfaction is the most commonly cited reason for job turnover (Gullatte & Jirasakhiran, 2005).

- In 2004, the American Association of Colleges of Nursing (AACN) reported a 14.1% enrollment increase in baccalaureate programs in nursing. Yet nursing programs in 2004 turned away 32,797 qualified applicants because of limitations in sufficient numbers of faculty, clinical sites, classroom space, clinical preceptors, and money for programs (Fest, 2004).

- Government estimates state that in 2000 the average age of a working RN was 43.3 years. In 2000, the RN population under age 30 fell from 25.1% in 1980 to 9.1%. By 2010, 40% of all RNs will be age 50 or older.

- In 2000, the total RN population was 2,696,540, the lowest total number of nurses since 1980. An estimated 58.5% work full time in nursing, 23.2% work part time, and 18.3% do not work in nursing.

- Demographic changes, such as an aging population, more baby boomers, and longer life expectancy, continue to increase the need for more licensed nurses.

- A survey of nurses published in 2001 reported that 40% of nurses working in hospitals report dissatisfaction with their work. One of every three hospital nurses under age 30 plans to leave his or her job in the next 12 months (AACN, 2005).

- Nursing is often a second career, entered in the third or fourth decade of life (Miller-Murphy et al., 2005).

- A 2004 survey of ambulatory oncology nurses reports that 85% of those surveyed say that interaction with patients kept them working in their practice setting; the nature of their job is what they liked about their work (Ireland, DePalma, Arneson, Stark, & Williamson, 2004).

STRESS AND THE CAREGIVER

Professional Burnout

Burnout is a familiar problem to health care professionals. An estimated 61% of American families have both parents working outside of the home. Together, two parents work 81 hours a week outside of the home (Miller-Murphy et al., 2005). Down time is coveted. Nurses, like other professionals, share in the desire for nonwork time.

In oncology, the nature of the work exposes nurses to ongoing emotional, intellectual, and physical demands. Professional stress requires adaptation in the performance of a person's profes-

sional role. The impact of stress is intensified by a person who:

- is overly dedicated and committed
- needs control
- overidentifies with patients and families
- has strong dependency needs
- is a perfectionist
- has high expectations and goals
- has unclear personal boundaries
- is idealistic.

Coping effectively with stress is important not only for maintaining the health of individual caregivers but also for providing better nursing care for patients. Table 24-2 provides some common signs and symptoms of burnout (Gullatte & Jirasakhiran, 2005; Gwede, Johnsson, Roberts, & Cantor, 2005). Table 24-3 lists best practices for retention.

Caring for the Professional Caregiver

Because cancer is an experience that demands a great deal from both patients and caregivers, stress is inevitable. Finding ways to cope and deal with stress as a caregiver can contribute greatly to the length and satisfaction of a career in oncology nursing.

Coping involves recognizing job stressors. A variety of stress management strategies can be used once stressors are recognized. An understanding of these strategies is essential for both health care professionals and health care organizations. Strategies to address and manage both individual and organizational stress are listed in Table 24-4.

An important component of professional practice is addressing the stresses of the profession as a community—to maintain a healthy nursing workforce that is an integral part of a healthy society. Therefore, all nurses need to participate in stress-reduction efforts, advocating for their own health and the health of their colleagues (Gwede et al., 2005). Table 24-5 lists self-care behaviors for nurses.

TABLE 24-2: SIGNS AND SYMPTOMS OF BURNOUT

- Inability to concentrate
- Indecision
- Forgetfulness
- Sudden increased sensitivity to criticism
- Excessive defensiveness or anger when questioned about work performance
- Fatigue
- Exhaustion unrelated to actual lack of sleep
- Spike in sick days
- Regular complaints of feeling ill
- Indifference
- Noticeably decreased desire to get involved with new projects in areas that formerly were of interest
- Little or no interest in group activities
- Irritability
- Inability to cope with daily duties
- Expression of sense that everything is spinning out of control

TABLE 24-3: BEST PRACTICES FOR RETENTION

- Cultivate an interesting and accepting culture.
- Implement professional clinical and career ladders.
- Develop flexible work arrangements.
- Offer encouragement, praise, and recognition.
- Encourage direct manager-to-employee communication.
- Offer competitive compensation and benefits.
- Develop mentoring and preceptorship programs.
- Streamline paperwork.

(AACN, 2006; Friese, 2005; Gullatte & Jirasakhiran, 2005)

TABLE 24-4: STRATEGIES TO REDUCE STRESS

Strategies to address and manage both individual and organizational stress
- Having a sense of competence, control, or pleasure in work
- Having control over aspects of practice
- Managing one's lifestyle in a healthy way
- Developing a personal philosophy of illness, death, and professional role
- Leaving the work situation
- Distancing oneself from patients and their families
- Increasing education
- Having an outside support system and a sense of humor

Organizational strategies for managing stress
- Team philosophy and support building
- Staffing policies
- Administrative policies
- Collegial relationships
- Formalized ways of handling decisions
- Good orientation and educational programs
- Job flexibility
- Support groups

(Gwede et al., 2005)

EVIDENCE-BASED PRACTICE

Evidence-based practice (EBP) incorporates evidence from research, clinical expertise, and preferences into decisions about the health care of individual patients. EBP is a way to approach clinical decision making to improve day-to-day patient care and outcomes, underscored by evidence and state-of-the-art treatment recommendations (Cooke et al., 2004).

Nursing-sensitive patient outcomes (NSPOs) now drive practice in the work of oncology nurses at the bedside, in clinics, in research, in education,

TABLE 24-5: SELF-CARE FOR THE ONCOLOGY NURSE

- Identify behaviors that lead to burnout.
- Develop coping activities to change those behaviors.
- Develop self-support structures.
- Manage potential burnout by getting in touch with feelings.
- Learn to say no; prioritize important tasks.
- Find time for exercise and relaxation.
- Admit when overcommitted.
- Strive for balance in personal and professional life.

(Gwede et al., 2005)

and in policy (Friese, 2005). The intent of EBP and NSPOs is to define results based on nursing care, uniform the delivery of care, ensure quality based on that uniformity, and improve the quality of care.

Considerable work continues to establish EBP as the foundation for oncology nursing practice (Friese, 2005; Friese & Beck, 2004; Krebs, 2005; Rutledge, DePalma, & Cunningham, 2004). Informing practice through EBP inquiry involves a multistep process of identifying and critiquing available data about the problem.

Figure 24-1 highlights the process of establishing EBP for any given patient outcome.

Among sources for EBP are:

- The Cochrane Library (accessible online at http://hiru.mcmaster.ca/cochrane/cochrane/cdsr .htm)
- Medline's PubMed (a free service that can be found at http://www.ncbi.nlm.nih.gov/ PubMed/)
- CINAHL database (http://www.cinahl.com/ cdirect/cdirect.htm)

Results of the Oncology Nursing Society 2004 research priorities survey (for 2005-2008) are listed in Table 24-6.

EDUCATION ISSUES

A 2002 survey revealed that 96% of Americans believe that nurses play a significant role in a patient's welfare and recovery. The survey also reported that 73% of consumers are more likely to select a hospital that employs a high percentage of nurses with additional specialty certifications (Miller-Murphy et al., 2005).

FIGURE 24-1: EVIDENCE-BASED EDUCATION GUIDELINES

Types of Evidence	Strength of Evidence
Research-Based Evidence	*Strongest*
• Meta-analysis of multiple controlled clinical trials	
• Experimental studies, such as well-controlled, randomized clinical trials	
• Systematic reviews of all types of research	
• Multiple nonexperimental studies, including descriptive, correlational, and qualitative research	
• Published EBP guidelines, such as those published by professional organizations	
Non-Research-Based Evidence	
• Case studies	
• Program evaluation, quality improvement data, or case reports	
• Opinions of experts (e.g., standards of practice guidelines)	*Weakest*

Note. From *Evidence-Based Education Guidelines* (n.d.) by Oncology Nursing Society.
Retrieved April 17, 2007 from http://www.ons.org/nursingEd/documents/pdfs/guidelines.pdf. Reprinted with permission.

TABLE 24-6: ONCOLOGY NURSING SOCIETY 2004 RESEARCH PRIORITIES SURVEY RESULTS

20 Top Research Priorities for 2005-2008
(Listed under each questionnaire category)

From Cancer Continuum of Care
- Screening and early detection of cancer
- Prevention of cancer and cancer risk reduction
- Palliative care
- Cancer recurrence
- Curative treatment and care
- Late effects of treatment
- Hospice and end of life
- Initial cancer diagnosis

From Health Promotion/Disease Prevention Behaviors
- Tobacco use and exposure

From Communication and Decision Making
- Participation in decision making about treatment in advanced disease
- Patient and family education
- Participation in decision making about treatment
- Nurses as advocates
- Ethical issues

From Cancer Symptom Management
- Pain
- Fatigue and lack of energy
- Cognitive impairment and mental status changes

From Behavioral/Psychosocial Aspects of Cancer
- Quality of life

From Health Services
- Evidence-based practice
- Patient outcomes of cancer care

(Berger et al., 2005)

Knowledge becomes obsolete at a record pace. It is estimated that half of the medical knowledge that a freshman in college learns is obsolete, revised, or taken for granted by the time he or she becomes a senior (Miller-Murphy et al., 2005). Therefore, lifelong learning is key to keeping current and safe in practice. Because of specialty knowledge, subspecialties become a focus to maintain competency in practice.

Recruitment and education of specialty nurses are often more challenging and expensive than recruitment and education of generalist nurses. Specialty nurses' expertise is generally gained from on-the-job experiences (Gullatte & Jirasakhiran, 2005). That on-the-job experience, coupled with a curriculum for the specialty, provides direction for the generalist nurse to become specialized and grow in that specialty. Table 24-7 lists the most recent Oncology Nursing Society (ONS) Educational Blueprint, which provides the foundation for oncology nursing practice. (Further information about the Oncology Nursing Society follows under "Advocacy").

Certification

The role of the oncology nurse as a subspecialty within nursing is crucial in the delivery of quality health care for cancer patients. Toward fostering that specialty and expanding the pipeline of educated oncology nurses, the profession has established certification standards. In 1984, the ONS chartered the Oncology Nursing Certification Corporation (ONCC). The ONCC was tasked with establishing criteria for oncology nursing certification so that a body of knowledge and associated competencies would be clear to nurses, the health care system, and the public.

Since the ONCC was established, many nurses have taken the OCN certification exam, which recognizes the nurse's basic knowledge of oncology nursing. The test blueprint for the OCN exam is outlined in Table 24-8. Nurses continue to promote the specialty of oncology nursing through certification, based on the knowledge base established in this blueprint.

In 1995, the Advanced Oncology Nursing Certification (AOCN) exam was established using, as the exam foundation, the AOCN blueprint. AOCN certification recognizes advanced practice

TABLE 24-7: ONCOLOGY NURSING SOCIETY EDUCATIONAL AGENDA FOR 2007

Professional Practice Issues
- Advanced practice
- Legislative and health policy process
- Evidenced-based practice
- International collaboration
- Technology
- Leadership development and career development
- Certification
- Fundamentals of oncology nursing

Clinical Care
- Prevention and early detection
- Safeguards of oncology care
- Cultural issues
- Genetics
- New agents and approaches
- End-of-life and palliative care
- Ethics
- Complementary and alternative medicine
- Symptom management and psychosocial issues

Care Delivery Issues
- Continuity of care
- Health care economics
- Navigating the system and accessing care
- Nursing shortage
- Consumer awareness

Note. From *Oncology Nursing Society 2007 Education Agenda* (2007) by Oncology Nursing Society. Retrieved June 11, 2007, from http://www.ons.org/cecentral/agenda.shtml. Reprinted with permission. For the most recent information, go to www.ons.org

nurses within the specialty of oncology nursing. AOCN certification is renewable for 4 years, and earned with completion of a required number of continuing education credits or by retaking the certification exam.

In 2005, advanced specialty exams for nurse practitioners (AOCNP) and clinical nurse specialists (AOCNS) were established (ONCC, 2006). (These two certifications replace the AOCN certification. However, those with AOCN certification have grand-fathered certification, as long as they update their certification by completing continuing education requirements.) A summary of the AOCNP/AOCNS test blueprint is listed in Table 24-9.

As of 2006, more than 24,000 nurses had achieved oncology nurse certification, including 21,195 OCNs; 1,261 CPONs; 1,381 AOCNs; 313 AOCNPs; and 128 AOCNs. (CPON stands for Certified Pediatric Oncology Nurse.)

Advocacy

As leaders in the community, nurses who care for cancer patients can partner with other constituencies to achieve legislative gains. A 2004 survey of ONS members identified these five areas as top legislative priorities:

- reforming the health care system to overcome barriers to quality care for all

- ensuring access to pain control and symptom management from diagnosis through end of life

- ensuring private insurance coverage for cancer screening and early detection

- increasing Medicare reimbursement for oncology nursing and practice expenses

- increasing federal funding for research, early detection, prevention, and risk reduction (Miller-Murphy et al., 2004).

That community involvement extends to the professional community of oncology nurses.

In the early 1970s, nurses with a vision to see oncology nursing as a specialty joined together to establish the ONS. The organization, incorporated in 1975, has grown in 2006 to more than 33,000 members, with 224 local chapters and 30 special interest groups. The ONS has been one of the major organizations that support nurses' quest of an ever-expanding knowledge base. That knowledge base is the foundation that provides quality patient care and influences the patient's experience of cancer treatment.

From its inception, ONS has published a wide variety of position papers (see Table 24-10). Its current strategic plan includes these goals:

text continues on page 376

TABLE 24-8: OCN BLUEPRINT (1 OF 4)

Weight 36%	Content Area
	I. Quality of Life

A. Comfort

(physiology, risk factors, prevention, and management utilizing the nursing process)
- Pain
- Fatigue
- Pruritus
- Sleep disorders
- Dyspnea
- Fever and chills

B. Coping

(risk factors, prevention, and management utilizing the nursing process)
- Spiritual distress
- Financial concerns
- Emotional distress
- Social dysfunction
- Loss and grief
- Anxiety
- Altered body image
- Alopecia
- Cultural issues
- Loss of personal control
- Depression
- Survivorship issues

C. Sexuality

(physiology, risk factors, prevention, and management utilizing the nursing process)
- Reproductive issues
- Sexual dysfunction

D. Symptom management and supportive care
- Dying and death
- Local, state, and national resources
- Blood products
- Enteral and parenteral nutrition
- Rehabilitation
- Vascular access devices
- Pharmacologic interventions
  - Antimicrobials
  - Anti-inflammatory agents
  - Antiemetics
  - Analgesic regimens
  - Psychotropic drugs
  - Growth factors
- Nonpharmacologic interventions (e.g., heat, massage, imagery)

TABLE 24-8: OCN BLUEPRINT (2 OF 4)

13% **II. Protective Mechanisms**
(physiology, risk factors, prevention, and management utilizing the nursing process)
- Alterations in mobility
- Neutropenia
- Thrombocytopenia
- Alterations in skin integrity
- Neuropathies
- Alterations in mental status
- Infection
- Hemorrhage

10% **III. Gastrointestinal and Urinary Function**
(physiology, risk factors, prevention, and management utilizing the nursing process)
A. Alterations in nutrition
- Dysphagia
- Anorexia
- Mucositis
- Xerostomia
- Esophagitis
- Nausea
- Vomiting
- Taste alterations
- Electrolyte imbalances
- Weight changes
- Cachexia
- Ascites

B. Alterations in elimination
- Incontinence
- Constipation
- Diarrhea
- Bowel obstruction
- Ostomies, urinary diversions
- Renal dysfunction

8% **IV. Cardiopulmonary Function**
(physiology, risk factors, prevention, and management utilizing the nursing process)
A. Alterations in ventilation
- Anatomical or surgical alterations
- Pulmonary toxicity related to cancer therapy
- Anemia
- Pleural effusions

B. Alterations in circulation
- Lymphedema
- Cardiovascular toxicity related to cancer therapy
- Fluid and electrolyte imbalances
- Thrombotic events

TABLE 24-8: OCN BLUEPRINT (3 OF 4)

7%   **V. Oncologic Emergencies**
(physiology, risk factors, prevention, and management utilizing the nursing process)
   A. Metabolic
- Disseminated intravascular coagulation (DIC)
- Syndrome of inappropriate antidiuretic hormone secretion (SIADH)
- Septic shock
- Tumor lysis syndrome
- Anaphylaxis
- Hypercalcemia

   B. Structural
- Cardiac tamponade
- Spinal cord compression
- Superior vena cava syndrome
- Increased intracranial pressure

12%   **VI. Scientific Basis for Practice**
   A. Carcinogenesis
   B. Immunology
   C. Genetics
   D. Specific cancers
- Pathophysiology
- Diagnostic measures
- Prognosis

   E. Classification
       – Tumor classification
       – Staging
       – Grading

   F. Major treatment modalities (goals and approaches, indications, mechanisms of action, safety, patient and family education)
- Surgery
- Radiation
- Biotherapy
- Antineoplastic agents
- Bone marrow transplant
- Unproven alternative therapies

3%   **VII. Health Promotion**
   A. Epidemiology
   B. Prevention
- Risk factors
- Prevention strategies

   C. Early detection
- Health history
- Physical exam
- Screening methods and recommendations

TABLE 24-8: OCN BLUEPRINT (4 OF 4)

11%	**VIII. Professional Performance**
	A. **Application of Statement on the Scope and Standards of Oncology Nursing Practice**
	B. **Appropriate sources of data for evidence-based practice**
	C. **Education process (teaching and learning principles)**
	D. **Legal issues**
	E. **Ethical issues**
	F. **Patient advocacy**
	G. **Quality assurance**
	H. **Professional development**
	I. **Multidisciplinary collaboration**

Note. From *2007 Oncology Nursing Certification Test Bulletin* by Oncology Nursing Certification Corporation (2007). Retrieved June 12, 2007 from http://www.oncc.org/getcertified/TestInformation/docs/bulletin07.pdf. Reprinted with permission.

TABLE 24-9: AOCNP/AOCNS TEST BLUEPRINT SUMMARY (1 OF 2)

Weight	Content Area
4%	**I. Cancer Screening, Prevention, Early Detection, and Genetic Risk**
	A. Risk factors and at-risk populations
	B. Prevention, risk reduction, screening and early detection guidelines
	C. Hereditary cancer evaluation and counseling
8%	**II. Cancer Diagnosis and Staging**
	A. History and physical
	B. Diagnostic testing and results (including pathology and tumor markers)
	C. Presentation, common metastatic sites, and prognosis
	D. Staging guidelines
20%	**III. Cancer Treatment Modalities**
	A. Chemotherapy (including hormonal and targeted)
	B. Surgery
	C. Radiation therapy
	D. Biological therapy (e.g., monoclonal antibodies, radioimmunotherapy, gene therapy)
	E. Blood and marrow transplantation
	F. Multimodality therapies
	G. Complementary and alternative therapies
	H. Implications of comorbid conditions
	I. Side effects of treatment
	J. Clinical trials
19%	**IV. Acute, Chronic, and Late Symptom Management**
	A. Etiology and patterns of symptoms (related to disease and treatment)
	B. Toxicity and symptom rating scales
	C. Pharmacological interventions (e.g., analgesics, antiemetics, laxatives, antimicrobials)
	D. Nonpharmacological interventions (e.g., relaxation techniques, hypnosis, biofeedback, art/music therapy)
	E. Procedural interventions (e.g., paracentesis, thoracentesis, radiation)
	F. Complementary and alternative therapies
	G. Delivery systems (e.g., PCAs, VADs, pumps)

TABLE 24-9: AOCNP/AOCNS TEST BLUEPRINT SUMMARY (2 OF 2)

12%	**V. Oncologic Emergencies** A. Risk factors B. Etiology C. Prevention D. Assessment E. Management
15%	**VI. Psychosocial Management** A. Risk factors for psychosocial disturbances (e.g., comorbidities, specific treatment, lack of social support) B. Assessment techniques C. Sexuality D. Pharmacological interventions (e.g., anxiolytics, antidepressants) E. Nonpharmacological interventions (e.g., relaxation techniques, hypnosis, biofeedback, art/music therapy) F. Coping methods G. Family dynamics H. Diversity (e.g., cultural, lifestyle, religious)
5%	**VII. Coordination of Multidisciplinary Care** A. Roles of health care team members B. Rehabilitation C. Survivorship D. Community resources
9%	**VIII. Professional Practice** A. Ethical and legal issues (e.g., informed consent, advance directives) B. Documentation requirements (e.g., legal, regulatory, insurance reimbursement) C. Diagnostic and procedural coding D. Patient and family education E. Continuous quality improvement methods F. Advanced practice standards G. Health care legislation H. Licensing, certification, and credentialing issues
5%	**IX. End-of-Life Care** A. End-of-life symptom management B. Family support and education C. Grief and bereavement process D. Settings for care (e.g., home, hospice, inpatient)
3%	**X. Research Utilization**

Note. From *2007 Oncology Nursing Certification Test Bulletin* by Oncology Nursing Certification Corporation. Retrieved June 12, 2007 from http://www.oncc.org/getcertified/TestInformation/docs/bulletin07.pdf Reprinted with permission.

- Promote the integration of new scientific information and technology into existing and emerging roles of the oncology nurse.

- Create an environment where all members develop leadership skills as an essential component of their practice.

- Promote a coordinated effort to ensure quality cancer care.

- Increase organizational vitality and visibility.

TABLE 24-10: SELECTED ONCOLOGY NURSING SOCIETY POSITION STATEMENTS

Nursing Practice
- Breast Cancer Screening
- ONS and Geriatric Oncology Consortium Joint Position on Cancer Care in the Older Adult
- Cancer Pain Management
- Cancer Predisposition Genetics Testing and Risk Assessment Counseling
- End-of Life Care (with Association of Oncology Social Work)
- Oncology Services in the Ambulatory Setting
- Patient Safety
- Prevention and Early Detection of Cancer in the United States
- Rehabilitation of People With Cancer (with Association of Rehabilitation Nurses)
- Use of Complementary, Alternative, and Integrative Therapies in Cancer Care

Education, Certification, and Role Delineation
- Education of the RN, Who Administers and Cares for the Individual Receiving Chemotherapy and Biotherapy
- Identification of Registered Nurses in the Workplace
- Oncology Certification for Nurses
- Role of the Advanced Practice Nurse in Oncology Care
- Role of the Oncology Nurse in Cancer Genetic Counseling
- Use of Unlicensed Assistive Personnel in Cancer Care

Ethics and Human Rights
- ONS, ONS Foundation, ONCC, ONSEdge Commercial Support
- The Nurse's Responsibility to the Patient Requesting Assisted Suicide

Cancer Research
- Cancer Research and Cancer Clinical Trials

Health Policy and Consumer Advocacy
- Ensuring High-Quality Cancer Care in the Medicare Program
- Global and Domestic Tobacco Use
- The Impact of the National Nursing Shortage on Quality Cancer Care
- Quality Cancer Care

Note. From *About Oncology Nursing Society Positions* (n.d.) by Oncology Nursing Society. Retrieved June 11, 2007, from http://www.ons.org/publications/positions/. Reprinted with permission. For the most recent information, go to www.ons.org

Strategic Plan

In an effort to define oncology nursing practice and clarify the nurse with this special knowledge to the public, ONS has published its strategic plan, a living document for moving oncology nursing and patient care forward. The main elements of the 2006 ONS strategic plan are listed in Table 24-11.

SUMMARY

To continue to provide excellent oncology patient care, oncology nurses need to be aware of the challenges of the profession as well as know methods to maintain professional standards in practice and behavior. Areas for professionalism include education, research, and workplace issues. To continue excellence in practice, each nurse caring for oncology patients should have a vigilant and open approach to taking care of himself or herself and his or her colleagues. Nurses should also strive to achieve high professional goals and maintain their ethical standards through ongoing, lifelong study, research, and advocacy.

TABLE 24-11: SELECTED ONCOLOGY NURSING SOCIETY STRATEGIES AND ACTIONS FOR 2006

- Advocate on behalf of the nursing profession, the multidisciplinary oncology team, people at risk for cancer, people with cancer, and their families and caregivers.

- Generate and disseminate essential knowledge for oncology nursing professionals.

- Develop leaders in ONS and the profession of oncology nursing.

- Expand public awareness of ONS's and oncology nursing's contributions to quality cancer care.

- Increase the recruitment and retention of ONS members.

- Strengthen ONS and cancer care through diversity initiatives.

- Continuously improve the experience of members and other customers in transactions with ONS.

- Strengthen partnerships with national and international external organizations.

- Promote healthy lifestyles for health promotion and disease risk reduction.

Note. From *Oncology Nursing Society Strategic Plan: 2006 through 2009* by Oncology Nursing Society (2005). Retrieved June 11, 2007, from http://www.ons.org/about/strategicplan 2006.shtml. Reprinted with permission. For the most recent information, go to www.ons.org

EXAM QUESTIONS

CHAPTER 24
Questions 97-100

Note: Choose the option that BEST answers each question.

97. An ethical assessment focuses on

    a. values.

    b. competencies.

    c. rules.

    d. interpersonal skills.

98. A significant workplace issue affecting nurses nationwide, including those caring for cancer patients, is

    a. a reduced patient load.

    b. an aging workforce.

    c. reduced admissions to the emergency room.

    d. limited opportunities.

99. A major content area in the OCN Blueprint is

    a. renal and hepatic dysfunction.

    b. hemorrhage and anemia.

    c. anaphylaxis and allergic responses.

    d. symptom management and supportive care.

100. A component of the 2006 ONS Strategic Plan is to

    a. advocate for safe housing of patients.

    b. strengthen ONS and cancer care through diversity initiatives.

    c. prepare cancer nurses for retirement.

    d. promote physician practices in rural communities.

This concludes the final examination.

Please answer the evaluation questions found on page v of this workbook.

REFERENCES

American Association of Colleges of Nursing. (2006). *Nursing shortage fact sheet.* Retrieved April 17, 2007, from http://www.aacn.nche .edu/Media/pdf/NursingShortageFactSheet.pdf

Berger, A., Berry, D., Christopher, K., Greene, A., Maliski, S., Swenson, K., et al. (2005). Oncology Nursing Society year 2004 research priorities survey. *Oncology Nursing Forum, 32*(2), 281–290.

Cooke, L., Smith-Idell, C., Dean, G., Gemmill, R., Steingass S., Sun, V., et al. (2004). "Research to Practice": A practical program to enhance the use of evidence-based practice at the unit level. *Oncology Nursing Forum, 31*(4), 825–832.

Fest, G. (2004). *Federal funds to ease shortage falling short.* Retrieved April 17, 2007, from http://www.nurseweek.com/news/features/04 -08/funds.asp

Friese, C. (2005). Nurse practice environments and outcomes: Implications for oncology nursing. *Oncology Nursing Forum, 32*(4), 765–772.

Friese, C., & Beck, S. (2004). Advancing practice and research: Creating evidence-based summaries on measuring nursing-sensitive patient outcomes. *Clinical Journal of Oncology Nursing, 8*(6), 675–677.

Gullatte, M., & Jirasakhiran, E. (2005). Retention and recruitment: Reversing the order. *Clinical Journal of Oncology Nursing, 9*(5), 597–604.

Gwede, C., Johnsson, D., Roberts, C., & Cantor, A. (2005). Burnout in clinical research coordinators in the United States. *Oncology Nursing Forum, 32*(6), 1123–1130.

Ireland, A., DePalma, J., Arneson, L., Stark, L., & Williamson, J. (2004). The Oncology Nursing Society ambulatory office nurse survey. *Oncology Nursing Forum, 31*(6), E155.

Krebs, L. (2005). Application of statement of scope and standards of oncology nursing practice and evidence-based practice. In J. K. Itano & K. N. Taoka (Eds.), *Core curriculum for oncology nursing* (4th ed., pp. 877–892). St. Louis: Elsevier.

Miller-Murphy, C., Ballon, L., Culhane, B., Mafrica, L., McCorkle, M., & Worrall, L. (2005). Oncology Nursing Society Environmental Scan 2004. *Oncology Nursing Forum, 32*(4), 742.

Nelson-Marten, P., & Glover, J. (2005). Selected ethical issues in cancer care. In J.K. Itano & K.N. Taoka (Eds.), *Core curriculum for oncology nursing* (4th ed., pp. 909–920). St. Louis: Elsevier.

Oncology Nursing Certification Corporation. (2006). *2006 certification bulletin.* Available from http://www.oncc.org

Oncology Nursing Certification Corporation. (2007). *2007 oncology nursing certification test bulletin.* Retrieved June 12, 2007, from http:// www.oncc.org/getcertified/TestInformation/ docs/bulletin07.pdf

Oncology Nursing Society. (n.d.). *About Oncology Nursing Society positions.* Available from from http://www.ons.org/publications /positions/

Oncology Nursing Society. (n.d.). *Evidence-based education guidelines.* Retrieved April 17, 2007, from http://www.ons.org/nursingEd/documents/ pdfs/guidelines.pdf

Oncology Nursing Society. (2005). *Oncology Nursing Society Strategic Plan 2006 through 2009.* Available from http://www.ons.org/about/strategies2006_1.shtml

Oncology Nursing Society. (2007). *Oncology Nursing Society 2007 Education Agenda.* Retrieved April 17, 2007, from http://www.ons.org/ceCentral/agenda.shtml

Rutledge, D., DePalma, J., & Cunningham, M. (2004). A process model for evidence-based literature syntheses. *Oncology Nursing Forum, 31*(3), 543–550.

Sheridan, C. (2000). Ethical dimensions in cancer care. In B. Nevidjon & K. Sowers (Eds.), *A nurse's guide to cancer care* (p. 469-478). New York: Lippincott Williams & Wilkins.

RESOURCES

Alliance for Lung Cancer Advocacy, Support, and Education (ALCASE)
Post Office Box 849
Vancouver, WA 98666
360-696-2436
1-800-298-2436
http://alcase.org

American Brain Tumor Association (ABTA)
Suite 146
2720 River Road
Des Plaines, IL 60018
847-827-9910
1-800-886-ABTA (1-800-886-2282)
http://abta.org

American Cancer Society (ACS)
1599 Clifton Road, NE
Atlanta, GA 30329-4251
404-320-3333
1-800-ACS-2345 (1-800-227-2345)
http://www.cancer.org

American Cancer Society (ACS) – Supported Programs:
- I Can Cope
- International Association of Laryngectomies
- Look Good. . .Feel Better
- Ostomy Rehabilitation Program
- Reach to Recovery
- Road to Recovery

American Foundation for Urologic Disease (AFUD)
1128 North Charles Street
Baltimore, MD 21201
410-468-1800
http://afud.org

American Institute for Cancer Research (AICR)
1759 R Street, NW
Washington, DC 20009
202-328-7744
1-800-843-8114
http://aicr.org

Association of Community Cancer Centers
11600 Nebel Street, Suite 201
Rockville, MD 20852
301-984-9496
http://accc-cancer.org

Association of Oncology Social Work (AOSW)
100 North 20th St., 4th Floor
Philadelphia, PA 19103
215-599-6093
http://aosw.org

Association of Pediatric Hematology/Oncology Nurses
4700 W. Lake Avenue
Glenview, IL 60025-1485
847-375-4724
http://apon.org

Brain Tumor Society
Suite 3H
124 Watertown, MA 02472
617-924-9997
1-800-770-TBTS
http://tbts.org

Cancer Care, Inc.
275 Seventh Avenue
New York, NY 10001
212-302-2400
1-800-813-HOPE (1-800-813-4673)
http://cancercare.org

Cancer Research Foundation of America

Suite 110
1600 Duke Street
Alexandria, VA 22314
703-836-4412
1-800-227-2732
http://preventcancer.org

International Myeloma Foundation (IMF)

12650 Riverside Drive, Suite 206
North Hollywood, CA 91607
818-487-7455
1-800-452-CURE (1-800-452-2873)
http://myeloma.org

Kidney Cancer Association

Suite 203
1234 Sherman Avenue
Evanston, IL 60202-1375
847-332-1051
1-800-850-9132
http://nkca.org

The Leukemia & Lymphoma Society

1311 Mamaroneck Avenue
White Plains, NY 10605-5221
914-949-5213
1-800-955-4572
http://leukemia-lymphoma.org

Multiple Myeloma Research Foundation (MMRF)

383 Main Avenue
5th Floor
Norwalk, CT 06851

203-229-0464
http://multiplemyeloma.org

National Alliance of Breast Cancer Organizations (NABCO)

10th Floor
9 East 37th Street
New York, NY 10016
212-889-0606
1-888-80-NABCO (1-888-806-2226)
http://nabco.org

National Asian Women's Health Organization (NAWHO)

Suite 1500
250 Montgomery Street
San Francisco, CA 94104
415-989-9747
http://nawho.org

National Brain Tumor Foundation (NBTF)

Suite 700
414 Thirteenth Street
Oakland, CA 94612-2603
510-839-9777
1-800-934-CURE (1-800-934-2873)
http://braintumor.org

National Coalition for Cancer Survivorship (NCCS)

Suite 505
1010 Wayne Avenue
Silver Spring, MD 20910-5600
301-650-9127
http://canceradvocacy.org

National Hospice and Palliative Care Organization (NHPCO)

Suite 300
1700 Diagonal Road
Alexandria, VA 22314
703-243-5900
1-800-658-8898 (Helpline)
http://nhpco.org

National Marrow Donor Program

Suite 500
3433 Broadway Street, NE
Minneapolis, MN 55413
612-627-5800
1-800-MARROW-2 (1-800-627-7692)
http://marrow.org

Oncology Nursing Society

501 Holiday Drive
Pittsburgh, PA 15220
412-921-7373
http://ons.org

Ovarian Cancer National Alliance

910 17th Street, NW

Suite 413

Washington, DC 20006

202-331-1332

http://ovariancancer.org

Susan G. Komen Breast Cancer Foundation

5005 LBJ Freeway, Suite 250

Dallas, TX 75244

972-855-1600

http://komen.org

United Ostomy Association of America, Inc.

Suite 200

19772 MacArthur Boulevard

Irvine, CA 92612-2405

949-660-8624

1-800-826-0826

http://uoa.org

GLOSSARY

adjunct therapy: A treatment used together with the primary treatment. Its purpose is to assist the primary treatment. Also called *adjunctive therapy*.

adjuvant therapy: Treatment given after the primary treatment to increase the chances of a cure. Adjuvant therapy may include chemotherapy, radiation therapy, hormone therapy, or biological therapy.

alternative medicine: Practices used instead of standard treatments. They generally are not recognized by the medical community as standard or conventional medical approaches. Alternative medicine includes dietary supplements, megadose vitamins, herbal preparations, special teas, acupuncture, massage therapy, magnet therapy, spiritual healing, and meditation.

analgesic: A drug that reduces pain. Analgesics include aspirin, acetaminophen, and ibuprofen.

anaphylactic shock: A severe and sometimes life-threatening immune system reaction to an antigen to which a person has been previously exposed. The reaction may include itchy skin, edema, collapsed blood vessels, fainting, and difficulty breathing.

angiogenesis: Blood vessel formation. Tumor angiogenesis is the growth of blood vessels from surrounding tissue to a solid tumor. This is caused by the release of chemicals by the tumor.

angiogenesis inhibitor: A substance that prevents the formation of blood vessels. In anticancer therapy, an angiogenesis inhibitor prevents the growth of blood vessels from surrounding tissue to a solid tumor.

anorexia: An abnormal loss of the appetite for food. Anorexia can be caused by cancer, acquired immunodeficiency syndrome, a mental disorder (e.g., anorexia nervosa), or other diseases.

antineoplastic: A substance that blocks the formation of neoplasms (growths that may become cancerous).

apoptosis: A type of cell death caused by a series of molecular steps in a cell. This is the body's normal way of getting rid of unneeded or abnormal cells. The process of apoptosis may be blocked in cancer cells. Also called *programmed cell death*.

aromatase inhibitor: A drug that prevents the formation of estradiol, a female hormone, by interfering with an aromatase enzyme. Aromatase inhibitors are used as a type of hormone therapy for postmenopausal women who have hormone-dependent breast cancer.

Ashkenazi Jews: One of two major groups of Jewish individuals whose ancestors lived in Eastern Europe (Germany, Poland, Russia). The other group is comprised of Sephardic Jews, whose ancestors lived in North Africa, the Middle East, and Spain. Most Jews living in the United States are of Ashkenazi descent. Also called *Eastern European Jews*. Ashkenazi Jews have been found to be at greater risk for certain subtypes of breast cancer and a familial link to colon cancer.

autosomal dominant: A type of gene expression in which a genetic condition occurs when a mutation is present in one copy of a given gene (i.e., the person is heterozygous).

autosomal recessive: A type of gene expression in which a genetic condition occurs only when the mutation is present in both copies of a given gene (i.e., the person is homozygous for a mutation or carries two different mutations of the same gene, a state referred to as *compound heterozygosity*).

axillary lymph node dissection: Surgery to remove lymph nodes found in the armpit region. Also called *axillary dissection*.

biological therapy: Treatment to stimulate or restore the ability of the immune system to fight cancer, infections, and other diseases. Also used to lessen certain side effects that may be caused by some cancer treatments. Also called *immunotherapy*, *biotherapy*, or *biological response modifier therapy*.

biomarker: A substance sometimes found in the blood, other body fluids, or tissues. A high level of biomarker may mean that a certain type of cancer is in the body. Examples of biomarkers include CA 125 (ovarian cancer), CA 15-3 (breast cancer), CEA (ovarian, lung, breast, pancreas, and gastrointestinal tract cancers), and PSA (prostate cancer). Also called *tumor marker*.

BRCA1: A gene on chromosome 17 that normally helps to suppress cell growth. A person who inherits an altered version of the BRCA1 gene has a higher risk of getting breast, ovarian, or prostate cancer.

BRCA2: A gene on chromosome 13 that normally helps to suppress cell growth. A person who inherits an altered version of the BRCA2 gene has a higher risk of getting breast, ovarian, or prostate cancer.

complementary medicine: Practices often used to enhance or complement standard treatments. They generally are not recognized by the medical community as standard or conventional medical approaches. Complementary medicine may include dietary supplements, megadose vitamins, herbal preparations, special teas, acupuncture, massage therapy, magnet therapy, spiritual healing, and meditation.

corticosteroid: A hormone that exhibits antitumor activity in lymphomas and lymphoid leukemias. Corticosteroids may also be used for hormone replacement and for the management of some of the complications of cancer and its treatments. Also called *steroids*.

COX inhibitor: A type of drug that is used to treat inflammation and pain and is being studied in the prevention and treatment of cancer. COX inhibitors belong to the family of drugs called *nonsteroidal anti-inflammatory drugs*. Also called *cyclooxygenase inhibitor*.

COX-2 inhibitor: Cyclooxygenase-2 inhibitor. A nonsteroidal anti-inflammatory drug used to relieve pain and inflammation. COX-2 inhibitors are being studied in the prevention of colon polyps and as anticancer drugs.

dendritic cell vaccine: A vaccine made of antigens and dendritic antigen-presenting cells.

Ductal carcinoma in situ (DCIS): A noninvasive condition in which abnormal cells are found in the lining of a breast duct. The abnormal cells have not spread outside the duct to other tissues in the breast. In some cases, DCIS may become invasive cancer and spread to other tissues, although it is not known at this time how to predict which lesions will become invasive. Also called *intraductal carcinoma*.

Epidermal growth factor receptor (EGFR): A protein found on the surface of some cells to which epidermal growth factor (EGF) binds, causing the cells to divide. It is found in abnormally high levels on the surface of many types of cancer cells, so these cells may divide excessively in the presence of EGF. Also known as *ErbB1* or *HER1*.

estrogen receptor negative (ER–): Describes cells that do not have a protein to which the hormone estrogen will bind. Cancer cells that are ER– do not need estrogen to grow and usually do not stop growing when treated with hormones that block estrogen from binding.

estrogen receptor positive (ER+): Describes cells that have a protein to which the hormone estrogen will bind. Cancer cells that are ER+ need estrogen to grow and may stop growing when treated with hormones that block estrogen from binding.

extravasation: When a vesicant agent leaks into the vein or surrounding tissue. Extravasations can permanently damage tissue.

familial adenomatous polyposis (FAP): An inherited condition in which numerous polyps (growths that protrude from mucous membranes) form on the inside walls of the colon and rectum. It increases the risk of colorectal cancer. Also called *familial polyposis.*

gene therapy: Treatment that alters a gene. In studies of gene therapy for cancer, researchers are trying to improve the body's natural ability to fight the disease or to make cancer cells more sensitive to other kinds of therapy.

genetic counseling: A communication process between a specially trained health professional and a person concerned about the genetic risk of disease. The person's family and personal medical history may be discussed, and counseling may lead to genetic testing.

genetic predisposition: Increased likelihood or chance of developing a particular disease due to the presence of one or more gene mutations or a family history that indicates an increased risk of the disease. Also called *genetic susceptibility.*

genetic testing: Analyzing deoxyribonucleic acid to look for a genetic alteration that may indicate an increased risk of developing a specific disease or disorder.

genomics: The study of the complete genetic material, including genes and their functions, of an organism.

granulocyte colony-stimulating factor (G-CSF): A colony-stimulating factor that stimulates the production of neutrophils (a type of white blood cell). It is a cytokine that belongs to the family of drugs called *hematopoietic* (blood-forming) *agents.* Also called *filgrastim.*

granulocyte-macrophage colony-stimulating factor (GM-CSF): A substance that helps make more white blood cells, especially granulocytes, macrophages, and cells that become platelets. It is a cytokine that belongs to the family of drugs called *hematopoietic* (blood-forming) *agents.* Also called *sargramostim.*

HER2/neu: Human epidermal growth factor receptor 2. The HER2/neu protein is involved in the growth of some cancer cells. Also called *c-erbB-2.*

hereditary nonpolyposis colon cancer (HNPCC): An inherited disorder in which affected individuals have a higher-than-normal chance of developing colorectal cancer and certain other types of cancer, often before the age of 50. Also called *Lynch syndrome.*

in situ cancer: Early, noninvasive cancer that has not spread to neighboring tissue.

infiltrating ductal carcinoma: The most common type of invasive breast cancer. It starts in the cells that line the milk ducts in the breast, grows outside the ducts, and commonly spreads to the lymph nodes.

inflammatory breast cancer: A type of breast cancer in which the breast looks red and swollen and feels warm. The skin of the breast may also show the pitted appearance called *peau d'orange* (like the skin of an orange). The redness and warmth occur because cancer cells block the lymph vessels in the skin.

Karnofsky Performance Status (KPS): A standard way of measuring the ability of cancer patients to perform ordinary tasks. The KPS can range from 0 to 100. A higher score means the patient is better able to carry out daily activities. KPS may be used to determine a patient's prognosis, to measure changes in a patient's ability to function, or to decide if a patient could be included in a clinical trial.

lobular carcinoma: Cancer that begins in the lobules (the glands that make milk) of the breast. Lobular carcinoma in situ (LCIS) is a condition in which abnormal cells are found only in the lobules. When cancer has spread from the lobules to surrounding tissues, it is called *invasive lobular carcinoma*. LCIS does not become invasive lobular carcinoma very often, but having LCIS in one breast increases the risk of developing invasive cancer in either breast.

nanotechnology: The field of research that deals with the engineering and creation of things from materials that are less than 100 nanometers (one-billionth of a meter) in size, especially single atoms or molecules. The role of nanotechnology in the detection, diagnosis, and treatment of cancer is being studied.

neoadjuvant therapy: Treatment given before the primary treatment. Examples of neoadjuvant therapy include chemotherapy, radiation therapy, and hormone therapy.

node-positive: Cancer that has spread to the lymph nodes.

overexpress: In biology, to make too many copies of a protein or other substance. Overexpression of certain proteins or other substances can occur on the surface of a cell.

p53 gene: A tumor suppressor gene that normally inhibits the growth of tumors. This gene is altered in many types of cancer.

pancytopenia: A shortage of all types of blood cells, including red and white blood cells and platelets.

pedigree: A record of one's ancestors, offspring, siblings, and their offspring that may be used to determine the pattern of certain genes or disease inheritance within a family.

peripheral neuropathy: A condition of the nervous system that can cause numbness, tingling, burning, and weakness. It usually begins in the hands or feet and can be caused by certain anticancer drugs.

positron emission tomography (PET) scan: A procedure in which a small amount of radioactive glucose (sugar) is injected into a vein and a scanner is used to make detailed, computerized pictures of areas inside the body where the glucose is used. Because cancer cells often use more glucose than normal cells, the pictures can be used to find cancer cells in the body.

progesterone receptor negative (PR–): Describes cells that do not have a protein to which the hormone progesterone will bind. Cancer cells that are PR– do not need progesterone to grow and usually do not stop growing when treated with hormones that block progesterone from binding.

progesterone receptor positive (PR+): Describes cells that have a protein to which the hormone progesterone will bind. Cancer cells that are PR+ need progesterone to grow and usually stop growing when treated with hormones that block progesterone from binding.

recurrence: Cancer that has returned after a period of time during which the cancer could not be detected. The cancer may come back to the same place as the original (primary) tumor or to another place in the body. Also called *recurrent cancer.*

sentinel lymph node mapping: The use of dyes and radioactive substances to identify the first lymph node to which cancer is likely to spread from the primary tumor. Cancer cells may appear first in the sentinel node before spreading to other lymph nodes and other places in the body.

sun protection factor (SPF): A scale for rating the level of sunburn protection in sunscreen products. The higher the SPF, the more sunburn protection. Sunscreens with an SPF value of 2 through 11 give minimal protection against sunburn. Sunscreens with an SPF of 12 through 29 give moderate protection. Those with an SPF of 30 or higher give high protection against sunburn.

tumor marker: A substance sometimes found in the blood, other body fluids, or tissues. A high level of tumor marker may mean that a certain type of cancer is in the body. Examples of tumor markers include CA 125 (ovarian cancer), CA 15-3 (breast cancer), CEA (ovarian, lung, breast, pancreas, and gastrointestinal tract cancers), and PSA (prostate cancer). Also called *biomarker.*

INDEX

PRETEST KEY

Cancer Nursing:
A Solid Foundation for Practice

1.	b	Chapter 2
2.	c	Chapter 3
3.	c	Chapter 3
4.	a	Chapter 5
5.	d	Chapter 6
6.	b	Chapter 6
7.	d	Chapter 9
8.	c	Chapter 11
9.	a	Chapter 11
10.	d	Chapter 12
11.	d	Chapter 12
12.	b	Chapter 14
13.	d	Chapter 14
14.	a	Chapter 16
15.	d	Chapter 17
16.	b	Chapter 17
17.	a	Chapter 17
18.	c	Chapter 20
19.	a	Chapter 21
20.	d	Chapter 24

Western Schools® offers over 2,000 hours to suit all your interests – and requirements!

Cardiovascular
Cardiovascular Nursing: A Comprehensive Overview
Cardiovascular Pharmacology
A The 12-Lead ECG in Acute Coronary Syndromes

Clinical Conditions/Nursing Practice
A Advanced Assessment
Ambulatory Surgical Care (2nd ed.)
Asthma: Nursing Care Across the Lifespan
Chest Tube Management
Clinical Care of the Diabetic Foot
A Complete Nurses Guide to Diabetes Care
Chronic Obstructive Lung Disease
Diabetes Essentials for Nurses
Death, Dying & Bereavement
Essentials of Patient Education
Genetic & Inherited Disorders of the Pulmonary System
Healing Nutrition
Helping the Obese Patient Find Success
Holistic & Complementary Therapies
Home Health Nursing (2nd ed.)
Humor in Healthcare: The Laughter Prescription
Management of Systemic Lupus Erythematosus
Orthopedic Nursing: Caring for Patients with Musculoskeletal Disorders (2nd ed.)
Pain & Symptom Management
Pain Management: Principles and Practice
A Palliative Practices: An Interdisciplinary Approach
— Issues Specific to Palliative Care
— Specific Disease States and Symptom Management
— The Dying Process, Grief, and Bereavement.
Pharmacologic Management of Asthma
Pneumonia in Adults
Pulmonary Rehabilitation
Seizures: A Basic Overview
The Neurological Exam
Wound Management and Healing

Critical Care/ER/OR
Acute Respiratory Distress Syndrome (ARDS)
Adult Acute Respiratory Infections
Auscultation Skills (4th ed.)
— Heart Sounds
— Breath Sounds
Basic Nursing of Head, Chest, Abdominal, Spine and Orthopedic Trauma
A Case Studies in Critical Care Nursing
Critical Care & Emergency Nursing
Hemodynamic Monitoring
Lung Transplantation
A Practical Guide to Moderate Sedation/Analgesia
Principles of Basic Trauma Nursing
Traumatic Brain Injury

Geriatrics
Alzheimer's Disease: A Complete Guide for Nurses
Alzheimer's Disease and Related Disorders
Cognitive Disorders in Aging
Depression in Older Adults
Early-Stage Alzheimer's Disease
Geriatric Assessment
Healthy Aging
Nursing Care of the Older Adult (2nd ed.)
Psychosocial Issues Affecting Older Adults (2nd ed.)

Infectious Diseases/Bioterrorism
Avian Influenza
Biological Weapons
Bioterrorism & the Nurse's Response to WMD
Bioterrorism Readiness: The Nurse's Critical Role
H1N1 Flu (2nd ed.)
Hepatitis C: The Silent Killer (2nd ed.)
HIV/AIDS
Immunization Review
Infection Control Training for Healthcare Workers
Influenza: A Vaccine-Preventable Disease
MRSA
Pertussis: Diagnosis, Treatment, and Prevention
Smallpox
Tuberculosis Across the Lifespan
West Nile Virus (2nd ed.)

Oncology
Cancer in Women
Cancer Nursing (2nd ed.)
Chemotherapy and Biotherapies
Lung Cancer

Pediatrics/Maternal-Child/Women's Health
A Assessment and Care of the Well Newborn
Birth Control Methods and Reproductive Choices
Birth Defects Affecting the Respiratory System
Diabetes in Children
Effective Counseling Techniques for Perinatal Mood Disorders
Fetal and Neonatal Drug Exposure
Induction of Labor
Manual of School Health (3rd ed.)
Maternal-Newborn Nursing
Menopause: Nursing Care for Women Throughout Mid-Life
A Obstetric and Gynecologic Emergencies
— Obstetric Emergencies
— Gynecologic Emergencies
Pediatric Health & Physical Assessment
Pediatric Obesity
Pediatric Pharmacology
Perinatal Mood Disorders: An Overview
A Practice Guidelines for Pediatric Nurse Practitioners
Pregnancy Loss
Respiratory Diseases in the Newborn
Women's Health: Contemporary Advances and Trends (3rd ed.)

Professional Issues/Management/Law
Documentation for Nurses
Medical Error Prevention: Patient Safety
Management and Leadership in Nursing
Ohio Nursing Law: How Practice is Regulated
Surviving and Thriving in Nursing

Psychiatric/Mental Health
A ADHD in Children and Adults
Attention Deficit Hyperactivity Disorders Throughout the Lifespan
Basic Psychopharmacology
Behavioral Approaches to Treating Obesity
A Bipolar Disorder
A Child/Adolescent Clinical Psychopharmacology
A Childhood Maltreatment
A Clinical Psychopharmacology
A Collaborative Therapy with Multi-stressed Families
Counseling Substance Abusing or Dependent Adolescents
Depression: Prevention, Diagnosis, and Treatment
Disaster Mental Health
A Ethnicity and the Dementias
A Evidence-Based Mental Health Practice
A Geropsychiatric and Mental Health Nursing
Group Work with Substance Abusing & Dually Diagnosed Clients
A Growing Up with Autism
Harm Reduction Counseling for Substance Abusing Clients
Identifying and Assessing Suicide Risk in Adults
A Integrating Traditional Healing Practices into Counseling
A Integrative Treatment for Borderline Personality Disorder
Intimate Partner Violence: An Overview
IPV (Intimate Partner Violence) (2nd ed.)
A Mental Disorders in Older Adults
A Mindfulness and Psychotherapy
A Multicultural Perspectives in Working with Families
Multidimensional Health Assessment of the Older Adult
A Obsessive Compulsive Disorder
Post-Divorce Parenting: Mental Health Issues and Interventions
Posttraumatic Stress Disorder: An Overview
A Problem and Pathological Gambling
Psychiatric Nursing: Current Trends in Diagnosis
Psychiatric Principles & Applications
A Psychosocial Adjustment to Chronic Illness in Children and Adolescents
A Psychosocial Aspects of Disaster
A Schizophrenia
Schizophrenia: Signs, Symptoms, and Treatment Strategies
Serious Mental Illness: Comprehensive Case Management
Substance Abuse
Suicide
A Trauma Therapy
A Treating Explosive Kids
A Treating Substance Use Problems in Psychotherapy Practice
A Treating Victims of Mass Disaster and Terrorism
Understanding Attachment Theory

Visit us online at westernschools.com for additional CE offerings!